# Phonogroup

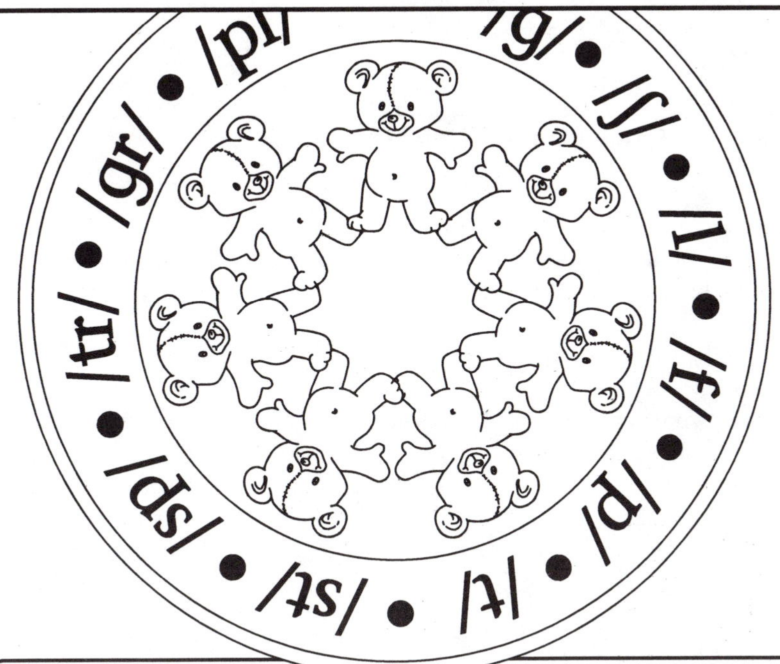


## A Practical Guide for Enhancing Phonological Remediation

**Margot E. Kelman, M.S., CCC-SLP**

**Mary Louise Edwards, Ph.D.**

Syracuse University

Syracuse, New York

**Thinking Publications**
Eau Claire, Wisconsin

03   02   01   00   99   98   97        10   9   8   7   6   5   4   3   2

**Library of Congress Cataloging-in-Publication Data**

Kelman, Margot E.
    Phonogroup : a practical guide for enhancing phonological remediation / Margot E. Kelman, Mary Louise Edwards ; [illustrated by Patti Argoff].
       p.  cm.
    Includes bibliographical references.
    ISBN 0-930599-30-6 (pbk.)
    1. Speech therapy for children.  I. Edwards, Mary Louise.  II. Argoff, Patti.  III. Title.
RJ496.S7K397   1994
618.9285'506—dc20
                   94-3456
                   CIP

*Printed in the United States of America*

Illustrations by Patti Argoff

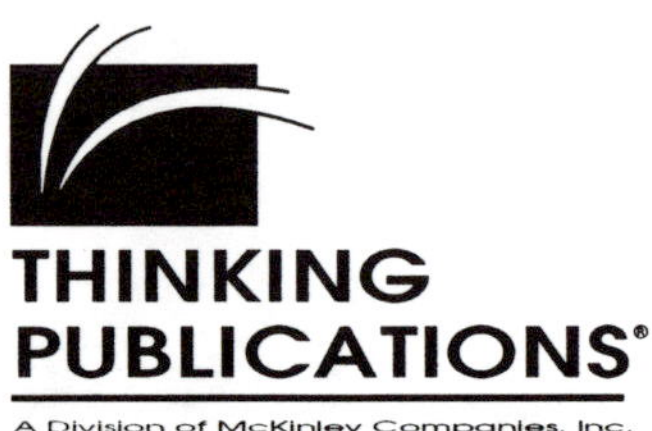

**THINKING PUBLICATIONS**®
A Division of McKinley Companies, Inc.

424 Galloway Street
Eau Claire, WI 54703
(715) 832-2488  •  FAX (715) 832-9082
E-Mail: custserv@ThinkingPublications.com

**To all the children
and parents who have
participated in the
Preschool Phonology Group
at Syracuse University**

# ABOUT THE AUTHORS

**Margot E. Kelman**, M.S., CCC-SLP, is an experienced speech-language pathologist who is currently director of the Gebbie Speech-Language Clinic and associate chair of the Communication Sciences and Disorders Program at Syracuse University. Before assuming the role as clinic director in 1989, she was employed as a speech-language pathologist serving infants, toddlers, and preschool children. In addition to her administrative duties and classroom instruction, Ms. Kelman supervises master's level student clinicians in the university clinic. Currently she codirects a therapy group for preschoolers with disordered phonology.

**Mary Louise Edwards**, Ph.D., received her doctorate in linguistics from Stanford University in 1979. She is associate professor and chair of the Communication Sciences and Disorders Program at Syracuse University. Her areas of specialization include normal and disordered phonology in children, as well as phonological assessment and remediation. Dr. Edwards has written books on both phonetics and phonology and has published numerous articles on various aspects of clinical phonology. She recently completed work on a 3-year NIH-funded research project investigating the co-occurrence of phonology and fluency disorders in young children. Currently, Dr. Edwards and Ms. Kelman codirect a therapy group for preschool children with disordered phonology.

vi

*Phonogroup: A Practical Guide for Enhancing Phonological Remediation* is an outgrowth of many years of clinical experience with young children. It combines theoretical underpinnings from phonology with practical application. Over 240 activities designed to remediate a number of different phonological processes are arranged in a user-friendly format, and are intended for speech-language pathologists working with young children who exhibit many misarticulations and reduced intelligibility.

*Phonogroup* is based on an indirect and naturalistic approach to phonological remediation developed at Syracuse University in the 1980s. Some of the major principles of this approach are directly related to the fact that it was originally developed for the simultaneous treatment of phonological errors and disfluencies in young children. These principles include the use of a slow speaking rate by the clinician and the use of extensive modeling of correct productions rather than direct correcting of inaccurate productions. We found this indirect approach to be effective in remediating children's phonological errors (Conture, Louko, and Edwards, 1993), which led us to form a similar group for young children with only phonology concerns.

In the past, we had occasionally observed the development (or "surfacing") of within-word speech disfluencies in preschool-aged children who were subjected to direct, drill-oriented phonology therapy (Comras, 1974; Conture, Louko, and Edwards, 1993), and, in fact, it appears that stuttering and disordered phonology frequently co-occur in children. Specifically, about one-third of young children who stutter also exhibit phonological concerns (Wolk, Conture, and Edwards, 1990; Wolk, Edwards, and Conture, 1993). Since we have no good way of predicting, at this point, which young children with disordered phonology may also be "at risk" for becoming disfluent, it seems prudent to use an intervention approach that facilitates improvement in phonology while minimizing communicative stress.

Since 1990, several presentations have been given at local, state, and national conventions that have described various aspects of this remediation approach. These include a 1990 presentation by Wolk, Edwards, and Louko at the annual convention of the New York State Speech-Language-Hearing

Association, as well as presentations by Edwards, Kelman-Maziuk, and Louko at the 1991 convention of the American Speech-Language-Hearing Association (ASHA) in Atlanta, Georgia, and by Edwards and Kelman-Maziuk at the 1993 ASHA convention in Anaheim, California. Largely because of the enthusiastic response received at these presentations, we decided to make the details of our remediation approach available to a wider audience. It is our hope that practicing speech-language pathologists and the children they serve will benefit from the approach described in *Phonogroup* and will enjoy the activities as much as the children and the student clinicians in our program have enjoyed them.

Our inspiration for *Phonogroup* came from many people. We owe much to the creative efforts of two doctoral students at Syracuse University, Linda Louko and Lesley Wolk, who were involved from the inception of the Preschool Phonology Group. We wish to express special appreciation to our colleague, Edward Conture, for sharing his insight and expertise regarding the use of an indirect approach to remediation with young children.

A great deal is owed to the preschool children who attended the Phonology Group and enriched our lives by their enthusiastic participation. We also wish to thank the parents who faithfully brought these children to the clinic and offered invaluable input as we developed and refined the remediation approach described here.

We sincerely appreciate the hard work and dedication of the graduate students in speech-language pathology at Syracuse University who contributed so much to this project: Laurie Albert, Anne Andrulonis, Ranya Awwad, Erin Black, Kristine Bowen, Jacqueline Bushell, Patricia Connors, Laura Dowling, Kara Dugan, Carolyn Ebner, Charlene (Adelmann) Franaszek, Kimberly Gallaugher, Lori Goldberg, Heather Hamilton, Caren Leamon, A. Carla Leotta, Amy Loan, Megan Lumia, Neeru Mahant, Margaret McQuillan, Michael McSheehan, Traci (Buskey) Micek, Lynne Miller, Dawn Murphy, Katie Murphy, Jori Pendergrast, Karen Persily, Kylie Puram, Danielle Rinaldi, Dorothy Schutta, Stacey Seiler, Leslie Sheldon, Shirley Silvers, Sharon Silvin, Darlene Stratton, Tina Tanner, Danni Thomas, Judy Thorne, Kathleen Walsh, Monica Willsey, Deborah Wilson, and Karen Zelter. Working with these student clinicians was a truly gratifying experience for us.

We extend sincere appreciation to Donna-Jean Marsulá, office assistant, for her word processing skill and considerable patience during the typing and retyping of many, many drafts. Thanks are also extended to Lynne Miller, graduate assistant, whose good cheer and competence helped us through the initial compilation of the activities, and Karen Prieto, clinic secretary, who assisted with word processing when time was short. Without their efforts, this manual would not have become a reality.

We wish to acknowledge Patti Argoff for her wonderful illustrations and her conscientious efforts in helping us meet our deadlines.

Special thanks to Linda Schreiber, Nancy McKinley, and other members of the staff at Thinking Publications as well as Ann Gorton, Marcia Krier, Peg Reichardt, and Jerry Vicino who enthusiastically reviewed our project and helped bring it to fruition.

We wish to extend our gratitude to our colleagues in the Communication Sciences and Disorders program, our families, and friends for their indulgence during the course of this project. Their patience and support have been invaluable.

Finally, the authors wish to thank each other for a stimulating and productive working relationship. Without an ample supply of perseverance, good humor, and moral support (in addition to snack food), this project would never have reached its final state.

*Phonogroup: A Practical Guide for Enhancing Phonological Remediation* is intended to assist speech-language pathologists in developing remediation goals and activities for groups of preschool/early school-age children with multiple speech sound errors. A phonological process approach is utilized to remediate children's error patterns. The purpose is to increase the intelligibility of children's speech by decreasing the application of phonological processes. A *phonological process* may be defined as a systematic sound change that affects a class of sounds (such as velars or fricatives) or a sound sequence (such as /s/ + stop clusters) (Edwards and Shriberg, 1983).

Unique characteristics of this resource include the use of an indirect, naturalistic approach to the remediation of phonological errors. This activity-oriented approach in which space, movement, and real objects are an integral part of intervention is motivating and stimulating for young children, especially those who may be resistant to traditional intervention or have concomitant problems (e.g., within-word speech disfluencies).

*Phonogroup* is organized so that speech-language clinicians can readily locate activities to remediate specific processes and target sounds, saving considerable planning time. Objects necessary for activities are easily obtainable from the home or classroom setting. Over 200 reproducible illustrations and patterns are included.

*Phonogroup* contains training words, behavioral objectives, probe lists, and a wealth of ideas for remediating common phonological processes in young children.

## Intended Population

*Phonogroup: A Practical Guide for Enhancing Phonological Remediation* is intended for use with groups of preschool/early school-age children (ages three to seven) who have moderate to severe phonological disorders. Because the approach described here is naturalistic and indirect, it is particularly useful with young children who have become self-conscious about their speech production and/or who may be at risk for other speech-language problems such as stuttering. It can also be used with children who exhibit language difficulties in addition to their phonological problems. This approach is compatible with the whole language philosophy and lends itself to use with an inclusive classroom intervention model.

Although the activities were designed for small groups of children (approximately four to six), modifications can be made for use with pairs of children or for individual therapy. Some activities can be adjusted for use with entire classes of students. *Phonogroup* activities are most effective when the severity level is comparable among the children, with some commonality among phonological errors. Adapting activities to meet the needs of children with physical limitations is also possible.

## Intended Users

Speech-language pathologists working in an early childhood setting, an elementary school, a clinic, or in private practice will find *Phonogroup* useful with groups of children who have phonological difficulties. Activities can easily be incorporated within the school day by educators, particularly those working in an integrated setting with a speech-language clinician. These activities also lend themselves to facilitating carryover to the home.

## Goals of *Phonogroup*

The overall goal of *Phonogroup* is to increase intelligibility by remediating entire patterns of errors (i.e., phonological processes) rather than perfecting individual error sounds one or two at a time. This general phonological goal is achieved through the following methods:

1. Heightening children's awareness of sounds by auditorily bombarding them with many productions of the selected target sound or sound sequence (e.g., consonant cluster) throughout the session.

2. When necessary, enhancing production of target sounds in isolation by incorporating them into naturalistic games and activities which encourage multiple repetitions.

3. Increasing accurate production of target sounds in carefully selected training words, first at the single-word level and then at higher linguistic levels as appropriate.

4. Promoting generalization through the use of a modified cycles approach.

5. Enhancing carryover of correct productions to other social/nonlinguistic contexts by incorporating naturalistic activities.

Additional desired outcomes or benefits of this approach include:

1. Building self-esteem and confidence in young children by enhancing their communication ability.

2. Enhancing children's ability to communicate with each other through the use of activities structured to promote peer interaction.

3. Providing an opportunity for caregivers/educators to learn and practice new skills that are appropriate in promoting phonological development.

4. Reducing communicative stress by reinforcing children for their participation in activities rather than for precise phonemic production and by allowing them to respond chorally rather than pressuring any individual child to provide a correct production.

5. Expanding vocabulary and word knowledge.

6. Incorporating gross and fine motor skill practice through the use of space and movement.

## Common Phonological Processes

This section is devoted to a brief review of common phonological processes found to be particularly relevant in working with preschool-age children. A more extensive list of processes with definitions and examples is provided in *Appendix A*. Although listings of processes are available elsewhere, terminology and definitions sometimes differ among various researchers/clinicians. The processes and definitions provided here are consistent with the activities and lesson plans described in *Phonogroup*. Note that this is not an exhaustive list of phonological processes. Given the variability among children, the speech-language clinician may occasionally encounter additional patterns that do not appear here or in any other published process list.

Processes listed in *Appendix A* are presented in their most general form. It should be noted that different children may apply processes differently. For example, one child may front velars to alveolars in all positions, while another child fronts only word-initial velars. Both children would be said to exhibit the process commonly referred to as Velar Fronting, although the process applies differently for each of them.

Preschool children typically exhibit a wide range of phonological processes, some of which are considered to be normal for their age, such as Vocalization of Liquids as in [kaʊ] for *car* and [tebu] for *table*. These age-appropriate processes are not included in this resource. Rather, you will find *age-inappropriate* processes, (i.e., processes that should have been eliminated at an earlier age), such as /s/ Cluster Reduction (e.g., [pun] for *spoon*, [noʊ] for *snow*); Liquid Cluster Reduction (e.g., [pen] for *plane*, [tʌk] for *truck*); and Gliding of Liquid /l/ (e.g., [wæmp] for *lamp*, [jaɪt] for *light*); Early Stopping (e.g., [ti] for *see*, [pæn] for *fan*); Initial Voicing (e.g., [bi] for *pea*, [du] for *two*); Velar Fronting (e.g., [tʊti] for *cookie*); Depalatalization (e.g., [su] for *shoe*, [fɪs] for *fish*). These particular age-inappropriate processes occur commonly enough to be frequent selections for remediation. (Note that square brackets are used to indicate the form actually produced by the child and slashes are used to indicate the adult phonemic form.)

## Historical Perspective

*Phonology* is the branch of linguistics that is concerned with sound systems and sound patterns. Attempts to clinically apply principles and concepts from phonology date back to the early 1970s when researchers such as McReynolds and Bennett (1972), McReynolds and Huston (1971), and others demonstrated that distinctive feature theory could be successfully applied in analyzing and treating the speech sound errors of young children with severe functional articulation disorders. At about the same time, there were a number of studies (Compton, 1970, 1975, 1976; Lorentz, 1974, 1976; Oller, 1973) aimed toward demonstrating the usefulness of a related theory of phonology called *generative phonology*. These studies described children's systematic sound errors in terms of *phonological rules*, often written in distinctive feature notation. The third theory of phonology to be applied clinically, for example by Edwards and Bernhardt (1973) and Ingram (1973/1976, 1974), was *natural phonology*. In this view, children's sound errors are accounted for by the operation of phonological processes, such as Cluster Reduction and Final Consonant Deletion. Despite differences among the three phonological theories that were applied clinically in the 1970s, all of these researchers were successful in showing that the "misarticulations" of children with many sound errors and low intelligibility could be accounted for within a phonological framework (i.e., by means of distinctive features, phonological rules, or phonological processes).

Several of these early researchers (Compton, 1975, 1976; McReynolds and Bennett, 1972) also showed that phonological descriptions could be used to plan remediation. This remediation was thought to be more efficient than traditional intervention for children with numerous sound errors because it focused on entire patterns of errors rather than individual sounds. In spite of the success of these early researchers, neither distinctive feature theory nor generative phonology really "caught on" clinically. Only one analysis procedure was published that was based on distinctive features (McReynolds and Engmann, 1975), and another was based on phonological rules (Compton and Hutton, 1978). Phonological process analysis, on the other hand, *did* catch on, at least in part due to the influence of Ingram's classic book on phonological disability, published in 1976. This was the first book on phonology written especially for speech-language pathologists. In it, Ingram showed how various principles and concepts from phonology, particularly phonological processes, could be used in analyzing and remediating children's sound errors.

### Phonological Process Analysis

The first published assessment procedure utilizing phonological processes was Weiner's (1979) *Phonological Process Analysis*, which incorporated some of the suggestions made by Ingram. This was followed just a year later by procedures by Hodson (1980, revised in 1986), and Shriberg and Kwiatkowski (1980). Ingram's own set of procedures was published in 1981. Additional process-based analysis procedures were published throughout the 1980s and into the 1990s, including those of Bankson and Bernthal (1990); Grunwell (1985); Khan and Lewis (1986). In addition, a number of programs for computer-assisted phonological analysis have also been published (e.g., Hodson, 1985; Long and Fey, 1988; Oller, 1990; Shriberg, 1986). Although the available procedures differ in the size and type of speech sample used, in the numbers and types of processes assessed, and in various other ways, they all attempt to find relationships among seemingly unrelated errors and to determine a child's major patterns of errors. In this way, they all go beyond traditional articulation tests, which simply tabulate a child's sound errors, perhaps classifying them in terms of substitutions, omissions, distortions, etc.

There are a number of basic assumptions that underlie the use of a phonological approach in assessing and treating children's speech sound errors. A few of these critical assumptions are summarized here:

1. If remediation is to fit the needs of the individual child, it must be based on a detailed phonological analysis.

2. Phonological analysis forms the basis for remediation by providing a means of describing the child's phonological system and isolating specific processes that need to be eliminated.

3. If a child is trained on carefully selected "key sounds" undergoing a process, there should be generalization to other (untrained) sounds undergoing the same process.

4. For a child with many sound errors, a phonological approach leads to more "principled" intervention that should be more efficient and effective because it focuses on entire patterns of errors rather than on single sounds.

Clinical phonologists carry out their phonological analysis and remediation methods in various ways. However, assumptions such as those just listed are shared by most experts who advocate using a phonological process approach with young children who exhibit many speech sound errors resulting in reduced intelligibility.

For children to benefit maximally from the phonological remediation techniques presented in *Phonogroup*, an understanding of each child's error patterns is necessary. That is, some sort of phonological process analysis must be carried out for each child. One of the numerous published assessment procedures may be used, or an informal phonological process analysis may be completed. *Appendix B* contains a brief summary of a few published phonological analysis procedures that are frequently used, as well as guidelines for completing a nonstandardized or "informal" phonological process analysis. (For additional information see Edwards [in press].)

## Remediation Techniques and Approaches

### *Minimal Pairs*

One of the major innovations in phonological remediation involves the use of minimal pairs (Weiner, 1979, 1981). The *minimal pairs approach* focuses on semantic contrasts. The idea is to use pairs of words that differ in just one sound (i.e., minimal pairs) to show children that their speech sound errors may result in the loss of a meaning difference. For example, if a child consistently reduces /s/ clusters, words such as *snow* and *no* may sound exactly alike. In this case, they might both be pronounced as [noʊ].

When minimal pairs are used clinically, games and activities are constructed in such a way that the child has to make some sort of sound difference if he or she is to succeed. For instance, if a game of "Go Fish" is being played, and the child wants the picture of *snow,* he or she must produce the word with an initial cluster. Otherwise, the clinician gives the child the picture representing *no*—not the one desired. Note that clinical phonologists differ as to whether or not they require the child to produce the *correct* sound. In many cases, any attempt on the part of the child to make a contrast is accepted, even if the production is not correct. In this example, if the child said [θnoʊ] instead of [snoʊ], that attempt would be accepted because it shows that the child is attempting to "suppress" the process of /s/ Cluster Reduction.

Although Weiner (1979) suggested using minimal pairs specifically to remediate processes which involve the omission of a sound, this approach is now well-accepted for remediating any process that results in the loss of a *phonemic contrast*, that is, any process that involves the deletion of a phoneme or the use of one phoneme in place of another.

A number of intervention materials and computer programs based on minimal pairs were published in the 1980s, including those by Elbert, Rockman, and Saltzman (1980), Kiernan and Zentz (1987), Martin and Ausberger (1981), Monahan (1984), Weiner (1982), and Young (1981). These materials are listed in the references.

In the approach to remediation presented in *Phonogroup*, minimal pairs that differ in just one parameter (place, manner, or voicing) are used when appropriate to focus the child's attention on the particular feature of concern. In addition, real words are used rather than nonsense words (compare to Gierut, 1989, 1990).

### Cycles Approach

Another significant innovation in phonological remediation is the *cycles approach* described by Hodson and Paden (1983, 1991). In this approach, intervention proceeds in "cycles," with each cycle lasting two to four months, and with several processes being targeted sequentially in each cycle. This approach is intended to provide the child with an opportunity to "generalize" correct patterns. Each process is targeted for two to four consecutive weeks, with a different phoneme being targeted in each session or each week (see Figure 1).

At the beginning and end of each session, two to three minutes are devoted to what Hodson and Paden (1983, 1991) call *auditory bombardment*. As they

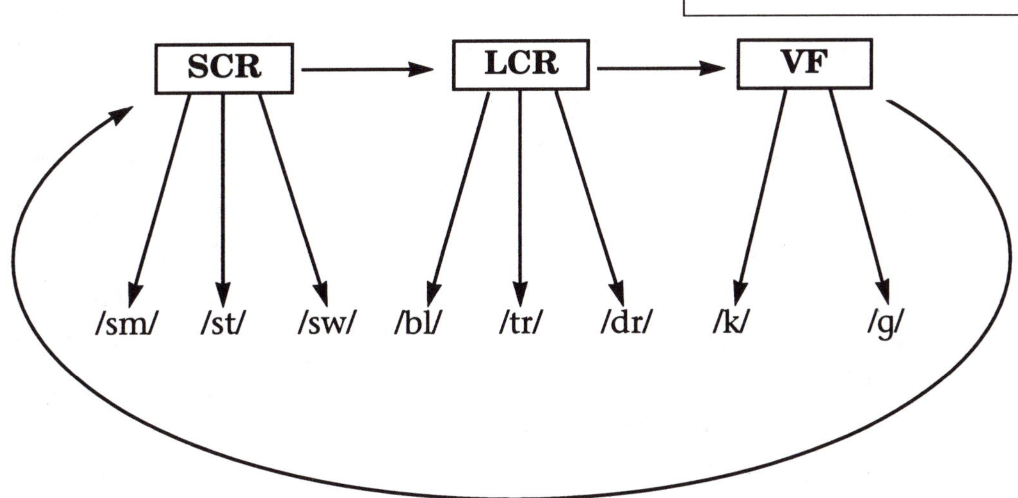



use this term, it refers to auditory stimulation with slight amplification. The child wears headphones and plays quietly while listening to a slightly amplified signal of the clinician reading lists of words that contain the target sound or cluster for that session.

In Hodson and Paden's (1983, 1991) approach, two to five "training words" are carefully selected to train each sound in each session. A "drill play" format is used. Minimal contrast training is not specifically incorporated.

*Phonogroup* utilizes Hodson and Paden's (1983, 1991) concept of cycles as a framework for structuring remediation. (Also see Tyler, Edwards, and Saxman, 1987.) In the *Phonogroup* approach, a number of processes are targeted in one "cycle," which lasts approximately two to three months. For instance, /s/ Cluster Reduction, Liquid Cluster Reduction, and Velar Fronting might be targeted in a cycle (as in Figure 1). One process is targeted for two to four consecutive sessions in each cycle, with a different phoneme or consonant cluster chosen for each session. In remediating /s/ Cluster Reduction, the specific targets might be /sm/, /st/, and /sw/. Two or three activities involving the target /sm/ cluster would then make up the first half-hour session. One advantage to the cycles approach is that if a child is not ready to progress with a particular sound or process, remediation continues to move forward and the target sound/process is focused on again during a later cycle. Also, use of cycles facilitates movement to another sound or process on which the child may experience more success.

### *Other Techniques/Approaches*

Several other phonological remediation techniques should also be mentioned here, although they have been less influential than minimal pairs and cycles. To eliminate assimilation processes (for example Velar Assimilation, as in [gʌk] for *duck*), Weiner (1979) suggested using a *modified paired-stimuli technique*. This involves pairing up a key word, such as *duck*, in which assimilation takes place, with another word that has the error sound in the same position, but which is not subject to assimilation because there is no sound in the word to "trigger" the assimilation, for instance *day* or *dime* (Weston and Irwin, 1971). For example, the child is presented with pairs of words such as *day-duck*, *dime-duck*, etc. In this example, the correct initial [d] in the first word of the pair should make it easier for the child to produce the correct initial [d] in the second member of the pair.

Weiner (1979) also recommended using a *modified sensory-motor approach* to remediate assimilation processes (McDonald, 1964). To illustrate, if *dog* is said as [gɔg], due to Velar Assimilation, *dog* is paired with (and produced directly after) a word with a correct final [d], such as *mad* or *sad*. If the two words are said as a compound word, with no break between the two parts, the correct final [d] should facilitate the production of a correct initial [d] in the word immediately following.

In the *metaphonological approach* to phonological remediation, activities are designed to heighten children's awareness of sounds and to help them think about the rules of the language (Chabon and Prelock, 1991; Jenkins and Bowen, 1994). In the past few years, there has been some discussion of using a *whole language approach* in the remediation of children's phonological problems. That is, phonology goals are addressed within the context of broader language goals (Hoffman, Norris, and Monjure, 1990).

Note that these procedures and approaches can be combined. For example, a cycles approach may be used in conjunction with minimal pairs. Or, after minimal pairs have been used to help the child realize that there are meaning differences that are not being conveyed, the words that have been trained may be used as "key words" to facilitate correct production in additional words. Some of these techniques are included in *Phonogroup* along with a few additional techniques that have been formulated specifically for use within the indirect and naturalistic approach to group remediation on which *Phonogroup* is based.

## How to Use *Phonogroup*

### General Procedures

This remediation approach can be employed in a variety of ways, depending on the needs of the children and the speech-language pathologist. For example, one group session may be used in conjunction with one individual session in each week, or two to three weekly group sessions may be conducted. Sessions occurring only once a week may not promote as rapid progress as more frequent sessions. The speech-language clinician is free to create other service delivery models as appropriate to fulfill the needs of the children. In inclusive settings, peers whose speech is not impaired may be involved in selected activities. Whenever possible, parents should participate in remediation sessions (see Parental Involvement, pages 20–23).

The first step in using *Phonogroup* is to select the target process to be remediated and the sound which will be the focus of that session. (See pages 12–17 for more specific guidelines for selection of target processes and sounds. Then refer to the activities that are appropriate to that target process and sound.)

*Phonogroup* activities include behavioral objectives, detailed procedures, and lists of necessary materials. Several target words appropriate for each activity are clearly identified, and words to specifically emphasize during auditory bombardment are italicized. Whenever possible, activities utilize materials that are easily obtainable and/or relatively inexpensive to purchase. Reproducible illustrations are provided.

Approximately two to three different activities can be implemented within a half-hour session (or four to five in a 60-minute session). If a sound is to be targeted for two to three consecutive sessions (as recommended), then activities should be selected to incorporate several different remediation techniques and procedures. The speech-language clinician should strive to utilize a variety of modalities in each session. For example, a quiet activity such as listening to a story might be followed by an activity that incorporates use of space and movement, such as searching for hidden objects with a flashlight.

### Selecting Remediation Targets

Decisions regarding the selection of remediation targets involve both the processes to be remediated as well as the specific sounds undergoing the processes. These are essentially separate decisions, although there is some overlap among the factors to be considered. Where to begin will depend on the individual children within the group, with consideration given to the characteristics of their phonological systems, as well as their age and behavior.

### *Selecting Target Processes*

Target processes are selected based on the children's error patterns. Whenever possible, processes should be selected that do not interfere with one another (e.g., because they affect different sounds or apply in different positions), such as Velar Fronting, Final Consonant Deletion, and Initial Voicing. A number of specific suggestions for the selection of target processes follow. Note that these suggestions are alternatives and may lead to different choices regarding which process to target first.

1. If children are just *delayed* phonologically (i.e., exhibit no unusual processes), focus on processes that are typical of early normal development or processes that affect early sounds, such as stops and nasals produced in the front of the mouth. Such "early" target processes include Final Consonant Deletion, /s/ Cluster Reduction, Liquid Cluster Reduction, Initial Voicing, Velar Fronting, and Stopping of /f, s/.

2. If immediate success is a primary concern, focus on *optional* processes (i.e., processes that apply less than 100% of the time, processes that apply only in certain positions, or processes that affect sounds which are in the children's phonetic inventories or for which they are stimulable).

3. If a process is *crucial* (i.e., because it is unusual or pervasive or contributes heavily to unintelligibility), then select it as an early remediation target.

4. If there are processes that *interact* (e.g., two or more processes apply to one sound), remediate each individually, so that the children are not expected to "undo" two or more processes at once. For example, if Velar Fronting interacts with both Initial Voicing and Final Devoicing, as in [daɪ] for *car* and [pɪt] for *pig*, Velar Fronting should be remediated by focusing on initial /g/ and final /k/ so that the voicing processes will not interfere. Similarly, remediate Initial Voicing by focusing on initial /p/ and /t/ to avoid interference from Velar Fronting.

5. In group remediation, consider the proportion of children in the group who exhibit each process, as well as personality variables and group dynamics. Processes that are exhibited by all or most of the children may be given highest priority. Sessions provide general speech practice for children whose specific errors are not being targeted; this reduces communicative stress and enhances sound awareness.

To determine the proportion of children in the group who exhibit each process, complete a Process Summary form using each child's phonological analysis. (A blank Process Summary form can be found in *Appendix C*.) List the processes down the left-hand side of the page, and list the children's names from left to right across the top. In the appropriate space below each child's name and across from the name of the process, briefly summarize how the process applies (i.e., word-positions, sounds affected, and frequency or percent of occurrence). (See *Appendix B* for instruction in calculating frequency of occurrence.) This makes it easy to see which processes are shared by all or most of the children, as well as how the children apply the processes.

In the sample form provided in Figure 2, the letters I, M, and F refer to initial, medial, and final word positions. Arrows are used to show the child's substitutions, with the adult sound to the left of the arrow and the child's production to the right of the arrow. The percent indicates percentage or frequency of

**Figure 2**

Date: _10/15_          **PROCESS SUMMARY**

| PROCESS: | Names | | | |
|---|---|---|---|---|
| | **Marc** | **Dana** | **Dominic** | **Elizabeth** |
| **Liquid Cluster Reduction** | 0%<br>r→w<br>/l/ correct | 19%<br>(I, M)<br>only in /b, g, f/ clusters | 44%<br>(I)<br>/r, l/ | 100%<br>(I, M, F)<br>/r, l/ |
| **/s/ Cluster Reduction** | 75% (I)<br>st→t, θ<br>sp→f | 18% (I)<br>/sm, sk, str/<br>(interacts with voicing) | 25% (I) | 38% (I, M, F) |
| **Final Consonant Deletion** | 14%<br>l, s→ø | 7%<br>z, s, d, l→ø | | 1x only |
| **Stopping** | 100% (I)<br>ð→d<br>v→b | 3% (I)<br>f→d<br>s→t | 1x only<br>ð→d | 58% (I, M, F)<br>f, v, θ, ð, z→ t, d<br>75% l→d |
| **Gliding of Liquids** | 31% (I, M)<br>r→w | 38% (I)<br>l, r→w | 67% (I, M)<br>+ clusters<br>l, r→w | 1 x only<br>str→sw |
| **Interdentalization** | 44% (I)<br>s→θ<br>z→ð | | 79%<br>(I, M, F)<br>s, z, ʃ, ʒ, ʧ, ʤ→θ, ð | |
| **Depalatalization** | | 9% (F)<br>ʃ, ʤ→s | 100%<br>(I, M, F)<br>ʃ→s→θ<br>ʒ→z→ð | 100%<br>(I, M, F)<br>ʃ→s<br>ʒ→s |

occurrence of the process. The symbol ø represents sounds deleted. As can be seen from this example, /s/ Cluster Reduction is exhibited by all four of the children, with frequencies of occurrence ranging from 18 percent to 75 percent. Similarly, Liquid Cluster Reduction is exhibited by three out of the four children.

### *Selecting Target Sounds*

Once the processes have been selected, choosing key sounds to remediate those processes is necessary. Select two or more sounds for each process, whenever possible, in order to promote generalization and to minimize the chances of overgeneralization. A number of suggestions for the selection of target sounds are presented below. These suggestions are based on traditional as well as more innovative criteria.

1. Select sounds that are already in the children's phonetic inventories (even if they are used only as substitutes).

2. Select sounds for which the children are stimulable.

3. Select early developing sounds.

4. Select sounds that will markedly improve intelligibility.

5. Select sounds that occur frequently in the language.

6. Select sounds of high value to the children (e.g., they occur in their names).

7. Select sounds that may promote generalization because they are from different classes (e.g., a labial sound and a lingual sound, or a fricative and a nasal).

8. Select sounds that are relatively easy to produce in the position of concern (e.g., voiceless sounds, particularly fricatives, are often easier to produce in final position). Keep in mind *process blocking* (Weiner, 1979). For example, Final Consonant Deletion may "block" or cover up the effects of Final Devoicing. Therefore, voiceless sounds should be selected as word-final targets whenever possible, unless the process being remediated is Final Devoicing.

### *Selecting Linguistic Level*

In addition to selecting the target process and sound, selecting the most appropriate linguistic level is necessary. When working with young children, training most often takes place at the meaningful word level. In those instances when it is necessary to focus on the sound in isolation, this can be accomplished through the use of "fun" auditory associations. For example, the /ʃ/ sound can be addressed in isolation by having the children say *shhhh* when the speech-language clinician purposefully makes unwarranted noise during an activity (refer to activities in the Depalatalization section beginning on page 161). Training at higher linguistic levels (i.e., carrier phrases and sentences) may take place after success has been achieved at the word level. The activities in *Phonogroup* should be adjusted to fit the linguistic level of the children in the group. In a group situation, the linguistic level that is most appropriate may differ for the different children. In those cases, the children should be encouraged to respond at the level that is most appropriate for them (e.g., the word or phrase level).

### *Selecting Training Words*

Once the target process, target sound, and linguistic level have been chosen for a session, determining the most appropriate word position is necessary. In some cases, there is no choice; for instance, Initial Voicing can only be targeted by working on sounds in word-initial position. When there is a choice, focus on a word position in which the following elements apply:

1. The process applies for all or most of the children.

2. At least a few of the children experience early success (e.g., because the process does not apply with 100 percent consistency).

3. Other processes do not interfere.

4. The target sound is relatively easy to produce (see item 8, Selecting Target Sounds, page 15).

After the process, sound, linguistic level, and position have been determined, carefully select two to five training words for each activity. Typically 6 to 10 different words are included in a 30-minute session, with some overlap in training words across activities. Whenever possible, it is advisable to choose words that do not contain error sounds other than the one being trained. Select training words that are:

1. Semantically appropriate for the child's age and developmental level.
2. Phonetically appropriate in terms of length, syllable structure, and difficulty of the sounds contained.
3. Relevant to the activities (e.g., choose at least a few verbs).

## Principles of *Phonogroup*

The approach to phonological remediation on which *Phonogroup* is based (Edwards, Kelman-Maziuk, and Louko, 1991) is an indirect one utilizing naturalistic activities to target specific phonological processes with relatively small groups of preschool/early school-age children. In *indirect* therapy (Conture, 1990), drill work and phonetic placement are *not* used, and the child's speech is not explicitly, directly, or overtly criticized or corrected. Rather, there is extensive modeling of correct productions, and children are reinforced for their participation in the activities rather than for precise phoneme productions. Correct productions are not differentially reinforced.

In *naturalistic* phonological remediation, target sounds and words are presented and produced as a natural part of or consequence of the activity in which the children are involved. Note that fewer productions may be elicited in this indirect and naturalistic approach than in more traditional and direct articulation training, and it may take longer for some children to progress. Nonetheless, this approach has been used effectively with young children, especially those who may be resistant to intervention and/or who may exhibit additional problems. (Also see Camarata, 1993.)

Use of a slow speaking rate, modeled by the speech-language clinician, is an essential principle of this approach. A slow rate of speech with increased pause time between sentences gives the children more time to process and understand what the clinician is saying, as well as giving them more time to formulate their responses. (See also Conture, Louko, and Edwards, 1993.) The speech-language pathologist does not have to talk like a record at the wrong speed! Even a slight decrease in speaking rate is likely to be helpful.

General principles to follow when implementing this approach to phonological remediation include the following:

1. Use extensive clinician modeling with carefully selected training words to bombard children with the target sound for the session.

2. Employ a slow speaking rate with increased pause time between sentences.

3. Encourage peer interaction, with all the children in the group (usually four to six) simultaneously involved in each activity so that waiting time is minimized.

4. Encourage children to respond chorally, providing them with a sense of "team spirit." This also decreases the communicative stress on each individual child.

5. Use space and movement in some activities within each session to maintain the children's interest and to capitalize on their natural mode of exploration.

6. Actively involve parents/caregivers in the remediation process. Whenever possible, have them observe and participate in intervention sessions so that they have an opportunity to practice appropriate elicitation techniques, such as modeling.

## Intervention Techniques

Several different techniques are typically used within each session to remediate phonological errors. One or more of the techniques described here are incorporated within each *Phonogroup* activity. Although they are not mentioned for each activity, *clinician modeling* and *bombardment* by means of extensive productions of target sounds and words are integral parts of each session. Words that should be emphasized by the clinician for auditory bombardment are italicized within each activity procedure. (Note that in the *Phonogroup* approach, bombardment takes place in a naturalistic way, by means of multiple productions of target words rather than by reading lists of words to the children.)

Providing clear models of the target words *before* the child's production is important. In addition, if a child produces a target word incorrectly, the clinician should immediately provide the correct model in a conversational manner, without overtly correcting the child's production. If incorrect productions persist throughout the session, the clinician should continue to model and emphasize the target sound.

The following additional techniques are incorporated within *Phonogroup* activities. The first technique is used in all activities. The remaining techniques are used when appropriate to the target process and target sound. Choices and foils are also used in all sessions, but not necessarily in each activity. Because drill work is not used, these techniques provide a basic mechanism for eliciting productions from the children.

1. *Training Words:* Each activity focuses on a small number of carefully selected target words containing the target sound in the position of concern. (Target words are words to elicit from the children.)

    *Target Process:*    Depalatalization
    *Target Sound:*    /ʃ/ (final)
    *Target Words:*    trash, fish, wash, dish, hairbrush

2. *Choices:* Choices between two logical alternatives (both involving target words) are provided to elicit productions in a natural conversational context.

    *Target Process:*    Depalatalization
    *Target Sound:*    /ʃ/ (final)
    *Example:*    "Do you *wish* for a *fish* or a *dish?*"

3. *Foils:* Purposeful and obvious lexical errors are made by the clinician to elicit target words from the children.

    *Target Process:*    Liquid Cluster Reduction

    *Target Sound:*    /bl/ (initial)

    *Example:*    While preparing to make blueberry blizzards, the clinician purposely calls *blueberries* (target word) *cherries* so that the children respond with, "No, *blueberries*."

4. *Minimal Pairs:* Several pairs of words are contrasted in which one member of the pair contains the children's error sound and the other contains the target (correct) sound (Weiner, 1979, 1981).

    *Target Process:*    Initial Voicing

    *Target Sound:*    /p/ (initial)

    *Minimal Pairs:*    pea/bee, pear/bear, pen/Ben, pie/bye

5. *Modified Sensory-Motor Approach:* A word in which the target sound is correct in *final* position is paired with a word in which the same sound is in error in *initial* position, or vice versa (Weiner, 1979). Word pairs are produced without a pause between them.

    *Target Process:*    Initial Voicing

    *Target Sound:*    /p/ (initial)

    *Word Pairs:*    hop-pig, hop-pie, hop-paint

6. *Modified Paired-Stimuli Technique:* A word in which the target sound is correct is paired with words in which the target sound is in error in the same position (Weiner, 1979).

    *Target Process:*    Velar Fronting

    *Target Sound:*    /k/ (initial)

    *Word Pairs:*    key-car, key-cake, key-king

## Parental Involvement

For significant improvement in intelligibility to occur, parents or care-givers should be involved in the intervention process. A remediation program can be enhanced with a relatively small amount of effort by actively soliciting parental or caregiver participation and by training them to use the identified techniques within the home environment (Eiserman, Weber, and McCoun, 1992; Ruscello, Cartwright, Haines, and Schuster, 1993).

For the speech-language pathologist who works in a private clinic, parental involvement should be relatively easy to achieve because parents are generally present to observe therapy on a regular basis. Involving parents and caregivers in other settings (e.g., preschool programs) becomes more challenging because they are not typically present to observe sessions. A clinician who is able to enlist 100 percent parental participation is most fortunate. However, in reality, there will be parents who, for one reason or another, do not participate. In many communities, single-parent families are common and the parent works full-time. The parent may have other children to care for at home, no means of transportation, or speak a language other than English. These factors might make participation in the group difficult or impossible. The speech-language pathologist should consider ways of supporting parents and caregivers who may have special problems with participation (Perrone, 1989). With careful and creative planning, parental involvement can be successfully achieved.

If parental involvement is to be an integral part of the remediation process, some commitment on the part of the parents is essential. Initial contact with parents and caregivers can be accomplished in a variety of ways. By sending a letter home, making a phone call or home visit, or arranging an introductory meeting (e.g., informal coffee), the speech-language clinician can enlist parental and caregiver support and interest in becoming a participant in the child's remediation plan. In school settings, the initial contact may be made during an open house or parent-teacher conference. The key to initial contact is that it be personal and specific. This initial contact can be followed by a group meeting for all the parents and caregivers, at which time the principles of the group are explained and group objectives are described. Make the meeting setting as comfortable as possible, so that parents feel welcome and not intimidated. Explaining the group principles in terms the parents can understand (i.e., avoiding speech-language pathology jargon) is also helpful. Again, place emphasis on the importance of parental cooperation as a benefit to the children.

Once the group is formed and introductory information is conveyed, meeting with the speech-language clinician on a consistent basis (e.g., monthly or bimonthly) is beneficial for the parents, caregivers, and children. During these regular group meetings, describe and demonstrate techniques used with the children. The parents should have the opportunity to participate in the following ways:

1. Observe the techniques being incorporated.

2. Practice the techniques themselves.

3. Obtain feedback.

Group meetings can also provide an opportunity for parents and caregivers to ask questions, seek clarification, and discuss their children's speech problems. As the parents become familiar with each other, they may develop friendships and share information among themselves.

Parents can also play a significant role during remediation sessions. Listed below are a few ways in which to integrate parents in activities:

1. Rotate parental participation by incorporating one parent per session or per week.

2. Include all parents in a session once a week or once a month.

3. Involve one or more parents in one activity per session.

Feel free to develop other ways of integrating parents. Through creative use of time, surveying parental schedules, and reviewing classroom events and activities, parental involvement can be adapted to meet the needs of the children in the group. During intervention sessions, some activities lend themselves to parental involvement more than others. A list of suggested activities is provided in *Appendix D*. Also, *Phonogroup* activities that are most appropriate for involving parents have an asterisk (*) following the activity title.

Sustaining active parent participation and communicating with parents throughout the time their child is in intervention is crucial to the child's success. This can be accomplished by regularly sending notes or letters to parents which describe activities to be implemented at home. Sample letters are provided in *Appendix D*. These letters can be particularly helpful for parents who cannot actually attend and participate in the group. The speech-language clinician may also consider regular telephone calls as a way of maintaining contact, or consider sending a "communication notebook" back and forth between home and the intervention setting.

Parents can also assist their child in completing activities at home. For example, the speech-language pathologist can send home an art activity such as *Trucks with /tr/ Cargo* (page 95), with additional illustrations of /tr/ target words for the parent and child to glue onto the truck together. During this home activity, the parent incorporates techniques learned from the group, such as modeling and providing choices. Stories, game cards, and board games can be reproduced and sent home with instructions. Food preparation activities easily lend themselves to additional sound practice at home.

## Monitoring Progress

### *Tally Sheet*

To facilitate data collection, a blank *Tally Sheet* is provided in *Appendix E*. The *Tally Sheet* may be duplicated if the clinician chooses to record the responses of any or all children during the session. Figure 3 is an example of a completed *Tally Sheet*. Checkmarks in the sample represent correct productions of the target, and phonetic symbols represent substitutions. A dash (-) is usually used for an omission but is not shown in the example. Given that children's responses may vary from activity to activity and from one target word to another, it is advisable to keep a record of all productions for each word as shown in the sample *Tally Sheet*. If desired, this information can then be combined and summarized using the *Phonogroup Session Log*.

**Figure 3**

# Tally Sheet

Date: _____9/15_____          Process: _Liquid Cluster Reduction_

Target Sound/Cluster: _____/dr/_____

| | Training Words | Names | | | | | |
|---|---|---|---|---|---|---|---|
| | | Jon | Kim | Terrell | Elyse | | |
| **Activity 1** | drive | ✓✓✓✓✓✓ | ʤ ʤ | d d d d | ✓✓✓ | | |
| | drum | ✓✓✓ | ʤ ʤ ʤ | dw dw dw | ✓✓ dw | | |
| | drink | ✓ dw | ✓ ʤ | dw | ✓✓✓ | | |
| | dress | d ✓✓ | ✓✓✓ | dw dw | ✓✓✓ | | |
| | dry | | ʤ ʤ ʤ | d d | ʤ dw dw | | |
| | draw | ✓✓ | ʤ ʤ | dw | ✓ dw | | |
| **Activity 2** | drip | ✓ dw | d d | ✓✓✓ | | | |
| | drive | ✓✓✓✓✓ | ʤ | d d d d | ✓ ʤ | | |
| | dragon | ✓✓✓ | d d | d d d | dw | | |
| | drink | ✓✓✓ | ✓✓ ʤ | | ✓✓✓ | | |
| **Activity 3** | drawer | ✓ | d | dw | d | | |
| | dress | dw dw | ✓✓✓ | dw dw | dw ✓ dw | | |
| | drum | ✓✓✓ | | dw dw dw | dw dw | | |
| | drip | ✓ | ✓✓ d | d d | ✓✓ d | | |
| | drink | ✓✓ dw dw | ʤ ʤ ✓ | dw dw | ✓✓ | | |
| **Activity 4** | dragon | ✓✓ | d ʤ | d d | ✓✓ dw | | |
| | drops | ✓✓✓✓✓ | ʤ d d | d dw | ✓ dw | | |
| | drink | dw dw ✓ | ✓ ʤ | dw dw | ✓✓✓ | | |
| | Drake | ✓✓ | ʤ d | d d | | | |
| | Drew | dw | d ʤ | dw dw | dw ✓ | | |
| | | | | | | | |
| | | | | | | | |
| | | | | | | | |

### Session Log

The *Phonogroup Session Log* conveniently summarizes results from each session. Figure 4 is an example of a completed *Session Log*. A blank session log is provided in *Appendix F*. This information can be used for planning future sessions and making comparisons across children. Documentation about productions that may be incorrect but closer to the model can help the speech-language pathologist see progress toward the target sound. For example, if a child typically reduces /s/ clusters by deleting the /s/, it may be helpful to know that half of his or her productions in a given session involve use of the [θ] rather than deletion of the /s/, as in [θpun] for *spoon*. Such examples show that the child is learning to use clusters even though they are not yet produced correctly.

**Figure 4**

Date: _____9/15_____

## Session Log

| Process: | Names | | | |
|---|---|---|---|---|
| *Liquid Cluster Reduction* | *Jon* | *Kim* | *Terrell* | *Elyse* |
| Sound: /dr/ | *81* % | *30* % | *6* % | *65* % |
| Position: I | C/T *44/54* | C/T *13/44* | C/T *3/43* | C/T *30/46* |
| Level: Word | o.p. *dr→dw (9x)* *dr→d (1x)* | o.p. *dr→dʒ (20x)* *dr→d (11x)* | o.p. *dr→d, dw (20x each)* | o.p. *dr→dw (12x)* *dr→d, dʒ (2x each)* |

% = level of accuracy (C ÷ T x 100)     C/T = # of correct productions /# of total productions
o.p. = other production(s) (not correct)

### *Probing*

In addition to using a *Tally Sheet* for each individual session, periodic probing (e.g., every two to four months or when significant changes have been observed) is recommended to monitor progress. *Probing* is a way of assessing production of selected sounds in a variety of positions within words that have *not* been trained. Therefore, it documents the extent to which generalization of correct productions has occurred beyond the specific words that have been used in remediation. The child's productions are phonetically transcribed, so it is also possible to determine if a child's error productions are closer to the correct adult form.

A probe list can be developed for each child to sample all the processes that need to be monitored. Although it may not be possible to monitor all the child's processes, it is suggested that words to sample the most prevalent processes and/or those that contribute most to the child's unintelligibility be incorporated in the probe list. Several words should be included to assess each sound in each position, preferably varying phonetic context, word length, and syllable structure. For instance, *black, sidewalk, rake,* and *lipstick* might be included as probe words for final /k/ (e.g., for a child who exhibits Velar Fronting). Note that one word may be used to probe two or more processes, thereby shortening the length of the complete list (e.g., *black* could be included to probe Liquid Cluster Reduction and Gliding of Liquids, as well as Velar Fronting).

Probe words should be elicited spontaneously (i.e., not by imitation). An object or picture-naming task is suggested as an appropriate elicitation method. In some cases, it may be necessary to provide a model and elicit a *delayed* imitation. Since the objective of probing is not to teach the probe words, no feedback regarding correctness of the productions should be provided. However, the child should be praised for cooperating during the task. A list of suggested probe words is included in *Appendix G*.

### *Re-evaluation*

Another way of monitoring progress is to periodically re-evaluate each child's phonology. For example, this may be done by obtaining a new speech sample and completing an informal phonological process analysis (see *Appendix B*), by administering a published phonological assessment procedure such as the *Assessment of Phonological Processes-Revised* (Hodson, 1986) or the *Khan-Lewis Phonological Analysis* (Khan and Lewis, 1986), or by using a computer program such as Shriberg's (1986) *Programs to Examine Phonetic and Phonologic Evaluation Records* (PEPPER). (Note that some "translation" will be necessary if Hodson's [1986] assessment procedure is used, since her process terminology is somewhat different.)

## Description of Activities for Group Remediation

*Phonogroup* includes activities to be used in phonology group sessions with young children. Many of the activities can be used with a variety of processes and sounds. To illustrate, an activity in which the children search for cards hidden around the room lends itself to use with virtually any remediation target. Note that activities for Liquid Cluster Reduction can also be used for Gliding of Liquids within clusters. Weak Syllable Deletion can be incorporated with other processes by including multisyllabic target words.

For ease in using these materials, the activities are organized by target process and, within each process, by target sound or consonant cluster. For example, all of the activities for /s/ Cluster Reduction are in one clearly labeled section and, within that section, all of the activities for /sn/ are together. In addition, activities for each target sound or cluster are organized so that stories are presented first, followed by art activities, snacks, songs, activities involving movement, and games.

At the beginning of the section for each target sound, the linguistic level and word position are specified. Many of the activities can be modified for various linguistic levels, depending on the ability of the children.

A sample behavioral objective is provided for each target sound. Percentages for accuracy levels are not specified in this group objective since these will vary for each child. Specific percentages can be included when writing each child's individualized educational program.

For each target sound, suggestions for nametags are listed. These assist in setting the sound/theme of the session and contribute to the children's perceptual training.

Each activity includes a title, appropriate target words, materials, and procedures. Although specific target words are included for each activity, these are merely suggestions. Other words can be added that may be particularly relevant to the geographical area or to other activities in which the children are involved. Typically two to six target words are included in each activity. Occasionally an activity may focus on just one target word, such as *float*. In general, however, productions can be elicited from the children much more naturally if there are at least two target words so that choices can be provided. Although stories often contain numerous relevant words to "bombard" the children with many exemplars of the target sound, most activities focus on a small number of carefully selected target words. Sometimes words are used in novel ways. For example, in a snack activity focusing on the /sn/ cluster, string cheese is used to make *snails* and fruit roll-ups are formed into *snakes*.

Because some processes are selected as targets much more frequently than others with this preschool/early school-age population, there are different numbers of activities for the various processes and sounds. Note that some processes that may be evident for young children with disordered phonology are not included at all. Clinicians are encouraged to develop naturalistic activities for processes not included here.

Most materials are readily accessible or inexpensive to purchase. Use real objects whenever possible. For some target sounds, appropriate stories are provided. *Appendix H* includes instructions and patterns for constructing materials (e.g., bingo board, fishing poles, feely box) that are used throughout the resource. Reproducible illustrations, organized by target sound and then alphabetized, are included in *Appendix I*. These illustrations may be duplicated for clinical and teaching purposes. The speech-language clinician is encouraged to supplement these with additional illustrations as needed.

Activities are designed in such a way that the children have some input and responsibility for implementing them. For example, while playing *Clyde*

*Says*, the children take turns being leader and deciding which action is to be performed. To give another example, the children take turns being "helper" by distributing illustrations to be used in an art activity. The helper offers the other children a choice of illustrations to include in their art project. This type of involvement encourages peer interaction.

Food preparation and eating activities are wonderful opportunities for naturalistic incorporation of target words. Multiple productions of target words can be easily elicited by providing very small portions of food and drink so that the children must request items frequently, without having a large mouthful of food. Also, placing food just out of reach of the children requires them to request the item from the speech-language clinician, parent or caregiver, or another child, thus producing the target word.

Children at this age need to have a sense of independence. During food activities, children can take turns being the "server." Foster independence by providing serving implements (e.g., small pitcher) that are easily handled by the children on their own. Some children enjoy wearing an apron to officially designate their role as server.

Before any food preparation or eating takes place, have all children wash their hands. Target words such as *wash* or *soap* may be incorporated if they are appropriate for that session. Adhere to health precautions during all activities involving food. For example, have the server use a spoon or plastic food gloves rather than fingers when providing portions to the children.

Parents or caregivers may express concern about particular types of snacks, and some children may have food allergies. Thus, parents should be consulted before any snack items are selected. Try to limit sugary snacks and encourage healthy eating practices.

Target only one sound or cluster in each intervention session so that ample opportunity for modeling and bombardment is provided. If the session is 30 minutes long, choose two to three activities using the same target sound or cluster, such as /fl/. Some of the activities for a particular target sound may lend themselves to a "theme" around which an entire session can be organized (e.g., seven /sp/ activities provided in *Phonogroup* pertain to the theme of *space*).

Since this approach is *indirect*, begin the session by indirectly introducing the sound for the day with nametags. Offer a choice of two nametags (e.g., "Do you want a *train* or a *truck?*"), thus providing another opportunity for modeling and sound practice. Suggested choices for nametags are listed for each target sound. Reproducible illustrations are provided for most of these words but using stickers that illustrate the target sound is also an option. Add the child's name to the nametag and attach with tape. Have the children tell you which nametag they have chosen. Ask them again at the end of the session.

Once the children's nametags are put on, give the children a brief description of the activities planned for the session. If the ordering of the activities in a particular session is not important, let the children (or one child per session) decide the order of the activities, thus providing an opportunity for child input.

The length of an intervention session may vary from 20 minutes to 1 hour, depending on the setting, the schedule, and children's needs. Regardless of the length of the session, include a variety of sensory modalities and movement. For example, a 30-minute session may include sitting in a circle to choose nametags, searching around the room for hidden objects or illustrations, and eating a snack at a table. In this way, there is a balance of active and sedentary tasks. The sample sessions provided here give ideas of ways in which to structure the sessions:

**30-minute sample session**

| | |
|---|---|
| Process: | /s/ Cluster Reduction |
| Target Sound: | /sp/ |
| Linguistic Level: | Word/Phrase/Sentence |
| Position: | Initial |
| Nametags: | Choice of *spaceship* or *spoon* |
| Activities: | *Spunky in Space* (page 60) |
| | *Space Snack* (page 57) |

**45-minute sample session**

| | |
|---|---|
| Process: | Depalatalization |
| Target Sound: | /ʃ/ |
| Linguistic Level: | Isolation/Word/Phrase/Sentence |
| Position: | Isolation and Final |
| Nametags: | Choice of *starfish* or *leash* |
| Activities: | *Tish the Dog* story (page 162) |
| | *Spraying and Washing* (page 168) |
| | *Banana Mush* snack with parents (page 164) |

**60-minute sample session**

| | |
|---|---|
| Process: | Initial Voicing |
| Target Sound: | /p/ |
| Linguistic Level: | Word/Phrase/Sentence |
| Position: | Initial |
| Nametags: | Choice of *pig* or *panda* |
| Activities: | *Picnic in the Park* story (page 212) |
| | *Pink and Purple Paint* (page 215) |
| | *Peaches or Pears* snack (page 217) |
| | *Shopping for* /p/ (page 224) |

The next section presents *Phonogroup* activities. Recall that activities are organized by target process and, within each process, by target sound or consonant cluster. Materials needed for these activities can be found in the appendices or are common objects available in most classrooms or homes.

Note: Activities suitable for parental involvement are denoted with an asterisk (*) following the title of the activity.

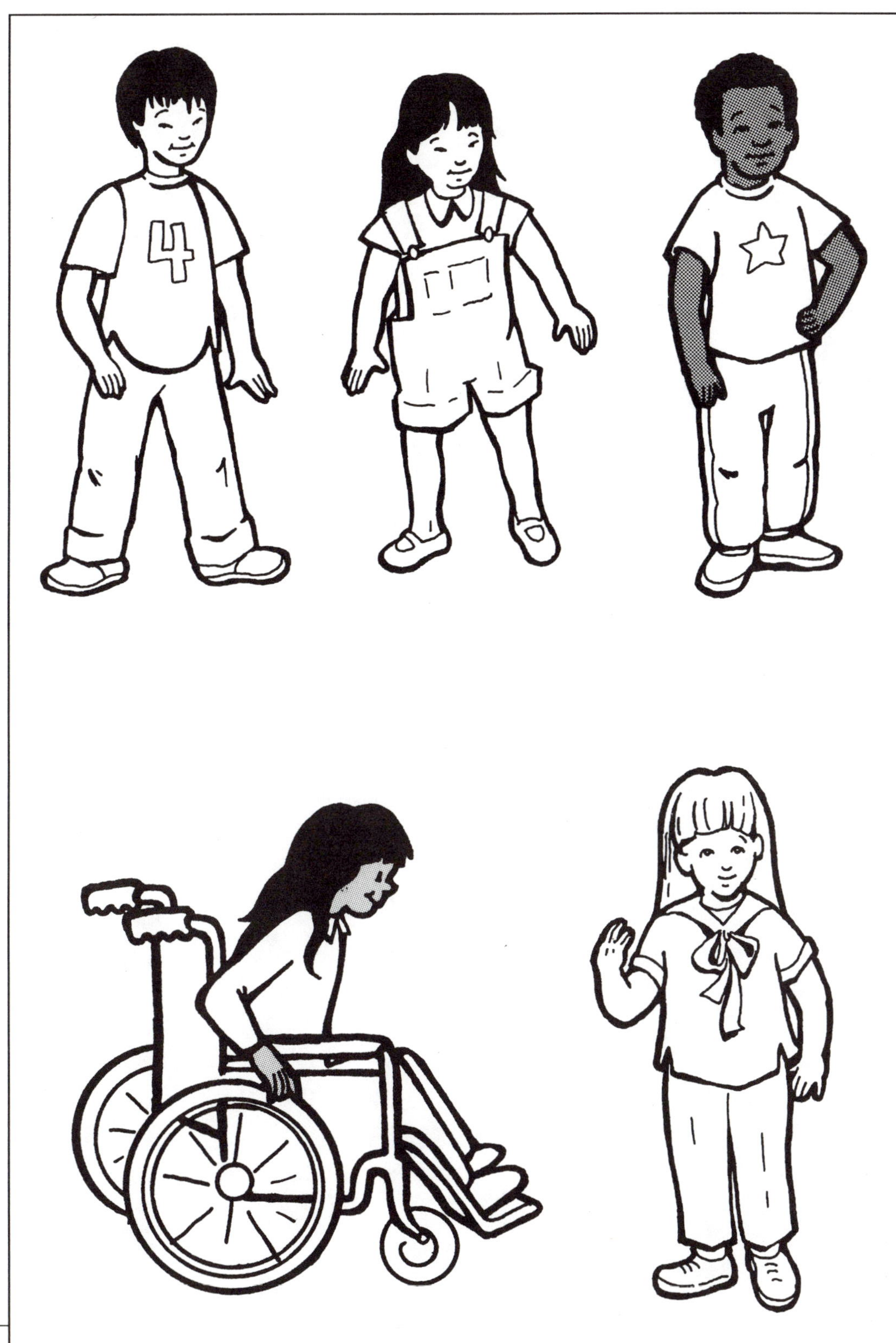

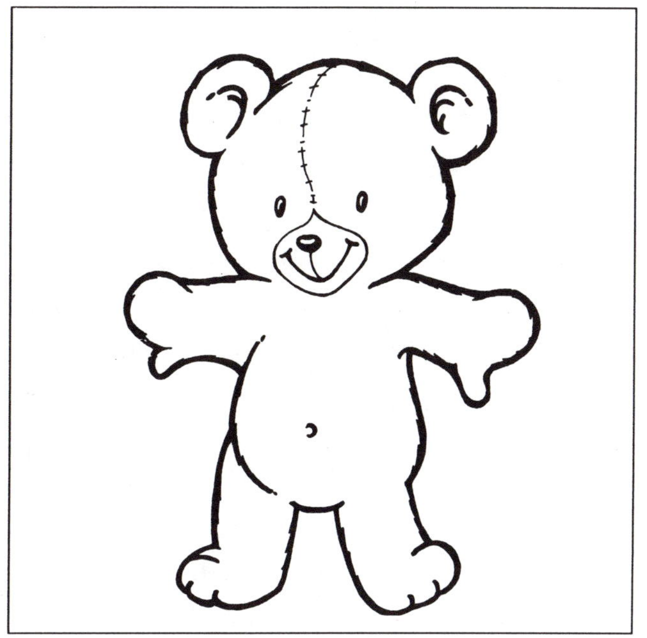

**Target Sound:**
/st/

**Linguistic Level:**
Word/Phrase/Sentence

**Position:**
Initial

**Objective:**
To decrease the application of /s/ Cluster Reduction, the children will produce word-initial /st/ clusters with varying levels of accuracy following the clinician's model or spontaneously.

**Suggestions for Nametags:**
In each session, provide a choice between two nametags to elicit productions of the target sound. Suggestions for the word-initial /st/ cluster include: *stairs, star, starfish, Sticky Bear.*

## Sticky Stan

**Target Words:** Stan, stepped, stick, sticky, stop, stopped, stuff

**Materials:** illustration of a boy (See pages 323–324.)
*Sticky Stan* story

**Procedure:** Duplicate the illustration of the boy *(Stan)*. Tell the story *Sticky Stan* about a boy named *Stan*. As the story is told, demonstrate the movements *Stan* makes using the illustration of *Stan*. Have the children join you in the actions, eliciting the target words as you do them.

**Story:** *Sticky Stan*
*Stan* went out to play in his backyard. He saw a pile of *stuff* near his mother's garden. *Stan* decided to *stick* his fingers in the *stuff*. It felt *sticky*. *Stan's* mother saw him and said, "Please *stop*. You'll get *sticky!*" But *Stan* didn't listen. He *stepped* in the *stuff*. *Stan* got all *sticky! Stan* should have *stopped* when his mother told him to.

## Sticky Bear

**Target Words:** star, steak, sticker, sticky, stockings, stomach, stove

**Materials:** initial /st/ illustrations (e.g., star, steak, stove)
Sticky Bear illustration          foil stars
double-sided contact paper      stickers

**Procedure:** Duplicate *Sticky* Bear and /st/ illustrations and cut them out. Cut bear shapes out of contact paper using the *Sticky* Bear pattern. Remove the backings of the contact paper and attach to the bear pattern leaving a *sticky* side of the paper exposed. Have the children participate in an art activity making a *Sticky* Bear by *sticking* /st/ illustrations, *stickers*, and *stars* on their *Sticky* Bear's *stomach* or *stockings* (legs). To elicit target words, offer a choice of items to affix to the bear.

## Peanut Butter Stickies*

**Target Words:** sticks, sticky, stir, stones

**Materials:**

| | |
|---|---|
| peanut butter | hot plate or stove |
| honey | dry milk powder |
| measuring spoon | spoon |
| saucepan | small plates |

**Procedure:** Make peanut butter *stickies* (recipe follows) with the children using a hot plate or stove. Give each child a turn to add ingredients and *stir*. Elicit choral productions of *stir, stir, stir* as the children take turns mixing the ingredients. Shape the *stickies* into *sticks* (small cylinders) and *stones* (little balls) before eating. Ask the children if their hands are *sticky* or not *sticky*.

**Recipe:** *Peanut Butter Stickies* (by Carolyn Ebner)
1–18 oz. jar of peanut butter
6 tablespoons of honey
dry milk powder

Combine peanut butter and honey in a saucepan. Cook over low heat until barely melted. Add dry milk powder a little at a time, until desired consistency is reached. After the mixture is cooled, mold into desired shapes.

## Sticks and Stones Stew*

**Target Words:** stew, sticks, stir, stones

**Materials:**
| | |
|---|---|
| stew pot | bowls |
| pretzel sticks | large spoon |
| round ball-like cereal (such as Kix) | |

**Procedure:** Using a *stew* pot, prepare a *stew* made of *sticks* (pretzel *sticks*) and *stones* (round cereal) with the children. Give each child an opportunity to add *sticks* and/or *stones* to the *stew*, *stir* it, then eat it for a snack. Have the children take turns serving the *stew* to the others and asking group members if they want *sticks* or *stones*. Encourage the children to provide very small portions so that frequent productions of the target words are elicited.

## /st/ Jigglers*

**Target Words:** star, stocking

**Materials:**
two flavors of JELL-O
cookie cutters

**Procedure:** In advance of this activity, prepare JELL-O Jigglers in two different flavors. (Find the directions for making JELL-O Jigglers on a box of JELL-O.) Using cookie cutters selected to elicit the target words, such as *star* or *stocking,* have the children cut shapes in the JELL-O. Provide a choice of cookie cutters for the children to use by asking, for example, "Do you want a *star* or a *stocking?*" Provide several cookie cutters so that waiting time is minimized for the children. Once the shapes are cut, have the children eat the JELL-O.

(Adapt this activity for any target sound.)

## Step and Stomp

**Target Words:**  start, step, stinky, stomp, stop

**Materials:**  stinky bug illustration
construction paper
footprints illustration (optional) (See page 312.)
cassette player
musical cassette tape

**Procedure:**  Before this session, duplicate several *stinky* bug illustrations and cut them out. Also cut footsteps out of construction paper. (Use the footprints illustration as a pattern if necessary.) Distribute cutouts of footsteps and *stinky* bugs randomly on the floor. Give each child the choice of *stepping* on the footsteps or *stomping* on the *stinky* bugs. Model *step, step, step*, as the children *step* on the footsteps, and *stomp, stomp, stomp*, as the children *stomp* on the bugs. To add interest, use music as a cue to indicate when to *start* and *stop*.

## Musical Stepping Stones*

**Target Words:**  stairs, stand, starfish, steak, step, still, stone, stop

**Materials:**  stairs, starfish, and steak illustrations
gray construction paper          cassette player
musical cassette tape          glue or glue stick

**Procedure:**  Duplicate illustrations of the *stairs, starfish*, and *steak*. Cut large *stones* out of gray construction paper and glue a picture of a *stairs, starfish,* or *steak* on one side of the *stones*. Place them in a circle on the floor. Have the children *step* on the *stones* in the circle as music is played. *Stop* the music intermittently. When the music *stops*, have the children turn over their *stone* and *stand still* as they name their picture.

## /st/ Store*

**Target Words:** stamp, star, stick, stickers, stocking, stone, store, store-keeper

**Materials:** toy cash register
pretend money
small shopping baskets
initial /st/ items
   (e.g., postage stamps, pretzel sticks, round ball-like
   cereal, star stickers, stickers, [children's] stockings)

**Procedure:** Arrange the room to look like a *store* with /st/ items in various places. Assign each child a role to play (such as shopper, cashier, or *storekeeper*). Recreate a shopping trip by acting out each role. Place the items for purchase just beyond reach of the shoppers, so they must ask the *storekeeper* for the item they wish to purchase. Have the *storekeeper* provide the shoppers with a choice of /st/ items to purchase (e.g., *stamps, stones* [round cereal], *stars, sticks* [pretzels], *stockings,* or *stickers*). Have the cashier name the items as the shoppers go through the checkout. Give each child an opportunity to play each role.

## /st/ **Activity Stations***

**Target Words:** stack, stars, station, stick, sticker, stir, stockings, stones, stuff

**Materials:** blocks
stockings
tissue paper
pretzel sticks
round ball-like cereal
large bowl
large spoon
stars
stickers
8½ x 11" sheets of paper

**Procedure:** Set up the following activity *stations* in various parts of the room:

1. Blocks (to *stack*).

2. *Stockings* and tissue paper (to *stuff stockings* with the tissue paper).

3. *Sticks* (pretzels) and *stones* (round cereal) in a bowl with a spoon (to *stir*).

4. *Stars*, *stickers*, and paper (to *stick stars* and *stickers* on paper).

Lead children through the *stations* in pairs. Have the children take turns telling each other what to do at each *station*. Encourage parents to accompany their children as they go from *station* to *station*.

## Fishing for /st/

**Target Words:** stairs, star, starfish, steak, stove

**Materials:** fishing poles (See *Appendix H*.)
construction paper
initial /st/ illustrations
   (e.g., stairs, star, starfish, steak, stove)
paper clips
bucket

**Procedure:** In preparation for this activity, create one fishing pole for each child. Cut several fish out of construction paper. Duplicate and attach illustrations of /st/ words to the construction paper fish with paper clips. Spread the paper fish out on the floor. Have the children fish for /st/ illustrations using the fishing pole. Allow several children to fish at the same time. Once the fish are caught, have the children bring them to you, name them, and put them into a bucket. As the children bring the fish to you, ask, for instance, "Did you catch *stairs* or a *star?*" After all the fish are caught, review the illustrations with the group. For the illustrations that are familiar to the children, provide a foil by saying, for example, "This is a hot dog," so that the children respond, "No, it's a *steak!*"

(Adapt this activity for any target sound.)

## Star Says*

**Target Words:**  star, start, steer, stir, stomp, stop

**Materials:**  star badge

**Procedure:**  This game is similar to "Simon Says." Act as the leader first, demonstrating different actions the children can perform (*stomp*, *stir*, or *steer*). Instruct the children when to *start stomping, stirring,* or *steering* by chanting (e.g., *stomp, stomp, stomp*) as the action is carried out. *Stop* the action by saying *stop!* Give each child an opportunity to lead the group. Have the leader wear a *star*.

## Start/Stop*

**Target Words:**  start, step, stop

**Materials:**  red and green construction paper

**Procedure:**  Before this activity, cut circular *start* and *stop* signs out of red and green construction paper. Have the children take turns being the leader and telling the other children when to *start* and when to *stop stepping* in this "Red Light/Green Light" game. Use the *start* and *stop* signs to indicate to the leader when to say *start* and *stop*. As the children take *steps* closer to the leader, have them chant *step, step, step*.

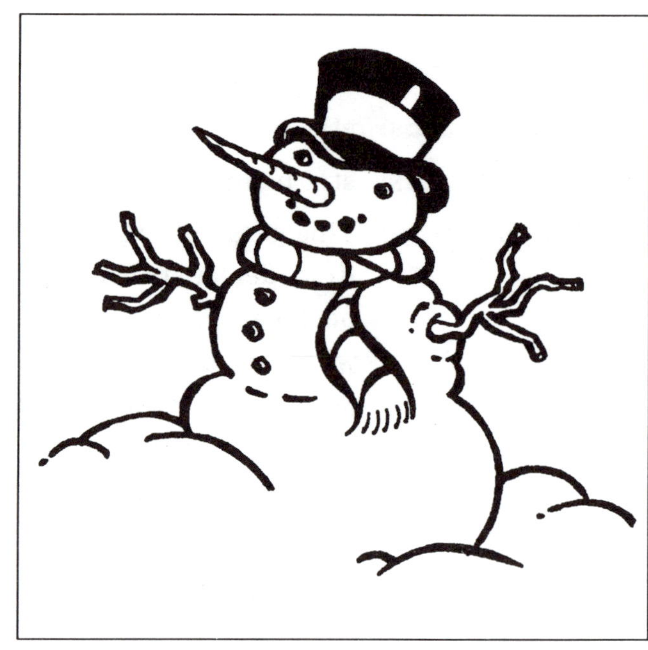

**Target Sound:**
/sn/

**Linguistic Level:**
Word/Phrase/Sentence

**Position:**
Initial

**Objective:**
To decrease the application of /s/ Cluster Reduction, the children will produce word-initial /sn/ clusters with varying levels of accuracy following the clinician's model or spontaneously.

**Suggestions for Nametags:**
In each session, provide a choice between two nametags to elicit productions of the target sound. Suggestions for the word-initial /sn/ cluster include: *snail, snake, sneakers, snowperson.*

## Snippy Story and Song

**Target Words:** snake, snap, sneak, sneeze, snip, Snippy, snore

**Materials:** *Snippy the Snake* story

**Procedure:** Read the story *Snippy the Snake* to the children, bombarding them with initial /sn/ words. Lead the group in a song to the tune of "Are You Sleeping?"

**Story:** *Snippy the Snake*

*Snippy* the *Snake* lived in a house with tall grass around it. He liked to *sneak* around in the tall grass. One day while *Snippy* was *sneaking* in the grass, he began to *sneeze*. *Snippy sneezed* and *sneezed* and *sneezed*. *Snippy sneezed* so hard he broke the *snap* on his pants! *Snippy* started to slither home to change his pants. On his way home, *Snippy* felt very sleepy. He decided to *snip* some of the tall grass so he could lie down and take a nap. Very soon *Snippy* was fast asleep. He even began to *snore!*

*Snippy Song*
(Incorporate actions to illustrate target words while singing.)

    *Snippy's snoring,*
    *Snippy's snoring,*
    *Snore, snore, snore!*
    *Snore, snore, snore!*
    *Snippy* is *snoring,*
    *Snippy* is *snoring,*
    *Snore, snore, snore,*
    *Snore, snore, snore.*

(Repeat with *snap, sneak, sneeze,* and *snip.*)

## Snazzy Snakes

**Target Words:** snake, snazzy

**Materials:** Play-doh
sequins
small decorative eyes

**Procedure:** Demonstrate how to make a *snazzy snake* out of Play-doh. Have the children roll the Play-doh into a *snake* shape and decorate it with sequins, eyes, etc. As the *snakes* are being made, model and elicit *snazzy* and *snake* from the children.

## Snowperson Art*

**Target Words:** snowballs, snow boots, snowflakes, snow hat, snowperson

**Materials:** construction paper
cotton balls
glue or glue sticks

**Procedure:** Draw an outline of a *snowperson* (three circles graduated in size) on construction paper. Create *snowflakes* and appropriately sized *snow hats* and *snow boots*, one set per child, out of construction paper. Cut them out. Give each child a *snowperson* outline. Have each child decorate the *snowperson* by choosing from among the four target /sn/ items—*snowballs* (cotton balls), *snow hats*, *snow boots*, and *snowflakes*. Put the objects for the art work slightly out of reach (e.g., lined up on the chalk tray or pinned to a bulletin board) so the children must request them verbally.

## Snowsnakes and Snowpeople

**Target Words:** snake, snow, snowballs, snowperson

**Materials:** snake and snowperson illustrations
construction paper
cotton balls
glue or glue sticks

**Procedure:** Enlarge, duplicate, and cut out illustrations of the *snake* and *snowperson*, one per child. Glue onto construction paper. Give the children the choice of making a *snowperson* or a *snowsnake* by gluing *snowballs* (cotton balls) on the chosen picture. To obtain a cotton ball, have the children say, "*Snowball* please," "*Snowball*," or "*Snow*," depending on their linguistic ability.

## Snake and Snail Snack

**Target Words:** snack, snail, snake

**Materials:** fruit roll-ups
string cheese

**Procedure:** Introduce this *snack* activity by telling the children they have a choice of making a *snake* or a *snail* to eat. Provide a premade sample of each one so the children can visualize the final product. Have the children verbally choose which one they want to make and eat. Make the *snake* by rolling a fruit roll-up into a long cylindrical shape. Make the *snail* by using strips of string cheese that are wound in a coil shape. As the children are forming their *snakes* and *snails,* encourage discussion that elicits the target words.

## Snow Cones

**Target Words:** snack, snow, snow angel, snow cones, snow fort, snow-people

**Materials:** crushed ice
blender
frozen juice concentrate
spoons
small cups

**Procedure:** Bring in *snow* (crushed ice) and blend it in the blender with frozen fruit juice concentrate to make *snow* cones. Eat the *snow cones* for a *snack* while talking about *snow* and different things to do in the *snow,* such as making *snow angels, snowpeople,* and *snow forts.*

## Snap the Toy

**Target Words:** snap, snapped

**Materials:** carpet squares
child's toy that snaps or clicks

**Procedure:** Seat the children on carpet squares in a circle. Have one of the children sit in a chair facing away from the group or sit facing the group with his or her eyes closed. Have the rest of the children place their hands behind their backs. Place a *snapping* toy in one of the children's hands. Have the child with the toy *snap* it, then have the child who is "it" open his or her eyes and guess who has the toy by saying, "(Suzie) *snapped* the toy." For children with limited linguistic ability, modify the response to *snap* while pointing to the child who *snapped* the toy.

## Snow Tub

**Target Words:**   snow, snowball, snowflake, snowpeople

**Materials:**   tub filled with snow
mittens

**Procedure:**   (This activity is best done in the winter in a cold climate; if snow is not available, use crushed ice instead.) Fill a tub with *snow*. Have the children wear mittens and engage in a sensory-play activity by making *snowballs* and small *snowpeople*. Model target words and encourage productions through the use of foils and conversation.

## Sneak and Find

**Target Words:**   snail, snake, sneak, sneakers, snowball

**Materials:**   snail and snake illustrations
pairs of large sneakers
cotton balls
flashlights or pen lights

**Procedure:**   Before the session, duplicate and cut out illustrations of *snails* and *snakes* and gather pairs of large *sneakers*. Hide paper *snails, snakes,* and *snowballs* (cotton balls) around the room. Have the children put on the oversized *sneakers*. Dim the lights and have children *sneak* around to find the hidden objects using a flashlight. Tell the children to chant *sneak, sneak, sneak* as they search. After each object is found, instruct them to bring it back to you (or a designated member of the group) and name it. Provide a correct model of the target word after the child's production. Once all the objects are found, have the children come together and sort all the *snails, snakes,* and *snowballs,* naming each one.

## /sn/ **Activity Stations**

**Target Words:** snap, sneeze, snore, snowball

**Materials:** spinner (See *Appendix H.*)
facial tissues      cotton balls
clothing with snaps    container to catch cotton balls
pillow      bell

**Procedure:** Create a spinner with the words *snap, sneeze, snore,* and *snowball* as spinner options. Set up the following activity stations in various parts of the room:

1. (*Snap*) a jacket, sweater, or pants with *snaps* (to *snap* or un*snap*).

2. (*Sneeze*) facial tissue on a table (to simulate a *sneeze*).

3. (*Snore*) a pillow on a table (to feign sleeping and to *snore* loudly).

4. (*Snowball*) a container and cotton balls (to throw the *snowball* [cotton ball] into the container).

Demonstrate the activity required at each station. Have the children take turns spinning the spinner to see which station to go to. Instruct the child to name the station, run to it, and complete the action while the other children chant the target word. Once the action is completed, tell the child to return and ring the bell.

## Sneakers and Flashlights

**Target Words:**  sneak, sneakers

**Materials:**  adult-size sneakers
flashlights

**Procedure:**  Hide pairs of large *sneakers* around the room. Give each child a flashlight. Turn off the lights and have the children chant *sneak, sneak, sneak* while looking for the *sneakers*. When all the children have located a pair, have them put on the sneakers while saying, "I found the *sneakers*" or "*Sneakers.*"

## /sn/ Bingo*

**Target Words:**  snail, snake, sneaker, snowball, snowflake, snowperson

**Materials:**  bingo boards (See *Appendix H.*)
initial /sn/ illustrations
   (e.g., snail, snake, snowperson)
cloth grab bag (See *Appendix H.*)
cotton balls

**Procedure:**  Before the session, prepare bingo boards with four to six initial /sn/ illustrations on them. Make an identical set of illustrations to use as calling cards and place them in the cloth bag. Give each child a bingo board. Have the children take turns being the "caller" by drawing an /sn/ calling card from the bag and naming it for the others. If the picture named is on a child's board, instruct him or her to cover it with a *snowball* (cotton ball) while repeating the name of the picture. Continue the game until all the children have covered all of their illustrations.

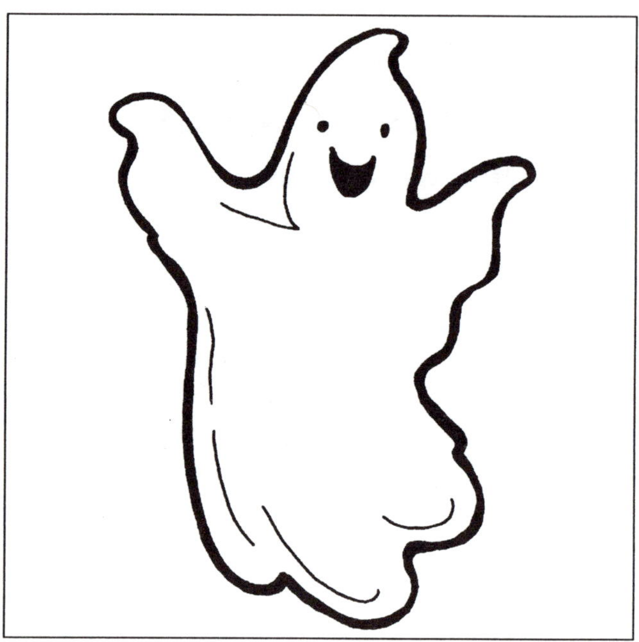

**Target Sound:**
/sp/

**Linguistic Level:**
Word/Phrase/Sentence

**Position:**
Initial

**Objective:**
To decrease the application of /s/ Cluster Reduction, the children will produce word-initial /sp/ clusters with varying levels of accuracy following the clinician's model or spontaneously.

**Suggestions for Nametags:**
In each session, provide a choice between two nametags to elicit productions of the target sound. Suggestions for the word-initial /sp/ cluster include: *spaceship, spider, spook, spoon.*

## Space Spaghetti*

**Target Words:**   space food, spaghetti, spinach

**Materials:**   white yarn
green tissue paper
paper plates
glue or glue sticks

**Procedure:**   Before the session, cut strands of yarn and crumple pieces of green tissue paper. Have the children make *space food* by gluing *spaghetti* (strands of yarn) and *spinach* (crumpled green tissue paper) onto a paper plate. Parents can easily participate in this activity by providing choices for their child of *spaghetti* or *spinach* to glue onto the plate. Glue each strand of *spaghetti* and *spinach* separately to elicit many productions from the children.

# Spying for Space Food

**Target Words:** spaghetti, spinach, spy

**Materials:** white yarn
green tissue paper
glue or glue sticks
paper plates

**Procedure:** Before the session, cut strands of white yarn and crumple pieces of green tissue paper. Hide them around the room. Have the children *spy* (search) for *space* food consisting of *spinach* (crumpled pieces of green tissue paper) and *spaghetti* (strands of yarn) which are hidden. As they search, have the children chorally chant *spy, spy, spy.* Once the *space* food is found, instruct the children to gather and glue their *spinach* and *spaghetti* onto a paper plate. (See *Space Spaghetti* on the preceding page for a variation of this activity.)

## Sponge Painting

**Target Words:** spider, spin, spinner, sponge, spook, spoon

**Materials:** initial /sp/ illustrations (e.g., spider, spook, spoon)
spinner (See *Appendix H.*)
glue or glue stick
large sheets of paper
paint smocks (or large shirts)
sponge wedges
paint

**Procedure:** Before the session, make multiple copies of several /sp/ illustrations. Use one of each to create the *spinner* and glue the others to large sheets of paper. Prepare each child for *sponge* painting by rolling up their sleeves and putting on smocks. Provide each child with a *sponge* wedge and one of the large sheets of paper with the /sp/ illustrations glued on it. Have the children take turns *spinning* the *spinner* and naming the picture it lands on. Provide a choice such as, "Did you land on the *spider* or the *spoon?*" to elicit the target word. Then have the children *sponge* paint the picture identified by the *spinner*. Incorporate foils such as calling a *spoon* a fork instead, so the child responds, "No, *spoon!*"

## Space Treats

**Target Words:** space drink, space treat, sparkles

**Materials:** small boxes of fruit juice
aluminum foil
round vanilla wafers
frosting
colored sugar crystals

**Procedure:** Before the session, cover small boxes of fruit juice with aluminum foil. Have the children eat *space treats* (round vanilla wafers) and a *space drink* (juice boxes covered with aluminum foil). Give each child a turn to serve the other children. Have the children frost their *space treat*. After the cookies are frosted, encourage the children to request *sparkles* (colored sugar crystals) to put on top of their *space treats*.

## Space Snack

**Target Words:** space drink, space food, space hat, spaceship

**Materials:** hats
aluminum foil
small boxes of fruit juice
blanket
table
fruit snacks (such as fruit roll-ups)

**Procedure:** Before this activity create *space hats* (hats covered with aluminum foil), *space drinks* (juice boxes covered with foil), and a *spaceship* (a blanket draped over a table). Instruct the children to put on *space hats* before entering their *spaceship* to have a snack. The snack consists of *space food* (fruit roll-ups) and a *space drink* (juice boxes covered with aluminum foil). Have the children take turns asking each other if they would like *space food* or a *space drink*.

## I Spy

**Target Words:** spider, spook, spoon, spy

**Materials:** initial /sp/ illustrations (e.g., spider, spook, spoon)
tape
toilet paper tube

**Procedure:** Duplicate multiple copies of /sp/ illustrations and tape them on the walls around the room. Give each child a turn to *spy* for the illustrations by using a *spy* glass (toilet paper tube). As the child *spies* the picture, have him or her say, "I *spy* a (*spider*)." For children with limited linguistic skills, modify the response to just the target word (e.g., *spoon*).

## I Am Special

**Target Words:** sparkle, special, spin, spy

**Materials:** none

**Procedure:** Introduce the actions of *spy* (form a circle with your thumb and index finger and place it over one eye), *spin* (turn around in a circle), and *sparkle* (wiggle your fingers in the air). Sing the following song to the tune of "Are you Sleeping?" Insert a different target word each round.

*I Am Special*
(Incorporate actions while singing.)
   I am *special,* I am *special,*
   I can *spy,* I can *spy.*
   I am *special,* I am *special,*
   I can *spy,* I can *spy.*
(Repeat with *sparkle* and *spin.*)

## Feed the Spider or Space Dog

**Target Words:** space dog, spaghetti, spider, spinach, sponge, spook, spoon

**Materials:** initial /sp/ illustrations or objects
   (e.g., spaghetti, spider, spinach, sponge, spook, spoon)
dog illustration (See page 322.)    tape
two grocery bags

**Procedure:** Duplicate /sp/ illustrations or obtain real /sp/ objects. Also, enlarge and duplicate the *spider* and dog (*space dog*) illustrations. Tape them on open grocery bags. Have the children choose an /sp/ picture (or object), name it, and tell the group if they are going to feed the *spider* or the *space dog*. Once the choice is made, assist the child in placing the picture (or object) in the appropriate bag while modeling the child's choice.

## Pin the Spot on Sparky or Spike

**Target Words:** Sparky, Spike, spot

**Materials:** construction paper
illustrations of two dogs (See page 322.)
tape

**Procedure:** Cut small circles (*spots*) out of construction paper. Enlarge and duplicate illustrations of two different-looking dogs (*Sparky* and *Spike*). Mount them on the wall or chalkboard. Have each child take a *spot* and indicate whether he or she wants to tape it on *Sparky* or *Spike*. Once the choice is made, have the child tape the *spot* on the dog selected.

# Spunky in Space

**Target Words:** space, spaceship, spaghetti, spider, spinach, spoon, Spunky, spy

**Materials:** hats
aluminum foil
blanket
table
initial /sp/ items
(e.g., boxes of spaghetti, plastic spiders, cans of spinach, spoons)

**Procedure:** Before the session, create *space* hats (hats covered with aluminum foil) and a *spaceship* (a blanket draped over a table). Hide /sp/ items around the room. Tell the children that *Spunky* is packing for a trip in *space* by putting *space* food and a *space spoon* into the *spaceship*. Allow one child, designated as *Spunky,* to wear the *space* hat and sit by the *spaceship*. Instruct the children to *spy* for *Spunky's space* food and *spoon* by searching throughout the room for the items. Model by saying, "I *spy* (*spinach*)" then bringing the object to *Spunky* by the *spaceship*. Instruct *Spunky* to identify the *space* item before placing it in the *spaceship*. Follow this sequence for each object that is found. While searching, have the children say *spy, spy, spy*. Encourage the children to take turns being *Spunky*.

## Spin and Pin*

**Target Words:** Sparky, spider, spider web, spin, spot

**Materials:** spider illustration
construction paper
dog illustration (See page 322.)
tape
blindfold
chalk and chalkboard

**Procedure:** Before this activity, duplicate several *spider* illustrations and cut several small circles (*spots*) out of construction paper. Enlarge and duplicate the dog (*Sparky*) illustration and tape it to the chalkboard. Also draw a *spider web* on the chalkboard. Give the children a choice of taping a *spot* on *Sparky* or a *spider* on the *spider web*. Encourage the children to take turns being blindfolded and *spun* around gently while the other children chant *spin, spin, spin.*

## Spot Toss*

**Target Words:** spider, spook, spoon, spot

**Materials:** construction paper
initial /sp/ illustrations (e.g., spider, spook, spoon)
bean bags

**Procedure:** In advance of this activity, cut large circles (*spots*) out of construction paper. Duplicate the initial /sp/ illustrations. Place the large *spots* on the floor in one section of the room. Place an /sp/ picture under each *spot*. Have the children take turns tossing bean bags onto the *spots* and naming the pictures underneath them.

## Space Spin

**Target Words:** space dog, spaceship, spider, spin, spook, spoon

**Materials:** dog illustration (See page 322.)
initial /sp/ illustrations
   (e.g., spider, spook, spoon)
large spinner (See *Appendix H*.)
blanket
table
tape

**Procedure:** Duplicate two copies of the dog (*space dog*) and several /sp/ illustrations. Use one of each to create a large *spinner*. Place the remaining illustrations on the floor. Create a *spaceship* in the room by placing a blanket over a table. Have half of the children in the group sit in the *spaceship*. Have the other half of the children sit around the *spinner*. Encourage each child to take a turn *spinning* (while all other children chorally produce *spin, spin, spin*). When the *spinner* stops, have one child from inside the *spaceship* come out to see the picture identified by the *spinner*. Instruct the child to name the picture, find the matching picture, and bring it into the *spaceship*. After each child outside the *spaceship* has had a turn, allow the groups to switch places.

## Yarn Spider Webs*

**Target Words:** space, spatula, spider, spider web, spinach, spook, spoon, spot

**Materials:** list of questions
ball of yarn (or string)

**Procedure:** Before the session, prepare questions that contain a choice of two of the target words (e.g., "Do you eat soup with a *spoon* or a *spatula?*"). Have the children sit in a circle on the floor. Ask each child one of the prepared questions. After a child answers a question, pass a ball of yarn to him or her. Then ask another child a question. After the second child responds, direct the first child to pass the ball of yarn to the next child, but tell the first child to hold on to one strand of the yarn. As the activity continues, have each child hold several strands of yarn that are connected across the circle to the others to form the shape of a *spider web.* Instruct the children not to let go of the yarn in their hands. Have the children talk about the *spider web* they are making.

## Spying with Spotlights

**Target Words:** space dog, spider, spook, spoon, spotlight, spy

**Materials:** dog illustration (See page 322.)
initial /sp/ illustrations (e.g., spider, spook, spoon)
flashlight

**Procedure:** Duplicate the dog (*space dog*) and several /sp/ illustrations and hide them around the room. Darken the room before the session. Have the children *spy* for /sp/ illustrations with a *spotlight* (flashlight). As the children find the illustrations, encourage them to name the illustration or say, "I *spy* a (*spoon*)." Provide the children with choices (e.g., "Did you *spy* a *spider* or a *spoon?*").

## Making a Spider Web

**Target Words:** spider, spider web, spin, spinner, spook, spoon

**Materials:** spider illustration
/sp/ illustrations (e.g., spider, spook, spoon)
spinner (See *Appendix H.*)
tape
chalk and chalkboard

**Procedure:** Enlarge and duplicate several *spider* illustrations and cut them out. Also duplicate /sp/ illustrations making two copies of each. Tape one of each to the *spiders*. Attach the duplicate illustrations to the spinner. Tape the *spiders* with /sp/ illustrations on them within a large outline of a *spider web* drawn on the chalkboard. *Spin* the *spinner*. Draw a line from the outline of the *spider web* to the picture selected. As the children take turns, have them *spin* the *spinner* and name the /sp/ picture. Direct the children to draw a line from the previous picture to the picture indicated on the *spinner*. Continue the activity until a *spider web* is created on the chalkboard.

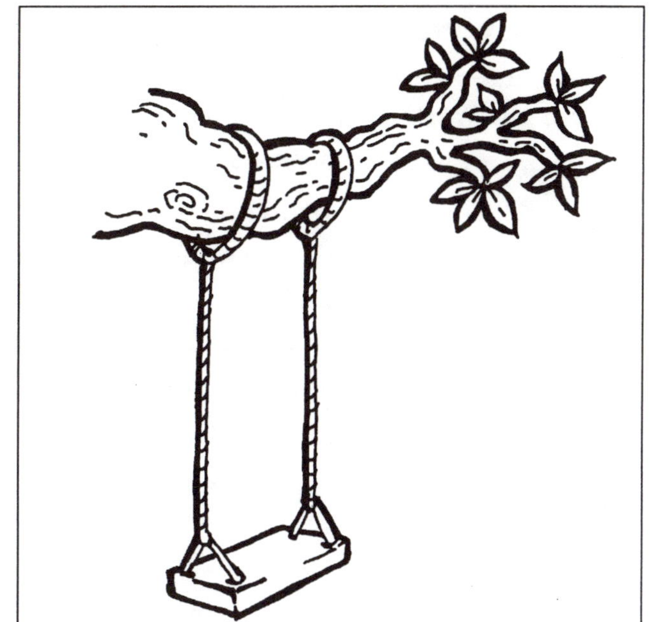

**Target Sound:**
/sw/

**Linguistic Level:**
Word/Phrase

**Position:**
Initial

## Objective:
To decrease the application of /s/ Cluster Reduction, the children will produce word-initial /sw/ with varying levels of accuracy following the clinician's model or spontaneously.

## Suggestions for Nametags:
In each session, provide a choice between two nametags to elicit productions of the target sound. Suggestions for the word-initial /sw/ cluster include: *swan, sweater, swing*.

## Sweat, Sweat, Sweat!

**Target Words:** Swami, sweatband, sweatshirt, sweat shorts, sweat socks, sweaty

**Materials:** sweat clothes
(e.g., sweatbands, sweatshirts, sweat shorts, sweat socks)
*Sweat, Sweat, Sweat!* story

**Procedure:** Before the session, gather one of each item of *sweat* clothing for each child. If necessary, send requests for clothes home or ask coworkers to help by sharing their *sweat* clothes for this activity. Arrange piles of *sweat* clothes in various areas of the room (e.g., all *sweatshirts* in one corner, all *sweat socks* in another corner, etc.). Read the *Sweat, Sweat, Sweat!* story to the children, bombarding them with initial /sw/ words. After each article of clothing is mentioned in the story, hold it up to show the children. Read the story again, but this time have the children act out the story by dressing up at each area of the room until they are completely dressed in *sweat* clothes. Move around the room with the children, telling them one part of the story at a time, then wait for them to act it out. Refer back to the story to elicit the target words. (See *Swami Sweats* on the next page for an alternative activity.)

**Story:** *Sweat, Sweat, Sweat!*
It was a beautiful day and *Swami* Bear decided to go outside. His mother told him to put on his *sweat* clothes. *Swami* Bear put on his *sweat socks* first. Then *Swami* Bear put on his *sweat shorts*. Next, he put on his favorite *sweatshirt*. *Swami* was ready to go outside! His mother reminded him to bring his *sweatband*. *Swami* Bear went outside in his *sweat* clothes. He ran down the street very fast. *Swami* was very *sweaty* from running.

## Swami Sweats

**Target Words:** Swami, sweatband, sweatshirt, sweat shorts, sweat socks

**Materials:** Swami Bear and sweat clothes illustrations
*Sweat, Sweat, Sweat!* story

**Procedure:** Before this activity, duplicate the *Swami* Bear illustration and *Swami* clothing so that each child will have one set. Cut *Swami* Bear and the clothing out. Read the story *Sweat, Sweat, Sweat!* Have the children create an art picture by dressing *Swami* in his *sweat* clothes.

## Swimming or Swinging Swan*

**Target Words:** swamp, swan, swim, swing

**Materials:** swamp, swan, and swing illustrations
colored paper
large sheets of paper
glue or glue sticks

**Procedure:** Before the session, duplicate several illustrations of the *swan* on different colors of paper and cut them out. Enlarge and duplicate the *swing* and *swamp* illustrations, making one per child. Provide the children with the large picture of the *swing* glued to the left side of a large sheet of paper and a *swamp* glued on the right half. Have the children request a paper *swan* cutout and say whether they want the *swan* to *swing* or to *swim* in the *swamp*. Once the choice is made, instruct the child to glue the *swan* on the appropriate illustration and to request another *swan*. Emphasize the word *swan* rather than the color names.

## Swami Bear Artwork

**Target Words:** Swami, swim fins, swim mask, swimmies, swimming, swimsuit, swim trunks

**Materials:** illustrations of Swami Bear and swimming accessories
glue or glue sticks
sheets of construction paper, larger than 8½ x 11"

**Procedure:** Duplicate one *Swami* Bear illustration and one set of *swimming* accessories per child. Cut out *Swami* Bear and the *swimming* accessories. Direct the children to glue *Swami* Bear onto a piece of construction paper. Have the children verbally choose which *swimming* accessories they want to glue on *Swami*.

## Sweetheart Snack*

**Target Words:** sweet, sweetheart, swirl

**Materials:**

| | |
|---|---|
| heart-shaped cookies | napkins |
| food coloring | small cups |
| frosting | fruit punch |
| plastic knives or popsicle sticks | |

**Procedure:** Provide unfrosted *sweetheart* cookies (heart-shaped cookies). Instruct the children to *swirl* food coloring into frosting and then *swirl* it onto their cookies with plastic knives or popsicle sticks. Have the children ask for a *sweet* drink (fruit punch) when they are thirsty. Serve the drink in very small amounts so that the children have to frequently request, "More *sweet* drink, please."

## Swirl Snack*

**Target Words:**  sweet, swirl

**Materials:**  celery sticks
small bowls
peanut butter
sweet juice
small cups

**Procedure:**  Give the children celery sticks and a bowl with a small amount (approximately one tablespoon) of peanut butter in it. Encourage the children to chant *swirl, swirl, swirl* as they *swirl* their celery sticks in the peanut butter. Give each child a small amount of a *sweet* drink, such as grape juice. Have the children request, "More *sweet* juice, please."

## Sweet Treat

**Target Words:**  sweet, swirl

**Materials:**  small plates
apple slices
honey in squeeze bottle

**Procedure:**  Before the session, gather small plates for the children to prepare their treat on and cut apples into slices. Help the children make a *sweet* treat of apple slices and *swirls* of honey. Encourage the children to chant *swirl, swirl, swirl* as they squeeze honey onto their apples using a circular motion. Use only a bit of honey at one time so children ask to *swirl* again.

## Sweeping Relay

**Target Words:** sweep

**Materials:** large, soft ball or crumpled paper
brooms
pom-poms

**Procedure:** Instruct the children to take turns (in pairs) *sweeping* a large, soft ball or a ball of paper across the room with a broom while the other children shake pom-poms and cheer *sweep, sweep, sweep!* After one child has *swept* the ball to the other side of the room, direct the child's teammate to take a turn.

## Sweet Pea Says

**Target Words:** sway, sweep, Sweet Pea, swim, swing

**Materials:** none

**Procedure:** Lead a session of "*Sweet Pea* Says" (similar to "Simon Says"), utilizing /sw/ action words as commands. Model the target words and actions of *swim*, *sweep*, *swing*, and *sway*. Once the children understand the game, encourage them to take turns being *Sweet Pea*.

## Sweeping and Swatting

**Target Words:** swamp, swan, swat, sweater, sweat socks, sweep, swing

**Materials:** initial /sw/ illustrations
(e.g., swamp, swan, sweater, sweat socks, swing)
broom
fly swatter

**Procedure:** Before the session, duplicate /sw/ illustrations and place them around the room. Have each child in turn select a picture by naming it. Give the child a choice of *sweeping* the picture with a broom or *swatting* the picture with a fly *swatter*. Have the other children cheer *sweep, sweep, sweep* or *swat, swat, swat!*

## Swans and Swings

**Target Words:** swan, swan pond, swing, swing set

**Materials:** swan and swing illustrations
chalk and chalkboard
tape

**Procedure:** Duplicate several illustrations of the *swan* and *swing* and cut them out. Before the session, draw a *swan pond* and a *swing set* (without the *swings*) on a chalkboard and hide pictures of *swans* and *swings* around the room. Have the children search for the *swans* and *swings* that were hidden. Instruct the children to find one picture at a time and return it to you, identifying what they found. Instruct them to tape the *swans* onto the *swan pond* and the *swings* on the *swing set*, telling the others where they have placed their *swans* or *swings*.

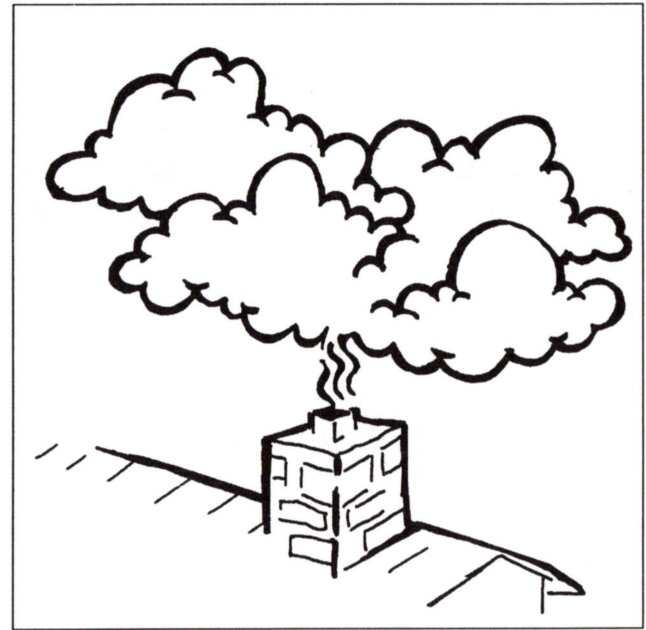

### Target Sound:
/sm/

### Linguistic Level:
Word/Phrase/Sentence

### Position:
Initial

### Objective:
To decrease the application of /s/ Cluster Reduction, the children will produce word-initial /sm/ clusters with varying levels of accuracy following the clinician's model or spontaneously.

### Suggestions for Nametags:
In each session, provide a choice between two nametags to elicit productions of the target sound. Suggestions for word-initial /sm/ clusters include: *smile, smock, smoke.*

## Smooth Leaves for Smitty

**Target Words:** small, smart, smelly, smile, Smitty, smooth

**Materials:** wax paper
sandpaper
*Smooth Leaves for Smitty* story

**Procedure:** Prepare three or four leaf cutouts per child, with a mix of *smooth* leaves and leaves that are not *smooth* (using wax paper and sandpaper). Distribute the leaves around the room. Also prepare two trees, one made of wax paper and one made of sandpaper. Mount both on a wall or chalkboard. Read the story *Smooth Leaves for Smitty* to the children, bombarding them with initial /sm/ words. Use the cutouts of leaves and trees as props. Direct the children to search around the room to find leaves that are *smooth* and leaves that are not *smooth*. When the children return with leaves, have them match the leaves to the tree that is *smooth* or the tree that is not *smooth*. Recall events in the story with the children.

**Story:** *Smooth Leaves for Smitty* (by Kylie Puram)
One day, *Smitty* went for a walk. He was looking for *smooth* leaves. He went to the park and picked up a leaf. How did the leaf feel? It wasn't *smooth*. *Smitty* wanted only *smooth* leaves. He looked under a *small* tree and picked up another leaf. Was it *smooth*? No, it was not *smooth*. Then he looked behind a *smelly* garbage can. There was another leaf! It was *smooth*! *Smitty* wanted one more *smooth* leaf. He was *smart* and looked in a tree. There was another *smooth* leaf! *Smitty smiled* because he found *smooth* leaves.

## Ms. Smith's Flowers

**Target Words:** small, smell, smile, Smith, smoke, smooth

**Materials:** illustrations of a girl (See pages 324–326.)
smile and smoke illustrations
flower illustration (See page 297.)
*Ms. Smith's Flowers* story

**Procedure:** Before this activity, duplicate the illustrations. Make two copies of the flower. Color one red and one yellow. Read the story *Ms. Smith's Flowers* to the children, bombarding them with initial /sm/ words. As the story is read, have the children place the pictures along the chalkboard or wall in sequence as they occur in the story. After the story is read, mix up the pictures and have the children assist in putting them back in order. As this is being done, discuss the story including as many productions of the target words as possible.

**Story:** *Ms. Smith's Flowers*
One spring day, Ms. *Smith* was outside *smelling* her flowers. They *smelled* good! The red one *smelled* like cherries, and the yellow one *smelled* like lemons. Suddenly, Ms. *Smith smelled* something different. Ms. *Smith smelled smoke!* The *smoke* made Ms. *Smith's smile* go away. Ms. *Smith* forgot to take her *smooth* pudding off the stove and it burned. There was *smoke* all around her *small* house. When the *smoke* was gone from the *small* house, Ms. *Smith smiled* again and made more *smooth* pudding. It *smelled* wonderful.

## Smokey the Bear

**Target Words:** small, smart, smashed, smell, smoke, Smokey

**Materials:** bear illustration (Use the grizzly bear, page 297, or draw Smokey.)
*Smokey the Bear* story

**Procedure:** Before this session, duplicate the bear illustration or draw one. Read the story *Smokey the Bear* to the children, bombarding them with initial /sm/ words. Show the bear illustration to the children as the story is read. Since there is an important lesson to be learned from this story, talk about what happened to *Smokey*, incorporating the target words.

**Story:** *Smokey the Bear* (by Danni Thomas)
*Smokey* the Bear lived in the forest. *Smokey* didn't like to get up in the morning. One day, *Smokey* got out of bed and *smashed* his head on the ceiling. *Smokey's* room was too *small* for him to stand up. *Smokey* took a walk through the forest. *Smokey* began to *smell smoke.* As *Smokey* walked closer to the *smoke,* he saw fire. *Smokey* helped his friends put out the fire. *Smokey* said, "Be *smart!* Don't play with matches." Then *Smokey* said, "Playing with matches can start a big fire."

## Smooth Pudding

**Target Words:** smiles, smock, smooth

**Materials:** pudding
tape
aluminum foil
spoon
smocks

**Procedure:** Prepare *smooth* pudding with or without the children's help. Tape a piece of aluminum foil to the table in front of each child. Place a large spoonful of pudding on each piece of aluminum foil. While wearing *smocks*, have the children *smooth* the pudding out on the aluminum foil, drawing *smiles* in it. As the children participate in this activity, engage them in conversation to model these words frequently and to elicit the target words. If extra pudding remains, have a snack activity in which the children talk about the pudding they are eating (e.g., "Is it *smooth* or not *smooth?*"; "More *smooth* pudding, please!").

## Small Pudding Pies*

**Target Words:** small, smash, smell, smooth

**Materials:** pudding
graham crackers
zipper plastic bags
wooden mallet (optional)
small bowls or cups
small spoons

**Procedure:** Before this activity, prepare pudding to make *small* pudding pies. Instruct the children to *smash* graham crackers in a zipper plastic bag (pounding the graham crackers with their fists or a wooden mallet) while chanting *smash, smash, smash*. Once the graham crackers are *smashed*, give each child a *small* bowl or cup to sprinkle the crumbs into. Then direct the children to add spoonfuls of *smooth* pudding. Encourage the children to *smell* the *smooth* pudding. Provide a *small* spoon to eat the pudding pie.

## Smacks or Smarties

**Target Words:** Smacks, small, Smarties, smock

**Materials:**

| | |
|---|---|
| small bowls | smock or oversized shirt |
| Sugar Smacks cereal | napkins |
| Smarties candies | small serving spoon |
| serving tray | |

**Procedure:** Place a *small* bowl of Sugar *Smacks* cereal and a *small* bowl of *Smarties* candies on a tray. Have each child take a turn wearing the *smock* and serving the snack to the other children with a *small* spoon. Instruct the server to ask each child, "Would you like *Smacks* or *Smarties?*" Encourage the server to serve *small* portions of food, so that frequent productions of the target words can be elicited.

## Smooth Grab Bag

**Target Word:** smooth

**Materials:** cloth grab bag (See *Appendix H.*)
items that are not smooth
   (e.g., nail file, sandpaper, textured piece of material)
items that are smooth
   (e.g., aluminum foil, smooth rock)

**Procedure:** Collect items such as those suggested in the materials list and place them in a cloth grab bag. Have the children select items, one at a time, from the cloth bag and say whether each item is *smooth* or not *smooth*. Place emphasis on the target word *smooth*, rather than the actual name of the object. Have the children sort items into their respective categories, helping as needed. To vary this activity, ask the children to bring items from home that are *smooth* or not *smooth*.

## Musical Smoke and Smiles*

**Target Words:** smile, smoke

**Materials:** smile and smoke illustrations
cassette player
musical cassette tape

**Procedure:** Duplicate one *smile* and one *smoke* illustration per child. Place pictures of *smiles* and *smoke* face down in a circle on the floor. Have the children march or walk around the circle to music. Stop the music intermittently. When the music stops, instruct the children to identify the picture they stopped at or next to.

# Show and Smell*

**Target Words:** smell, smells

**Materials:** fragrant or aromatic objects
(e.g., candle, cinnamon, coffee, perfume)
nonfragrant or nonaromatic objects
(e.g., cotton balls, paper, rocks)
cloth grab bag (See *Appendix H*.)

**Procedure:** In advance of this activity, request that the children bring something from home that *smells* and something that doesn't *smell*. Supplement with additional items. Place all items in a cloth grab bag. (All items can be placed in small plastic bags ahead of time to keep the smells separate.) Direct the children to take turns reaching into the bag and selecting one item. Have the group discuss whether the item *smells* or doesn't *smell*, placing emphasis on the target word *smell* rather than the name of the object. Pass around each item for the children to see whether it *smells* or not. The target word can be practiced at the sentence level by having the children say, "I *smell* (<u>cinnamon</u>)" as the object is passed to them.

## Musical Smiles*

**Target Words:** smile, smiling

**Materials:** smiling face illustrations
nonsmiling face illustrations
magazines or catalogs
musical cassette tape
cassette player

**Procedure:** Before this activity, cut out of magazines illustrations that are *smiling* or not *smiling*. Then, arrange enough chairs for all children in the group to sit in a circle, with the backs of the chairs facing into the circle. Place either a *smiling* illustration or an illustration that is not *smiling* face down on each chair. Instruct the children to march around the circle as music is played. Stop the music intermittently. When the music stops, direct each child to find a chair to sit on and say whether he or she sat on a *smiling* face or one that was not *smiling*. Have the children take turns turning the music on and off and asking the other children if they sat on a face that was *smiling* or not *smiling*. Do not eliminate a chair after each round, as in the traditional "musical chairs" game; rather, have all children participate in this activity each round.

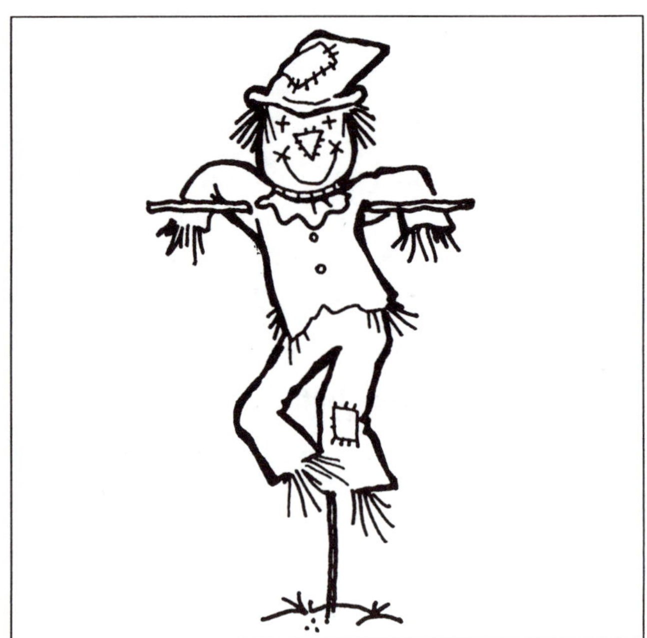

**Target Sound:**
/sk/

**Linguistic Level:**
Word/Phrase

**Position:**
Initial

**Objective:**
To decrease the application of /s/ Cluster Reduction, the children will produce word-initial /sk/ clusters with varying levels of accuracy following the clinician's model or spontaneously.

**Suggestions for Nametags:**
In each session, provide a choice between two nametags to elicit productions of the target sound. Suggestions for word-initial /sk/ clusters include: *scarecrow, school bus, skeleton, skunk.*

## Scott the Skunk

**Target Words:** Scarecrow, skip, scoot, Scotland, Scott, skunk, Skylar

**Materials:** *Scott the Skunk* story

**Procedure:** Read the story *Scott the Skunk* to the children, bombarding them with initial /sk/ words. At appropriate places in the story, have the children chorally chant *scoot, scoot, scoot!*

**Story:** *Scott the Skunk*

Once there was a *skunk* named *Scott*. *Scott* was looking for a friend to play with. He *skipped* over to *Skylar's* house. *Skylar's* mother came to the door. She said, "*Skylar* isn't home, so *scoot, scoot, scoot!*" *Scott* the *Skunk skipped* to Mr. *Scotland's* house. Mr. *Scotland* came to the door. He said, "*Skylar* isn't here, so *scoot, scoot, scoot!*" *Scott* the *Skunk* saw Mrs. *Scarecrow* and she said, "*Skylar* isn't here, so *scoot, scoot, scoot!*" So *Scott* the *Skunk skipped* to the *school*. There he found his friend *Skylar skipping* in the *school* yard.

## Skip, Skate, and Score*

**Target Words:** scarecrow, school bus, score, skate, skeleton, skip, skunk

**Materials:** initial /sk/ illustrations
(e.g., scarecrow, school bus, skeleton, skunk)
tape
chalkboard
foam ball

**Procedure:** In advance of this activity, duplicate four /sk/ illustrations and tape them on the chalkboard. Have the children sit facing the chalkboard, but a slight distance away. Instruct each child to take a turn *skipping* or pretending to *skate* up to the chalkboard. Once close to the chalkboard, give the child a chance to *score* by tossing a foam ball at one of the illustrations. Before tossing the ball, require the child to say which picture she or he wants to aim for.

## Fill the School Bus

**Target Words:** scarecrow, scarf, school bus, skates, skirt, skunk

**Materials:** initial /sk/ illustrations
(e.g., scarecrow, scarf, school bus, skates, skirt, skunk)
tape

**Procedure:** Before the session, duplicate and then hide /sk/ illustrations around the room. Also enlarge and duplicate the *school bus* and post it on the chalkboard or wall. Have the children go around the room gathering the /sk/ illustrations to put on the *school bus*. As each child finds a picture, have him or her bring it back to you and name it. Then instruct the child to tape the picture to the *school bus*. After all the illustrations are found, talk about what things are on the *school bus*.

## Skip/Skate to My Lou*

**Target Words:** skate, skip

**Materials:** none

**Procedure:** Demonstrate the actions of *skip* and *skate* to the children. Then sing the song "*Skip* to My Lou" as the action is performed. (For the first verse use *skip;* for the second verse use *skate*.)

*Skip to My Lou*
    *Skip, skip, skip* to my Lou,
    *Skip, skip, skip* to my Lou,
    *Skip, skip, skip* to my Lou,
    *Skip* to my Lou, my darling.
(Repeat with *skate*.)

**Target Sound:** 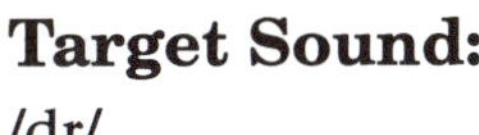
/dr/

**Linguistic Level:**
Word/Phrase

**Position:**
Initial

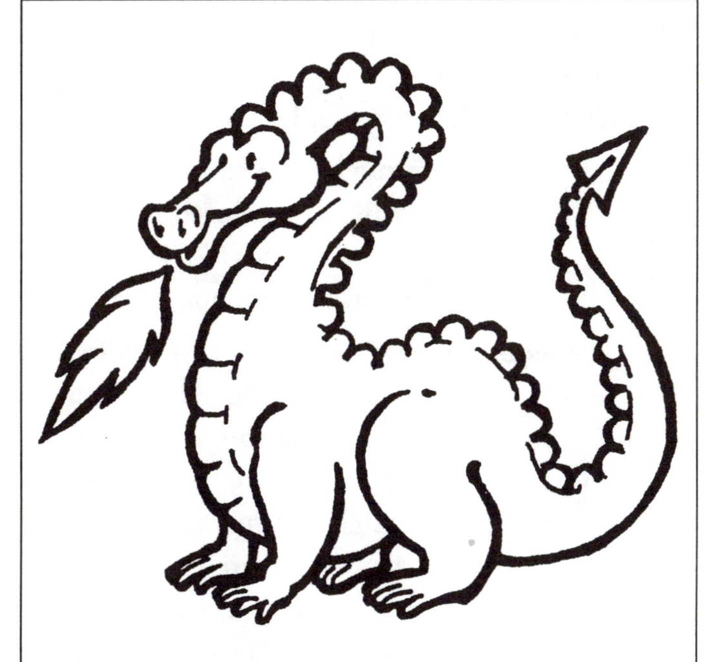

**Objective:**
To decrease the application of Liquid Cluster Reduction, the children will produce word-initial /dr/ clusters with varying levels of accuracy following the clinician's model or spontaneously.

**Suggestions for Nametags:**
In each session, provide a choice between two nametags to elicit productions of the target sound. Suggestions for the word-initial /dr/ cluster include: *dragon, dress, drill, drum*.

## Drippy Drew and Drake

**Target Words:** dragon, Drake, Drew, drip

**Materials:** dragon illustration
white and colored paper
paintbrushes
paint (liquid, nontoxic)

**Procedure:** Enlarge and duplicate two *dragon* illustrations per child, one on white paper and one on colored paper. Assist the children in *dripping* paint on the two *dragons* named *Drew* and *Drake*. Have the children identify which dragon they want to drip paint on. Encourage them to say *drip, drip, drip* as the paint is *dripping* from their paintbrush. To make this an outside activity, *draw dragons* on the playground with chalk and *drip* water on them.

## Dragon and Droopy Snack*

**Target Words:** dragon, Drake, drink, Droopy

**Materials:** cookie cutters in the shape of a dog and a dragon
bread
peanut butter and jelly
plastic knives or popsicle sticks
small cups
green juice or Kool-Aid
napkins

**Procedure:** Give the children a choice of making sandwiches cut out in the shape of either *Droopy* (a dog) or *Drake* (a *dragon*). Use cookie cutters to make cutouts of *Droopy* or *Drake*. Once the cutouts are made, have the children spread peanut butter and/or jelly on *Droopy* or *Drake*. To go along with the snack, have the children request small portions of a *dragon drink* (green juice).

## Dragon Drink or Drops

**Target Words:**  dragon, drink, drop

**Materials:**  construction paper
tape
blanket
table
cups
napkins
green juice or Kool-Aid
small gumdrops

**Procedure:**  Prepare a *dragon* tail for each child by cutting construction paper in a strip approximately 2 by 18 inches long. Fold it in accordion style. Tape a *dragon* tail to the lower back of each child. When the children have their *dragon* tails on, allow them to sit in a *dragon* cave (a blanket draped over a table). While in the *dragon* cave, have the children take turns asking each other if they want *dragon drink* (green juice) or *dragon drops* (gumdrops). Instruct the children to take turns passing the food to the others.

## Drippy and Dry

**Target Words:**  dragon, dress, drip, drippy, drum, dry

**Materials:**  chalk and chalkboard
plant sprayers
paper towels

**Procedure:**  Draw pictures of /dr/ items such as a *dragon*, *drum*, and *dress* on a chalkboard. Have each child verbally choose the picture on the chalkboard that he or she wishes to make *drippy* (by spraying it with a plant sprayer) and then *dry* (by wiping it with a paper towel).

## /dr/ Activity Stations*

**Target Words:** draw, drill, drink, drive, drum

**Materials:** drum and drumsticks
markers or crayons
drawing paper
juice
small cups
toy drill
toy car dash with steering wheel
spinner (See *Appendix H.*)

**Procedure:** Create a spinner board with numbers one through three on it. Then, set up the following activity stations in various parts of the room, boldly numbering as 1, 2, and 3:

1. A *drum* and *drumsticks* (to play the *drum*), and markers and paper (to *draw*).

2. Juice and cups (to *drink*), and a toy *drill* (to *drill* a hole).

3. A steering wheel (to *drive*), and crayons and paper (to *draw*).

Direct each child to select a /dr/ station by spinning the spinner. As the children approach each station, give them a choice of the two activities. Have them respond by verbalizing their choice.

## Drip, Drip, Dragon*

**Target Words:** dragon, drip

**Materials:** none

**Procedure:** Play a variation of the game "Duck, Duck, Goose" by substituting the words *"Drip, Drip, Dragon."* Tell the person who is "it" to walk around the outside of the circle, saying *drip* as she or he touches each player on the shoulder or head. When *dragon* is said, have the player who is touched chase the leader back to his or her place. This player then becomes "it."

## Dragon Bingo*

**Target Words:** dragon, draw, dress, drill, drum

**Materials:** bingo boards (See *Appendix H.*)
initial /dr/ illustrations (e.g., dragon, dress, drill, drum)
cloth grab bag (See *Appendix H.*)
dragon illustration

**Procedure:** Before the session, prepare bingo boards with four to six initial /dr/ illustrations on them. Make an identical set of illustrations to use as calling cards and place them in the cloth bag. Duplicate the *dragon* illustration to use as the bingo markers. Give each child a bingo board. Have the children take turns *drawing* a /dr/ calling card from the bag and naming it for the others. If the picture named is on a child's board, instruct him or her to cover it with a picture of a *dragon*. Continue the game until all children have covered all of their illustrations.

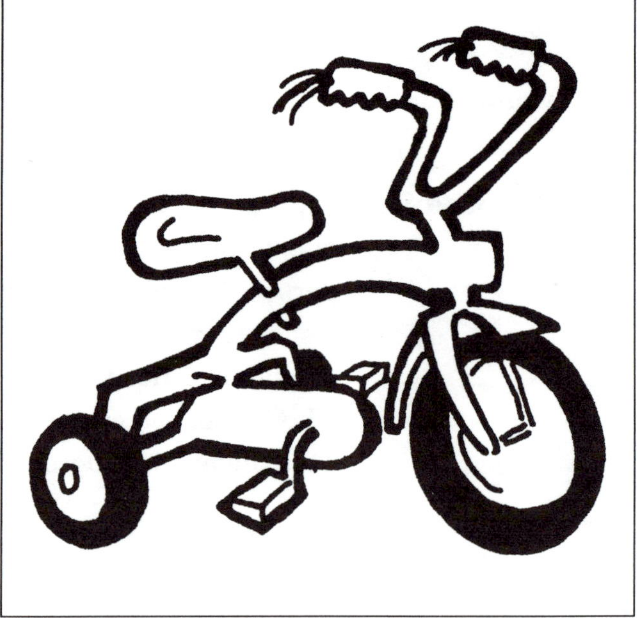

**Target Sound:**
/tr/

**Linguistic Level:**
Word/Phrase/Sentence

**Position:**
Initial

**Objective:**
To decrease the application of Liquid Cluster Reduction, the children will produce word-initial /tr/ with varying levels of accuracy following the clinician's model or spontaneously.

**Suggestions for Nametags:**
In each session, provide a choice between two nametags to elicit productions of the target sound. Suggestions for the word-initial /tr/ cluster include: *train, tree, tricycle, truck, trumpet.*

## Troy and Tracy Travel in a Truck

**Target Words:** tractor, Tracy, train, travel, tree, tricycle, trip, Troy, truck, trumpet

**Materials:** toy truck
initial /tr/ illustrations
  (e.g., tractor, train, tree, tricycle, trumpet)
*Troy and Tracy Travel in a Truck* story

**Procedure:** Duplicate the /tr/ illustrations. Make two copies of the *tricycle* illustration. Then read the story *Troy and Tracy Travel in a Truck* to the children, bombarding them with initial /tr/ words. Have the children put illustrations of /tr/ words in a toy *truck* and name them in unison as the story is read.

**Story:** *Troy and Tracy Travel in a Truck*

*Troy* and *Tracy* like to *travel* in their *truck*. When they *travel,* they take many things with them. For this *trip,* *Troy* decided to take a toy *train*. *Troy* put the *train* in the *truck*. *Tracy* wanted to take a *tree*. *Tracy* put the *tree* in the *truck*. *Troy* said, "Let's take my *tricycle*." *Troy* put his *tricycle* in the *truck*. *Tracy* put in her *tricycle* too. *Troy* decided he wanted to take his toy *tractor*. *Troy* put the *tractor* in the *truck*. *Tracy* wanted to bring her *trumpet*. She put her *trumpet* in the *truck*. *Troy* and *Tracy* were ready for their *trip!*

# Trouble for Trish and Travis

**Target Words:** track, tractor, train, travel, Travis, treasure, tricycle, trip, Trish, tropical, trouble, truck, truth, try

**Materials:** initial /tr/ illustrations of transportation vehicles (e.g., tractor, train, tricycle, truck)
*Trouble for Trish and Travis* story

**Procedure:** Duplicate illustrations of transportation vehicles. Then read the story *Trouble for Trish and Travis* to the children, bombarding them with initial /tr/ words. Show illustrations of the modes of *transportation* as they are mentioned in the story. Have the children recall the events in the story.

**Story:** *Trouble for Trish and Travis* (by Caren Leamon)

*Trish* and *Travis* were going on a *trip* to a *tropical* island. They were looking for buried *treasure*. *Trish* said, "Let's take a *train*. It is a fast way to *travel*." *Travis* agreed, "Let's *try* the *train*."

*Trish* and *Travis* got on the *train*. All of a sudden, they heard bump, bump, bump, and the *train* stopped on the *track*. They got off and *Trish* said, "Oh, no! *Trouble* with the *train!*" *Travis* said, "That's the *truth!* What should we *try* now?"

*Trish* said, "Let's *try* a *truck*. It is a fast way to *travel*." *Travis* agreed, "Let's *try* a *truck*." *Trish* and *Travis* hopped on a *truck*. All of a sudden, they heard bump, bump, bump. The *truck* stopped in its *tracks*. They got off and *Trish* said, "Oh, no! *Trouble* with the *truck!*" *Travis* said, "That's the *truth!* What should we *try* now?"

*Trish* said, "Let's *try* a *tractor*. It is a fast way to *travel*." *Travis* agreed, "Let's *try* a *tractor*." *Trish* and *Travis* hopped on a *tractor*. The *tractor* did not go bump, bump, bump. The *tractor* took *Trish* and *Travis* all the way to the *tropical* island! There they *tried* to find the buried *treasure*. *Trish* and *Travis* found it with no *trouble* at all!

## Trucks with /tr/ Cargo*

**Target Words:** train, tree, trout, truck, trumpet

**Materials:** truck illustration
initial /tr/ illustrations
   (e.g., train, tree, trout, truck, trumpet)
cloth grab bag (See *Appendix H.*)
glue or glue sticks
9 x 12" construction paper

**Procedure:** Duplicate several /tr/ illustrations per child. Also enlarge and duplicate one *truck* illustration for each child. Cut along the bottom and sides of the rectangular "cargo" portion of each *truck*. Glue each *truck* onto the large sheet of construction paper, leaving the cargo space free to glue /tr/ illustrations inside. Have each child pick a /tr/ picture from a cloth grab bag and name it for the rest of the group. Then have the children glue their /tr/ pictures inside their *trucks* by lifting up the cargo flap and affixing the pictures. After all illustrations are glued onto the *trucks,* encourage each child to tell the group about his or her picture.

## Making Treasure Boxes

**Target Words:** train, treasure, tree, truck, trumpet

**Materials:** initial /tr/ illustrations
  (e.g., train, tree, truck, trumpet)
glue or glue sticks
shoe boxes

**Procedure:** Duplicate multiple copies of initial /tr/ illustrations. Hide them around the room. Send the children on a *treasure* hunt to find the /tr/ pictures. As each child finds a picture, instruct him or her to bring it to you and name it. If the child does not respond to "What did you find?", give the child a choice. For example, ask, "Is it a *train* or a *truck?*" After the *treasure* hunt, have the children glue the illustrations on their own *treasure* box (a shoe box). To elicit target words, ask the children, "What are you putting on your *treasure* box?"

## Train Art*

**Target Words:** tractor, train, trash can, travel, tree, tricycle, truck, trumpet

**Materials:** initial /tr/ illustrations
(e.g., tractor, trash can, tree, tricycle, truck, trumpet)
large train illustration
glue or glue sticks

**Procedure:** Duplicate initial /tr/ illustrations. Also enlarge and duplicate the large train illustration for each child. Tell the children that to collect objects for their *train*, they have to *travel* to several *train* stations. Place parents, teachers, or other children around the room at each *train* station. Provide two different /tr/ illustrations (e.g., a *truck* and a *tree*, a *trumpet* and a *trash can*) at each *train* station. Instruct the station attendee to offer a choice of items when a child approaches the station (e.g., "*truck* or *tree?*"). After all the items are collected, have the adults assist the children in creating a *train* collage by giving the children choices between two pictures at a time to glue onto the *train*.

## Treats, Treats, Treats!

**Target Words:** train, treasure, treat, tree, truck, trumpet

**Materials:** initial /tr/ illustrations
(e.g., train, tree, truck, trumpet)
plastic eggs
treats (e.g., raisins or cereal)
serving tray

**Procedure:** Duplicate /tr/ illustrations. Prepare plastic eggs by taping one /tr/ picture to each egg and placing a treat inside. Hide the eggs in the room. Have all the children search for the eggs at once. After finding all the eggs, direct the children to put them on a *tray*. Have one child ask the others which egg they would like by giving choices (e.g, "*trumpet* or *tree?*"). Give each child the opportunity to ask the others what they would like. Afterwards, have them eat the *treats* from inside the eggs.

## Trix or Trolls*

**Target Words:** trade, Trix, trolls

**Materials:** Trix cereal
gummy bears
plastic wrap
plastic eggs
napkins

**Procedure:** Before the session, wrap a small amount of *Trix* cereal and *trolls* (gummy bears) in plastic wrap and place them in plastic eggs. Have the children select an egg, open it, and state whether they found *Trix* or *trolls*. Encourage the children to *trade* with each other by verbally requesting *Trix* or *trolls*.

## Treats and Tropical Drink*

**Target Words:** trade, tray, treat, tropical

**Materials:** treats wrapped in plastic
(e.g., small amounts of cereal, raisins, etc.)
serving tray
fruit punch
small cups
napkins

**Procedure:** For a snack, serve *treats* on a *treat tray* to the group. Allow each child a turn to be the server. Provide the children with a choice between a *treat* and a *tropical* drink (fruit punch). Give them the opportunity to *trade* with each other (as long as the *treats* are still wrapped).

## Collecting Trash and Treats

**Target Words:** trash, trash can, tray, treat

**Materials:** crumpled paper        trash can
treats (raisins or peanuts)   serving tray
plastic wrap

**Procedure:** Prepare for this activity by strewing *trash* (crumpled paper) and *treats* (raisins or peanuts wrapped in plastic wrap) around the room. Turn the lights off. Before the children enter the room, tell them there was a party last night and the people left a lot of *trash* and *treats*. Turn the lights on as the children enter the room. Have them collect the *trash* and *treats*. Instruct them to bring one item at a time to you and then name it. Ask them if they want to put the item in the *trash can* or on the *treat tray*. Let the children eat the *treats*.

## Truck Travel

**Target Words:** tractor, train, trash can, tree, tricycle, trout, truck

**Materials:** /tr/ illustrations
(e.g., tractor, train, trash can, tree, tricycle, trout)
toy trucks

**Procedure:** Enlarge and duplicate the /tr/ illustrations. Duplicate several additional sets of /tr/ illustrations but do not enlarge them. Set up areas in the room that have one large initial /tr/ illustration posted and several small ones that match. Have the children take turns choosing (verbally selecting) one of the areas to drive their toy *truck* to, then have them pick up a /tr/ picture. Tell the children to put the /tr/ illustrations in their *truck*. When they return, have them name each picture.

## Trash or Treat Grab Bag

**Target Words:** trash, trash can, tray, treat

**Materials:** treats wrapped in plastic
(e.g., small amounts of cereal or raisins)
crumpled paper
cloth grab bag (See *Appendix H.*)
serving tray
trash can

**Procedure:** Place *treats* and *trash* (crumpled paper) in a cloth grab bag. Have the children choose items from the bag. As each item is taken out, have the child tell the group if it is a *treat* or *trash*. Place the *treats* onto the *treat tray* and the *trash* in the *trash can*. The *treats* can later be eaten for a snack.

## Treasure Hunt

**Target Words:** tractor, train, tray, treasure, treasure chest, tree, truck, trumpet

**Materials:** initial /tr/ illustrations
 (e.g., tractor, train, tree, truck, trumpet)
shoe box
serving tray

**Procedure:** Before the session, duplicate the /tr/ illustrations and bury (hide) multiple copies of them around the room. Tell the children they will be going on a *treasure* hunt to search for illustrations that you tell them about. Provide a clue before each search such as, "Look for something that rides on railroad *tracks (train).*" Once the children determine that they must find a *train,* have them say *train, train, train* as they search. As each child finds a *train,* instruct him or her to bring it to you and then verbally choose whether to put it in the *treasure chest* (a shoe box) or on the *tray.*

## Human Train*

**Target Words:** train, train track, trash can, tree, trout, truck, trumpet

**Materials:** construction paper                     whistle
initial /tr/ illustrations
 (e.g., trash can, tree, trout, truck, trumpet)

**Procedure:** Create *train tracks* from large strips of construction paper. Tape /tr/ illustrations on the back of the *tracks* and then lay them on the floor. Instruct the children to place their hands on the shoulders (or waist) of the person in front of them to form a *train.* Have them march on the *train tracks,* and stop when the whistle blows. Then instruct the children to pick up the piece of *track* they are standing on and name the picture on the other side.

## Trout and Triangles

**Target Words:** train, tree, triangle, trout, truck, trumpet

**Materials:** construction paper
initial /tr/ illustrations
   (e.g., train, tree, trout, truck, trumpet)
paper clips
fishing poles (See *Appendix H.*)

**Procedure:** Cut several *triangles* and *trout* (fish) out of construction paper. Duplicate additional /tr/ illustrations and cut them out. Attach a /tr/ picture to each *triangle* and *trout* with a paper clip. Spread the *triangles* and *trout* on the floor of the room. Have each child take a turn fishing for *triangles* and *trout* using a fishing pole. Require the children to state whether they would like to catch a *trout* or a *triangle* before fishing. Then have them tell the group which picture is on their *triangle* or *trout*.

## /tr/ Concentration

**Target Words:** tractor, train, tree, trout, truck, trumpet, try

**Materials:** initial /tr/ illustrations
   (e.g., tractor, train, tree, trout, truck, trumpet)
glue or glue stick
index cards

**Procedure:** Make matching pairs of /tr/ picture cards by duplicating two sets of each /tr/ illustration and gluing them to index cards. Lay the cards face down on the table. Have the first child turn one card over, name it, and then turn another over to find a match. If a match is made, allow the child to keep the pair and turn another card over. If a match is not made, place the cards face down again and give the next child a turn. Model "*Try* again!"

**Target Sound:**
/br/

**Linguistic Level:**
Word/Phrase/ Sentence

**Position:**
Initial

**Objective:**
To decrease the application of Liquid Cluster Reduction, the children will produce word-initial /br/ clusters with varying levels of accuracy following the clinician's model or spontaneously.

**Suggestions for Nametags:**
In each session, provide a choice between two nametags to elicit productions of the target sound. Suggestions for the word-initial /br/ cluster include: *bread, brick, bridge, broom.*

## Breakfast for Brian

| | |
|---|---|
| **Target Words:** | bran, bread, breakfast, Brian, broccoli, brothers, brownies, Bruce |
| **Materials:** | illustrations of two boys (See pages 323–324.) <br> *Breakfast for Brian* story <br> containers of initial /br/ items <br> (e.g., slice of bread in a bag, box of brownies, box of bran cereal) <br> broccoli |
| **Procedure:** | Duplicate the illustrations of two different boys, *Brian* and *Bruce*. Read the story *Breakfast for Brian* to the children, bombarding them with initial /br/ words. Use the illustrations and /br/ items to add interest to the story. Have the children name items representing key words from the story. |
| **Story:** | *Breakfast for Brian* |

This is *Bruce*. This is *Brian*. They are *brothers*. *Brian* said, "I am hungry. I want to eat *breakfast*." *Bruce* said, "I will make *breakfast* for you. Do you want *bran* cereal or *bread*?" "I want *bran* cereal AND *bread*," said *Brian*. "I am very hungry!" *Bruce* made *bran* cereal and *bread* for *Brian*. *Brian* said, "Thank you for the *bran* cereal and *bread*. My *breakfast* was so good! But I am still hungry." "Do you want *broccoli* or *brownies*?" asked *Bruce*. "I want *broccoli* AND *brownies*," said *Brian*. "I am very hungry!" *Bruce* made *broccoli* and *brownies* for *Brian*. *Brian* said, "Thank you for the *broccoli* and *brownies*. My *breakfast* was so good! I'm not hungry anymore."

## Bright and Brown Bracelets*

**Target Words:** bracelet, bright, brown

**Materials:** yarn
tape
Cheerios (or any donut-shaped brown cereal)
Froot Loops (or any donut-shaped multicolored cereal)

**Procedure:** Give each child a piece of yarn large enough to be used as a *bracelet*. Tie a large knot on one end of the yarn and cover the other end with a small piece of tape to assist in guiding the cereal on. Introduce the Cheerios as *brown* cereal and Froot Loops as *bright* cereal. Have the children ask for *bright* or *brown* cereal to string on the yarn. Once several pieces of cereal have been strung onto the yarn, tie it on the child's wrist as a *bracelet*.

## Breakfast

**Target Words:** bran, bread, breakfast, brush

**Materials:** bread
bran cereal
small bowls
napkins
toothbrushes
toothpaste

**Procedure:** For *breakfast,* have the children choose between *bread* and *bran* cereal. Provide small portions so that the children request the target items frequently. Give each of the children a turn to serve the others. After *breakfast,* have the children *brush* their teeth.

## Break Time

**Target Words:** brittle, brownie, brush

**Materials:** brownies
peanut brittle
napkins
toothbrushes
toothpaste

**Procedure:** Prepare small portions of *brownies* and peanut *brittle* for the children to eat as a snack. Have the children ask each other if they want *brownies* or *brittle*. Since this is a sugary snack, have the children *brush* their teeth after they have finished eating. Model saying *brush, brush, brush*.

## London Bridge*

**Target Words:** breaking, bridge, broken

**Materials:** none

**Procedure:** Have two children join hands and hold them up high in the air to form a *bridge*. Have the other children parade under the *bridge* singing, "London *Bridge* is *breaking* down, *breaking* down, *breaking* down; London *Bridge* is *breaking* down, *BRIDGE, BRIDGE, BROKEN!*" Repeat, having new children form the *bridge* until everyone has had a chance to be part of the *bridge*.

# Brenda and Brad

**Target Words:** braces, Brad, braids, Brenda

**Materials:** illustrations of the boy face and the girl face
(See pages 327–328.)
yarn
tape
ribbon (optional)
tag board
aluminum foil
feely box (See *Appendix H.*)

**Procedure:** Duplicate the illustration of the boy face (*Brad*) and the girl face (*Brenda*). (Notice that *Brenda* is missing her *braids* and *Brad* is missing his *braces*.)

For this activity, also prepare *braids* and *braces*. To form *braids*, cut three pieces of yarn approximately 10 inches in length each. Combine the pieces and tape at one end. *Braid* the three pieces together and tape the other end or tie a ribbon around it. Create numerous small *braids*. To make *braces*, cut tag board into squares to fit into *Brad's* mouth. Cover the tag board with aluminum foil to simulate braces.

Show the illustrations of *Brad* and *Brenda* to the children. Introduce *Brad* by saying that he lost his *braces*. (Explain what *braces* are.) Introduce *Brenda* by saying that she wants to wear her hair in lots of little *braids*. Place *braces* and *braids* in a feely box. Have the children close their eyes and reach into the feely box. Provide them with a choice of putting the *braids* on *Brenda* or *braces* on *Brad*.

## Building with Bricks

**Target Words:** bread, bricks, bridge, broom, brush

**Materials:** cardboard bricks, cubes, or stacking cups
initial /br/ illustrations
  (e.g., bread, bridge, broom, brush)
tape

**Procedure:** Gather cardboard *bricks*. Duplicate and tape a /br/ picture on each *brick*. Have the children construct a building with the *bricks*. As each child adds a *brick* to the structure, instruct him or her to name the picture on the *brick*. Modify this activity by using smaller cubes or stacking cups if desired.

## Baker's Brew

**Target Words:** bracelet, bread, brew, bricks, broom, brush

**Materials:** /br/ illustrations (e.g., bread, bricks, brush)
poster board     child-size broom
large stew pot     bakers' hats
/br/ items
  (e.g., bracelets, bread, cardboard bricks, yarn braids, brush)

**Procedure:** Before this activity, duplicate /br/ illustrations and create simple drawings of *bracelets* and *braids*. Simulate a recipe card by listing the name of each ingredient, along with a picture representation on a large poster. Explain to the children that they are going to make a baker's *brew*. Use a large stew pot to hold all the ingredients. Have each child wear a baker's hat and verbally select a /br/ item from the recipe card to put in the *brew*. As each child names and places an item in the stew pot, allow them to stir the *brew* with a child-size *broom* while everyone chants *brew, brew, brew!*

## /br/ **Activity Stations***

**Target Words:** bracelets, braids, bread, breakfast, bright, brown, brownie, brush

**Materials:** four dolls
toothbrush
hairbrush
pretend (or real) brownies and bread
Froot Loops
Cheerios
yarn braids
bracelets

**Procedure:** Set up the following activity stations around the room with a doll at each station:

1. A tooth*brush* and a hair*brush* (to *brush* the doll's teeth or hair).

2. *Bread* and a *brownie* (to feed a *breakfast* of *bread* or a *brownie* to the doll).

3. Froot Loops and Cheerios (to feed *bright* [Froot Loops] or *brown* [Cheerios] cereal to the doll).

4. *Braids* and *bracelets* (to put on the doll).

Present the children with a choice of activities at each station. Require them to verbally state their /br/ item choice.

## Musical Bricks*

**Target Words:** bread, bricks, bridge, broom, brush

**Materials:** construction paper
initial /br/ illustrations
  (e.g., bread, bricks, bridge, broom, brush)
tape
cassette player
musical cassette tape

**Procedure:** Cut large *bricks* out of construction paper. Duplicate /br/ illustrations and tape them to the bottom of the *bricks*. Lay the *bricks* in a circle on the floor. Play music as the children march around the circle. Stop the music intermittently. When the music stops, have the children tell the group which /br/ picture is under their *brick*.

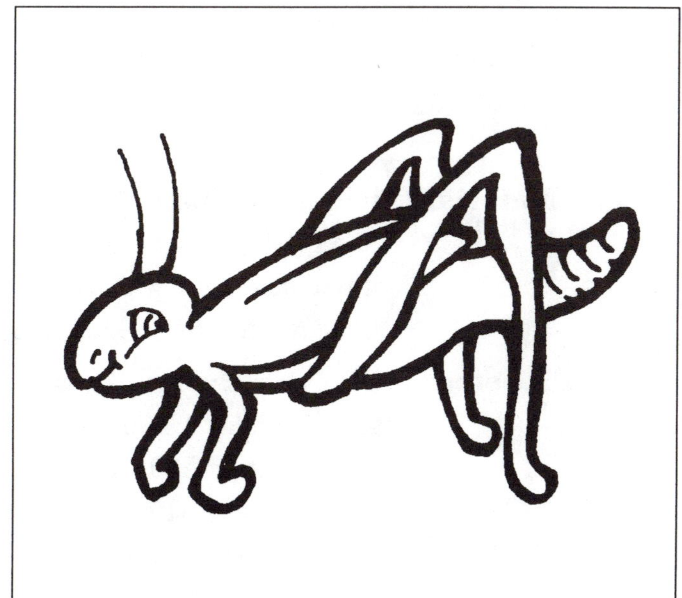

**Target Sound:**
/gr/

**Linguistic Level:**
Isolation/Word/Phrase/
Sentence

**Position:**
Isolation/Initial

**Objective:**
To decrease the application of Liquid Cluster Reduction, the children will produce word-initial /gr/ clusters with varying levels of accuracy following the clinician's model or spontaneously.

**Suggestions for Nametags:**
In each session, provide a choice between two nametags to elicit productions of the target sound. Suggestions for the word-initial /gr/ cluster include: *grapes, grasshopper, grizzly bear, groundhog.*

# Greg the Grumpy Grizzly Bear

**Target Words:** grass, grasshopper, green, Greg, Greta, Gretchen, grizzly bear, Groggy, groundhog, growling, grrrr, grumpy

**Materials:** initial /gr/ illustrations
(e.g., grass, grasshopper, grizzly bear, groundhog)
illustration of a girl (See pages 324–326.)
*Greg the Grumpy Grizzly Bear* story

**Procedure:** Duplicate the /gr/ illustrations and the illustration of a girl (*Gretchen*). Read the story *Greg the Grumpy Grizzly Bear* to the children, bombarding them with initial /gr/ words. Have the children say *grrrr!* each time *Greg growls* in the story. Afterwards, use the illustrations to help the children recall events in the story and to elicit target words.

**Story:** *Greg the Grumpy Grizzly Bear* (by Caren Leamon)

*Greg* the *Grumpy Grizzly Bear* was sleeping for his long winter nap. *Greg* was *grumpy* whenever someone woke him up from his nap. One day, *Greta* the *Grasshopper* was chirping very loudly. *Greg* the *Grumpy Grizzly Bear* came *growling* out of his cave. *"Grrrr!"* said *Greg* the *Grumpy Grizzly,* "You woke me up! *Grrrr!"* A few days later, *Groggy* the *Groundhog* was playing near *Greg's* cave. *Greg* woke up again and came out *growling.* *"Grrrr!"* said *Greg* the *Grumpy Grizzly,* "You woke me up! *Grrrr!"* A few weeks later, a girl named *Gretchen* was cutting the *green grass.* *Greg* woke up again and came *growling* out of his cave. *"Grrrr!"* said *Greg* the *Grumpy Grizzly,* "You woke me up! *Grrrr!"* But when *Greg* saw the *green grass,* he knew it was spring. It was time to wake up and stop being so *grumpy!* *Greg* the *Grumpy Grizzly* said, "What a *grrrreat* day to wake up!"

## Grocery Store*

**Target Words:** graham crackers, granola, granola bars, grapes, groceries, grocery store

**Materials:** /gr/ grocery items
(e.g., small bunches of grapes in plastic bags, granola bars, individually wrapped graham crackers, granola, etc.)
store clerk apron
pretend money
toy cash register or scanner
toy grocery baskets or other small baskets

**Procedure:** Place /gr/ *grocery* items on a table. Tell the children they are going to buy *groceries* for snack time. Have one child wear the *grocery store* clerk apron and act as the *grocery store* clerk. Instruct the *grocery* clerk to ask, "What *groceries* do you want?" Have the children name the items they are buying. After the items are purchased, encourage the children to offer each other some of their *groceries* to eat.

## Green/Gray Toss

**Target Words:** grapes, grass, grasshopper, gray, green, grizzly bear, groundhog, group

**Materials:** green and gray construction paper
initial /gr/ illustrations
  (e.g., grapes, grass, grasshopper, grizzly bear, groundhog)
bean bag
tape

**Procedure:** Before the session, duplicate the /gr/ illustrations. Cut amorphous shapes out of the *green* and *gray* construction paper and tape a /gr/ picture to the bottom of each shape. Lay the shapes on the floor. Have the children take turns tossing a bean bag onto a *green* or *gray* shape. Before tossing the bean bag, require them to verbally choose the color they will aim for. Direct them to turn over the *green* or *gray* shape the bean bag landed on and tell the *group* which /gr/ illustration is under it. (Emphasis should be placed on the /gr/ color in this activity rather than on the shape.)

## Grab Grizzly Bears or Grasshoppers

**Target Words:** grab, grass, grasshopper, grizzly bear

**Materials:** grasshopper and grizzly bear illustrations
green construction paper
cloth grab bag (See *Appendix H.*)

**Procedure:** Before the session, duplicate the *grasshopper* and *grizzly bear* illustrations and cut them out. Prepare an area in the room with real or pretend *grass* (shredded *green* construction paper). Place *grizzly bears* and *grasshoppers* in a cloth *grab* bag. Have one child tell another what to *grab* from the bag (e.g., "*Grab* a *grasshopper*"). Then have the children choose to place either the *grizzly bear* (or the *grasshopper*) in the *grass.*

## Hiding in Grass*

**Target Words:** grab, grapes, grass, grasshopper, great, grizzly bear, groundhog

**Materials:** chalk and chalkboard
green construction paper (optional)
initial /gr/ illustrations
    (e.g., grapes, grass, grasshopper, grizzly bear, groundhog)
cloth grab bag (See *Appendix H.*)

**Procedure:** Before this activity, duplicate the /gr/ illustrations. Then, draw a field of *grass* on the chalkboard or mount a strip of *green* construction paper fringed to look like *grass* on the wall. Have the children choose a /gr/ picture from the cloth *grab* bag, name it, then tape the picture on the *grass.* Before choosing, require the children to say, "I will *grab* (*grapes*)." Incorporate *great* as reinforcement for participating in the activity.

## Grandma Says*

**Target Words:** grab, Grandma, grapefruit, grass, grasshopper, grizzly bear, grow, growl, grrrr

**Materials:** gray wig
granny glasses

**Procedure:** Instruct the children to stand in a *group* facing you. Put on a *gray* wig and *granny* glasses and demonstrate the following /gr/ words and actions:

1. Hopping up and down like a *grasshopper*

2. *Growling* like a *grizzly bear*

3. *Grabbing* (picking) *grapefruit* from a tree

4. *Growing* like *grass* (reaching up high in the air)

After demonstrating all of these actions, say, "*Grandma says growl* like a *grizzly bear.*" (Have everyone *growl.*) After several turns, solicit volunteers to either be *Grandma* or assist *Grandma* (if they do not want to wear the *granny* glasses and *gray* wig) in choosing the next action. Encourage the children to use the target words when they are *Grandma* or *Grandma's* assistant.

## Bowling for /gr/

**Target Words:** grapes, grass, grasshopper, grizzly bear, groundhog

**Materials:** toy bowling set
initial /gr/ illustrations
  (e.g., grapes, grass, grasshopper, grizzly bear, groundhog)
tape

**Procedure:** Duplicate the /gr/ illustrations, then tape them to plastic bowling pins. Have the children knock down the pins with a plastic bowling ball and name the illustrations taped to the pins they knock down.

**Target Sound:**
/bl/

**Linguistic Level:**
Word/Phrase/Sentence

**Position:**
Initial

**Objective:**
To decrease the application of Liquid Cluster Reduction, the children will produce word-initial /bl/ clusters with varying levels of accuracy following the clinician's model or spontaneously.

**Suggestions for Nametags:**
In each session, provide a choice between two nametags to elicit productions of the target sound. Suggestions for the word-initial /bl/ cluster include: *black cat, block, bluebird, blue jeans.*

## Blaine and Blinky Pick Blueberries

**Target Words:** black, Blaine, blew, Blinky, blotches, blue, blueberries

**Materials:** illustration of a boy (See pages 323–324.)
illustration of a dog (See page 322.)
blue construction paper
blue and black markers or crayons (optional)
*Blaine and Blinky Pick Blueberries* story

**Procedure:** Duplicate the illustrations of the boy (*Blaine*) and the dog (*Blinky*). Color the dog *black*. Also cut *blueberries* out of *blue* construction paper. Read the story *Blaine and Blinky Pick Blueberries* to the children, bombarding them with initial /bl/ words. Show illustrations to the children as the story is read. Use the markers to add color to the illustrations, if desired. Afterwards, have the children recall events and incorporate target words in their discussion of the story.

**Story:** *Blaine and Blinky Pick Blueberries* (by Patricia Connors)

*Blaine and his black dog Blinky went out to pick blueberries. The wind blew and the rain fell when Blaine began to pick blueberries. Blinky ran through the puddles. Then Blinky jumped on Blaine and left black blotches on Blaine's shirt! Blaine laughed and then finished picking blueberries. On the way home, Blaine fed Blinky some blueberries. The blueberries made Blinky's tongue turn blue! Then Blinky licked Blaine's face and Blaine's face turned blue! When Blaine and Blinky got home, Blaine's mom laughed. She called them black and blue twins for the rest of the day!*

## Blake and Blair

**Target Words:** black, Blair, Blake, blast, blazer, blocks, blonde, blouse, blue

**Materials:** illustrations of a boy and a girl (See pages 323–326.)
yellow and black markers or crayons
illustrations of /bl/ clothing
(e.g., black socks, blazer, blouse, blue jeans)
catalogs
tape
blue suitcase
*Blake and Blair* story

**Procedure:** Enlarge and duplicate illustrations of a boy (*Blake*) and a girl (*Blair*). Color *Blake's* hair yellow and *Blair's* hair *black*. Cut pictures of /bl/ clothing out of catalogs. Tape *Blake* and *Blair* on the chalkboard or wall. Read the story *Blake and Blair* to the children, bombarding them with initial /bl/ words. Show illustrations depicting the target words as the story is read. Have the children help *Blake* and *Blair* pack their clothes in a *blue* suitcase.

**Story:** *Blake and Blair* (by Katie Murphy)

*Blake* and *Blair* are friends. *Blake* has *blonde* hair. *Blair* has *black* hair. *Blake* and *Blair* were going on a trip. *Blake* and *Blair* packed their *blue* suitcase. *Blake* and *Blair* put *blue* jeans, *black* socks, a *blouse*, and a *blazer* in their *blue* suitcase. In a *blizzard*, *Blake* and *Blair* drove to the airport which was three *blocks* away. *Blake* and *Blair* got on the airplane. The airplane *blasted* off toward the *blue* sky when the *blizzard* was over.

## Blake Goes Shopping

**Target Words:** black, Blake, blue

**Materials:** illustration of a boy (See pages 323–324.)
blue and black construction paper
initial /bl/ items
 (blue and black paint, blue and black cups)
*Blake Goes Shopping* story

**Procedure:** Duplicate the illustration of the boy (*Blake*). Cut *blueberries* and *blackberries* out of the *blue* and *black* construction paper. Read the story *Blake Goes Shopping* to the children, bombarding them with initial /bl/ words. Show the illustration of *Blake* and target word items while reading the story to the children. Ask the children the questions that are included in the story. After reading the story, have the children recall items bought by *Blake*.

**Story:** *Blake Goes Shopping* (by Darlene Stratton)

This is *Blake*. *Blake's* mom said, "I want you to go shopping. We need berries, paint, and cups." *Blake* rode to the store on his new *blue* bike. The first thing on *Blake's* list was berries. Did he buy *blueberries* or *blackberries*? (Allow the children to decide.) Next, *Blake* bought some paint. Did he buy *blue* paint or *black* paint? (Allow the children to decide.) The last thing on *Blake's* list was cups. Did he buy *blue* cups or *black* cups? (Allow the children to decide.) *Blake* went home. "Thank you for going shopping, *Blake*," his mom said. "What did you buy?"

## Blaine and Blossom Dress Up

**Target Words:** black, Blaine, blazers, blonde, Blossom, blue, blue jeans

**Materials:** illustrations of a boy and a girl (See pages 323–326.)
yellow and black markers or crayons
illustrations of blue jeans, black pants, blue blazers and black blazers, blue shoes and black shoes (cut from catalogs)
catalogs
glue or glue sticks

**Procedure:** Before the session, duplicate and cut out figures of a boy (*Blaine*) and a girl (*Blossom*), one of each per child. Cut the hair off of each figure but save these cutouts for this activity; color the hair yellow or leave *black*. Also cut out /bl/ clothing from catalogs. Give the paper-doll figures of *Blaine* or *Blossom* to each child. Have the children verbally select the items they want to put on the figures. Provide the children with choices such as *blonde* or *black* hair, *blue* or *black* shoes, etc. Then have the children glue the items on the figures.

# Blue and Black Snack*

**Target Words:** black, blanket, block, blue

**Materials:** blue JELL-O
blue blanket
blue apron
black jelly beans
blue Kool-Aid
bowls
serving spoons
small cups

**Procedure:** Before the session, prepare *blue* firm JELL-O (JELL-O Jigglers) and cut it into *block* shapes. At snack time, have all the children sit on a *blue blanket*. In turn, have each child wear a *blue* apron and act as the server for the group. Have the server offer the other children a choice of *blue* JELL-O *blocks*, *black* jelly beans, or a *blue* drink (Kool-Aid). Serve small portions so that frequent productions are elicited, and each child has a turn to be the server.

## Blueberry Blizzards*

**Target Words:** blanket, blend, blender, blizzard, blue, blueberries

**Materials:** blue blanket
blender
vanilla yogurt
blueberries (fresh or frozen)
bowls
spoons
napkins

**Procedure:** Seat the children on a *blue blanket* on the floor. Use a *blender* to mix a *blizzard* (vanilla yogurt and just enough *blueberries* to add blue color) for a snack. Give each child a turn to operate the *blender*. Have the others chant *blend, blend, blend* as each child turns the *blender* on. Give the children a small amount at a time to encourage requests for more *blueberry blizzard*.

## Blasting Blocks and Blizzards

**Target Words:** blackboard, blast, blizzard, blocks

**Materials:** chalk and blackboard
squirt bottle(s)

**Procedure:** Draw *blizzards* (lots of small snowflakes) and *blocks* on the *blackboard*. Give the children a choice of *blasting blizzards* or *blocks* from the *blackboard* with a squirt bottle. As one child *blasts* a *block* or *blizzard,* encourage the other children to cheer *blast, blast, blast!* If several children are participating in the activity, use more than one squirt bottle so that waiting time is minimized.

## Blue and Black Cats

**Target Words:** black, blue

**Materials:** blue and black eye liner
blue and black construction paper

**Procedure:** Using *blue* and *black* construction paper, cut out one set of cat ears and a tail of each color for each child. Tell the children they will be dressing up as cats. Give the children a choice of wearing *blue* or *black* ears, tails, and whiskers. (Use *blue* or *black* eyeliner to draw the whiskers.) This activity could also be incorporated into a unit on colors within the classroom.

## /bl/ Show and Tell

**Target Words:** black, blue

**Materials:** blue and black items

**Procedure:** In advance of the session, send a note to the parents requesting that their child bring in one *blue* and one *black* item from home. Supplement these items with your own *blue* and *black* materials. Engage in a "Show and Tell" activity. Identify each item as being either *blue* or *black*. Place emphasis on these target words rather than the name of the object.

## Blueberry Picking

**Target Words:** black, black pants, blue, blueberry, blue jeans

**Materials:** blue construction paper
/bl/ illustrations
  (e.g., black cat, black pants, blue jeans)
tape
blue bowl

**Procedure:** Before the session, cut large, circular *blueberries* out of construction paper. Duplicate and tape /bl/ illustrations on the back of the *blueberries* and tape them on the walls around the room. Direct the children to go *blueberry* picking, naming the illustrations as they find them. Tell the children to gather their *blueberries* and sit in a circle. Have a child walk around the circle with a *blue* bowl. Instruct the children to identify the illustrations and place their *blueberries* in the bowl.

## Blowing Bubbles

**Target Words:** blow, blow pipe, blow wand

**Materials:** bubble soap
bubble wands
bubble pipes
dish for bubble soap

**Procedure:** Place bubble soap in a dish. Have the children choose a *blow pipe* or *blow wand* and take turns *blowing* bubbles in teams of two. One team member chants *blow, blow, blow,* while the other team member *blows* bubbles.

## Blue and Black Blocks

**Target Words:** black, Blair, Blake, block, blue

**Materials:** illustration of a boy and a girl (See pages 323–326.)
blue and black construction paper

**Procedure:** Enlarge and duplicate the illustration of a boy (*Blake*) and a girl (*Blair*). Place the pictures on a chalkboard or wall. Cut several squares out of *black* and *blue* construction paper. Place a *block* (a *blue* or *black* square) next to *Blair* or *Blake* to start a tower. Have the children choose from *blue* and *black* squares to build a *blue* and *black block* tower for *Blake* or *Blair*.

## Blow Painting

**Target Words:** black, blow, blue

**Materials:** large sheets of paper
liquid, nontoxic paint (blue and black)
paint smocks
straws
child-size table

**Procedure:** Have the children wear paint smocks for this activity. Place large sheets of paper on a child-size table. Give each child a choice between *blue* or *black* paint. Pour paint onto the paper, and have two children at a time use straws to *blow* the paint around their paper. As the children *blow*, have the other children cheer *blow, blow, blow*.

## /bl/ Activity Stations*

**Target Words:** blanket, blink, blocks, blow

**Materials:** blocks
bubble soap
bubble wand
hand mirror
blanket
two chairs

**Procedure:** Set up the following four activity stations in various parts of the room:

1. *Blocks* ( to stack *blocks).*
2. Soap bubbles and *blowing* wands (to *blow* bubbles).
3. A hand mirror (for *blinking* eyes in the mirror).
4. A *blanket* draped over two chairs (for crawling under).

Describe to the children what can be done at each station. Have each child go from station to station with a partner (or parent) who tells her or him what to do.

## Musical Blocks

**Target Words:** black, blob, block, blue

**Materials:** blue and black construction paper
cassette player
musical cassette tape

**Procedure:** Cut *blue* and *black blocks* (squares) and *blobs* (amorphous shapes) out of construction paper. Place them in a circle on the floor. Play music as the children march around the circle. When the music stops, have the children tell the group what shape and/or color they are standing on or next to (e.g., "I'm on a *blue block*," or just "*Blue block*").

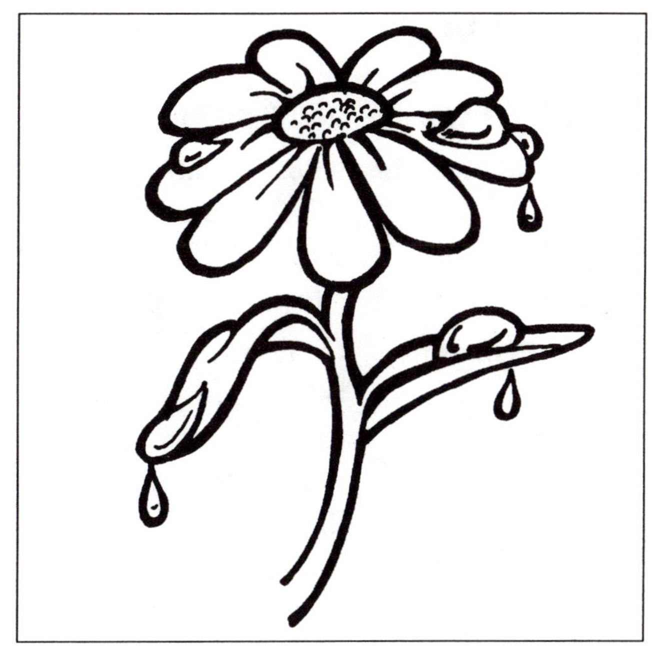

**Target Sound:**
/fl/

**Linguistic Level:**
Word/Phrase/Sentence

**Position:**
Initial

**Objective:**
To decrease the application of Liquid Cluster Reduction, the children will produce word-initial /fl/ clusters with varying levels of accuracy following the clinician's model or spontaneously.

**Suggestions for Nametags:**
In each session, provide a choice between two nametags to elicit productions of the target sound. Suggestions for the word-initial /fl/ cluster include: *flag, flashlight, flower, flute, fly.*

## We Are Floating*

**Target Words:** flashlight, flip-flops, float, floating, floss, flowers

**Materials:** a float or raft
flip-flop sandals
initial /fl/ items
  (e.g., flashlight, [dental] floss, flowers)

**Procedure:** In advance of the session, obtain and inflate a plastic raft, such as one used in a swimming pool. Also request that children bring a pair of *flip-flops* (sandals) from home. Have the children remove their shoes, put on *flip-flops,* and prepare to *float.* Allow them to choose /fl/ items to bring on the *float* with them. Gather the children on the *float,* and sing "We Are *Floating*" together.

*We Are Floating*
(Sing to the tune of "Are You Sleeping?")
  We are *floating,*
  We are *floating,*
  *Float, float, float!*
  *Float, float, float!*
  We are *floating,*
  We are *floating,*
  *Float, float, float!*
  *Float, float, float!*

## Shopping and Packing

**Target Words:** flag, flashlight, Fletch, flip-flops, Flo, Florida, floss, flower

**Materials:** illustrations of a girl and a boy (See pages 323–326.)
two suitcases
initial /fl/ items
  (e.g., flags, flashlights, flip-flops, [dental] floss, flowers)

**Procedure:** Before the session, duplicate the illustrations of the girl (*Flo*) and boy (*Fletch*). Tape one illustration on each of the suitcases. Tell the children that *Flo* and *Fletch* are going on a trip to *Florida*. *Flo* and *Fletch* need to buy some items at the store to take on their trip. Arrange /fl/ items around the room. Have one or two children act as storekeepers, while the other children buy these items (request them from the storekeeper) and choose to put them in *Flo's* or *Fletch's* suitcase.

## Flo Says*

**Target Words:** flap, flex, Flo, fly

**Materials:** none

**Procedure:** Introduce a modified version of "Simon Says," calling the game "*Flo* Says." Demonstrate each action that *Flo* can do: *flap* (bending arms and moving elbows up and down), *fly* (putting arms out like a bird), or *flex* (making a fist and bending the elbow). Have the children produce the target words, as they take a turn being *Flo*. As the children perform the actions, have them chorally repeat the action words (e.g., *flap, flap, flap*).

## Does It Float?

**Target Word:** float

**Materials:** objects that float
    (e.g., cork, Ivory soap, leaf, sponge)
objects that do not float
    (e.g., pencil, penny, rock, stick)
bucket or dish pan of water

**Procedure:** Gather a collection of *floating* objects and objects that do not *float*. Explain to the children that when some things are placed in water, they stay on top of the water or *float*, while other things do not *float*—they go under the water. Present objects one at a time. Before placing each object in the water, ask the children to guess whether the item will *float* or not *float*. Emphasize and repeat the target word *float*. Have the children take turns selecting an object and asking each other if it will *float* or not *float*. Encourage the children to chant *float, float, float* as the object is placed in the water.

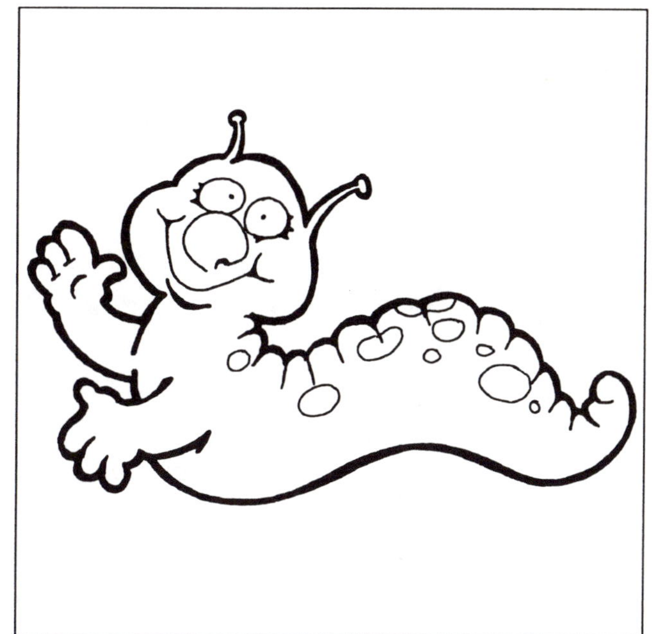

**Target Sound:**
/gl/

**Linguistic Level:**
Word/Phrase

**Position:**
Initial

## Objective:

To decrease the application of Liquid Cluster Reduction, the children will produce word-initial /gl/ clusters with varying levels of accuracy following the clinician's model or spontaneously.

## Suggestions for Nametags:

In each session, provide a choice between two nametags to elicit productions of the target sound. Suggestions for the word-initial /gl/ cluster include: *glasses, gloves, glowworm.*

## Glitter Gloves*

**Target Words:** glitter, glove, glow-in-the-dark, glue

**Materials:**

| | |
|---|---|
| paper | glitter |
| pen or pencil | glow-in-the-dark stickers |
| glue | |

**Procedure:** Set up the following four stations in various parts of the room:

1. Paper and pencils (to trace hands to form an outline for a *glove*).
2. *Glue* (to put on the outline).
3. *Glitter* (to sprinkle on the *glue*).
4. *Glow-in-the-dark* stickers (to put on the *glove*).

Instruct the children to go from station to station in sequence to make a *glitter glove*. Have an adult assist the children in tracing their hands at station #1. Incorporate the target words into the discussion of the action at each station.

## Glowworms in Glasses and Gloves

**Target Words:** glasses, glitter, gloves, glow, glowworm, glue

**Materials:** illustration of the glowworm, glowworm glasses, and glowworm gloves
glue or glue sticks
glitter

**Procedure:** Before the session, duplicate and cut out illustrations of the *glowworm, gloves,* and *glasses.* Give a *glowworm* to each child. Have the children *glue* the *glasses* and *gloves* on their *glowworms,* and add *glitter* to make their *glowworms glow.* Put these materials slightly out of reach to elicit the target words. Instruct the children to identify what their *glowworms* are wearing.

## Glowworm Search

**Target Words:** glasses, glitter, gloves, glowhouse, glowworm, glue

**Materials:** illustrations of the glowworm, glowworm glasses, and glowworm gloves
gloves (one pair per child)
glasses (one pair per child)
glue or glue sticks

**Procedure:** Before the session, draw an illustration of a *glowhouse* (a house that the *glowworm* could live in) and duplicate one for each child. Duplicate and cut out several illustrations of the *glowworm, gloves,* and *glasses. Glue* the *glasses* and *gloves* on the *glowworms* (or use the *glowworms* the children have made in the previous activity), then hide them around the room. Have the children ask for *gloves* and *glasses* to wear. Tell them to search the room for *glowworms* that are also wearing *gloves* or *glasses.* Instruct the children to identify what their *glowworms* are wearing before they *glue* them onto the *glowhouses.*

## Glitter T-Shirts*

**Target Words:** glasses, glitter, glove

**Materials:** T-shirts
tag board
tacks
corkboard
pen
cardboard
glitter paint

**Procedure:** Before the session, ask each child to bring in a plain T-shirt from home. Create two stencils out of tag board—one of *glasses* and one of a *glove*. First, have each child choose the *glasses* or the *glove* stencil for you to trace onto their shirt. Tack the T-shirt to the corkboard to hold the shirt firmly in place while tracing. Place a piece of cardboard inside the T-shirt to form a hard surface and then trace the stencil onto the T-shirt. Next, have the children trace over the stenciled outline with permanent *glitter* paint. Allow each child to put several stencil drawings on their T-shirts if they wish, while also encouraging them to tell whether *glasses* or *gloves* are in *glitter* on their T-shirts.

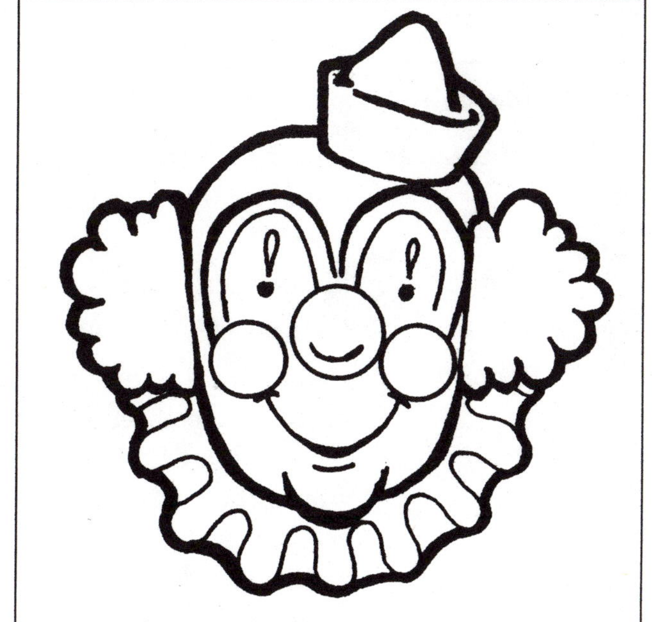

**Target Sound:**
/kl/

**Linguistic Level:**
Word/Phrase/Sentence

**Position:**
Initial

**Objective:**
To decrease the application of Liquid Cluster Reduction, the children will produce word-initial /kl/ clusters with varying levels of accuracy following the clinician's model or spontaneously.

**Suggestions for Nametags:**
In each session, provide a choice between two nametags to elicit productions of the target sound. Suggestions for the word-initial /kl/ cluster include: *clam, clock, clouds, clown.*

## Clifford's Closet

**Target Words:** clean, Clifford, clock, closet, clothes, clover, clown, clutter

**Materials:** 9 x 12" construction paper
initial /kl/ illustrations (e.g., clock, clothes, clover, clown)
tape
illustration of a boy (See pages 323–324.)
*Clifford's Closet* story

**Procedure:** Before the session, create a *closet* by cutting a straight vertical line three-fourths of the way up the center of a large piece of construction paper. Cut horizontal lines where the vertical cut ends so as to form a T. Fold back each side of the T and mount the closet on a board or wall. Duplicate several initial /k/ illustrations and tape them inside the *closet.* Duplicate the illustration of the boy *(Clifford)* to add interest to the story. Read the story *Clifford's Closet* to the children, bombarding them with initial /kl/ words. Have the children take turns removing an item of *clutter* from the *closet,* announcing to the group what they have removed. Afterwards, have the children recall the *clutter* that was in *Clifford's Closet.*

**Story:** *Clifford's Closet* (by Ranya Awwad)
This is *Clifford.* He has a *closet* in his room. One day, *Clifford* looked in his *closet. Clifford* said, "This *closet* is a mess! It is so *cluttered!* I must *clean* it." *Clifford* reached into his *closet.* He pulled out some *clothes. Clifford* looked in his *closet* again. "My *closet* is still *cluttered.* I must *clean* it some more." *Clifford* reached into his *closet.* This time he pulled out a *clock. Clifford* looked into his *closet* again. "It is still *cluttered,*" he said. "I must *clean* it some more." *Clifford* reached into his *closet.* He pulled out a *clown* face. *Clifford* said, "My *closet* is still *cluttered.* I must *clean* it some more." *Clifford* reached into his *closet.* This time he pulled out a four-leaf *clover. Clifford* looked in his *closet. Clifford* said, "My *closet* is finally *clean!*"

## Clothesline Art

**Target Words:** clam, clock, clothesline, clouds, clover, clown

**Materials:** initial /kl/ illustrations
  (e.g., clam, clock, clouds, clover, clown)
8½ x 11" cardboard or tag board
tape
yarn
glue or glue sticks
laundry basket
paper punch
clothesline and clothespins (optional)

**Procedure:** Before the session, duplicate several copies of /kl/ pictures. Cut pictures out but leave tabs to fold over the *clothesline*. Create a *clothesline* for each child by punching a hole at the outer edges and near the top of an 8½ x 11" piece of cardboard. String yarn loosely through the holes and tape in back. Gather /kl/ pictures in a laundry basket. Give the children a choice of what to hang on their *clotheslines*. If necessary, use the glue or glue sticks to "hang" the clothes. (As a variation, string a *clothesline* from one point in the room to another. Then have the children take turns choosing a /kl/ picture to hang on the *clothesline* with a *clothespin.)*

## Clown or Closet?*

**Target Words:** clam, clock, closet, clouds, clover, clown

**Materials:** clown illustration
construction paper
initial /kl/ illustrations
   (e.g., clam, clock, clouds, clover, clown)
tape

**Procedure:** Enlarge and duplicate the illustration of the *clown*. Cut out the mouth. Create a *closet* door out of construction paper (see page 138). Mount the *closet* and the large picture of the *clown* on the chalkboard or bulletin board. Offer the children a choice of giving /kl/ illustrations to the *clown* (by inserting them in its mouth) or taping them in the *closet*.

## Clyde Says*

**Target Words:** clap, climb, close, Clyde

**Materials:** spinner (See *Appendix H*.)
initial /kl/ action word illustrations

**Procedure:** Before the session, create a spinner. First, draw and then tape initial /kl/ action pictures (e.g., *clapping* hands, *climbing* a ladder, *closing* eyes) on it. Direct the child who is designated as *Clyde* to spin the spinner and tell the other children what action to carry out (e.g., "*Clyde* says, '*Clap* your hands'"). For children with limited linguistic ability, modify to say the action word only. Encourage everyone to act out the action while repeating the target word. Give each child a turn being *Clyde*.

## Clam Search

**Target Words:** clam, clock, closet, clouds, clover, clown

**Materials:** clam illustration
tape
initial /kl/ illustrations
(e.g., clock, clouds, clover, clown)
bucket

**Procedure:** Before the session, duplicate multiple illustrations of the *clam* and cut out. Duplicate and tape or glue /kl/ pictures on the back. Hide cutouts of *clams* around the room. Have the children *clean* the room by searching for the *clams*. As the children find each *clam* tell them to bring it to you and identify the /kl/ picture they found. Then tell the children to place the *clams* in the bucket.

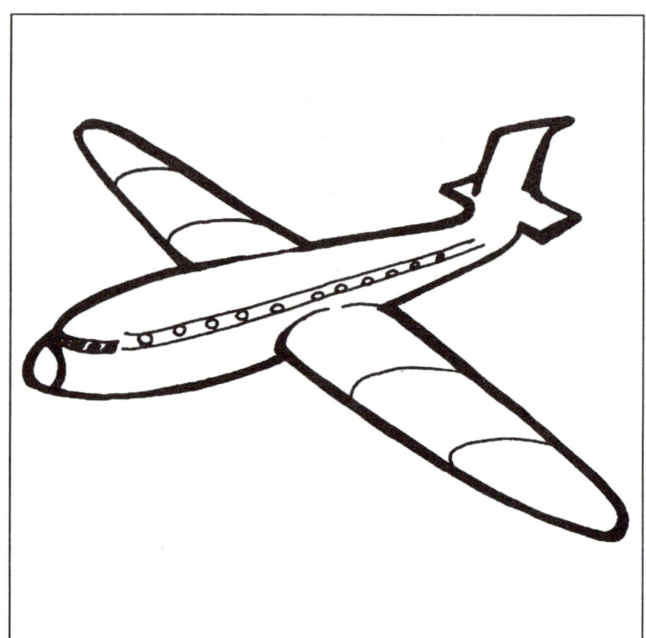

**Target Sound:**
/pl/

**Linguistic Level:**
Word/Phrase/Sentence

**Position:**
Initial

**Objective:**
To decrease the application of Liquid Cluster Reduction, the children will produce word-initial /pl/ clusters with varying levels of accuracy following the clinician's model or spontaneously.

**Suggestions for Nametags:**
In each session, provide a choice between two nametags to elicit productions of the target sound. Suggestions for the word-initial /pl/ cluster include: *plane, planet, plate, Pluto* (dog).

# Mr. Platt and the Plumber

**Target Words:** plan, plastic, Platt, pleasant, pliers, plink, plop, plumber, plunk

**Materials:** *Mr. Platt and the Plumber* story

**Procedure:** Read the story *Mr. Platt and the Plumber* to the children, bombarding them with initial /pl/ words. Have the children recall the events in the story (particularly the sounds made by the *plumbing*).

**Story:** *Mr. Platt and the Plumber* (by Caren Leamon)

Mr. *Platt* was a very *pleasant* man. He had a *pleasant* house and led a very *pleasant* life. One night, Mr. *Platt* woke up. He heard, *plop, plop, plop.* It was coming from the bathroom. "Oh, no!" said Mr. *Platt,* "I must call the *plumber!*"

So the next day Mr. *Platt* called the *plumber.* The *plumber* came right away. The *plumber* said, "Don't worry. I have a *plan.*" The *plumber* took out his *pliers* and twisted and turned. "There," said the *plumber.* "It is all fixed." What a *pleasure* it was!

That night, Mr. *Platt* woke up again. This time he didn't hear *plop, plop, plop.* He heard *plink, plink, plink.* Mr. *Platt* was not in a *pleasant* mood. "Oh, no!" said Mr. *Platt,* "I must call the *plumber!*"

So the next day, Mr. *Platt* called the *plumber.* The *plumber* came right away. The *plumber* said, "Don't worry. I have a *plan.*" The *plumber* took out his *pliers* and twisted and turned. "There," said the *plumber.* "It is all fixed." What a *pleasure* it was!

*(continued)*

*Mr. Platt and the Plumber—Continued*

That night, Mr. *Platt* woke up again. This time he didn't hear *plop, plop, plop*. He didn't hear *plink, plink, plink*. This time he heard *plunk, plunk, plunk*. Mr. *Platt* was not in a *pleasant* mood. "Oh, no!" said Mr. *Platt*, "I must call the *plumber!*"

So the next day, Mr. *Platt* called the *plumber*. The *plumber* came right away. The *plumber* said, "Don't worry. I have a *plan*." But the *plumber* didn't use his *pliers*. Instead he used *plastic* pipes.

Mr. *Platt* was very happy. He stayed in a *pleasant* mood for a long time.

## Making Turkeys with Plucked Feathers

**Target Words:** plane, plant, plate, plow, pluck

**Materials:** construction paper
initial /pl/ illustrations (e.g., plane, plant, plow)
glue or glue sticks
paper plates

**Procedure:** Before the session, cut feathers out of construction paper. Duplicate and glue /pl/ pictures onto the *plucked* feathers. Give each child a paper *plate*. Have the children trace their flattened hands on the paper *plates*. Instruct them to glue the *plucked* feathers with /pl/ pictures onto their turkeys (the paper *plates*). Ask the children to request the feathers they want to put on their turkeys (e.g., "I want a *plow*").

## Plane Placemats

**Target Words:** placemat, plane, plant, plate, plastic, plow

**Materials:** heavy stock paper          clear contact paper
initial /pl/ illustrations (e.g., plane, plant, plate, plow)
glue or glue sticks

**Procedure:** Enlarge and duplicate the *plane* onto heavy stock paper, creating one per child. (Enlarge the *plane* enough to be used as a *placemat* when cut out.) Cut the *planes* out. Duplicate multiple copies of the /pl/ illustrations. Give each child a *plane* to decorate. Offer choices of /pl/ illustrations to the children. Direct them to glue the pictures onto the *plane*. Have the children talk about the illustrations they selected. Incorporate foils in the discussion, for example, by calling the *plane* a car, to which the children respond, "No, *plane!*" Cover the pictures with clear contact paper (*plastic*) and use as *placemats*. This activity naturally leads to a snack.

## Plucking Turkey Feathers

**Target Words:** plane, plant, plate, plow, pluck

**Materials:** construction paper
initial /pl/ illustrations (e.g., plane, plant, plate, plow)
tape
paper plates

**Procedure:** Before the session, create a turkey out of construction paper and tape on the wall or chalkboard. Also, cut feathers out of construction paper. Duplicate the /pl/ illustrations and tape them to the feathers. *Place* the tail feathers on the turkey with the /pl/ pictures on them to be *plucked*. Give each child a choice of which tail feather to *pluck* from the turkey (e.g., "Do you want a *plate* or a *plane?*"). Once the tail feather is verbally chosen and *plucked*, *place* it on a paper *plate*.

## Plop, Plop, Pluck*

**Target Words:** plop, pluck

**Materials:** construction paper
real feathers (optional)

**Procedure:** Before the session, cut feathers out of construction paper, or use real feathers. Substitute in the "Duck, Duck, Goose" game the words *"Plop, Plop, Pluck."* Seat the children in a circle on the floor. Have everyone hold up a feather. Tell the person who is "it" (the leader) to walk around the outside of the circle, and to say *plop* as he or she taps each *player* on the head. When *pluck* is said, have the leader take the *player's* feather. Direct the *player* to chase the leader until the leader sits down in the circle. Continue the activity with the new *player* who is "it."

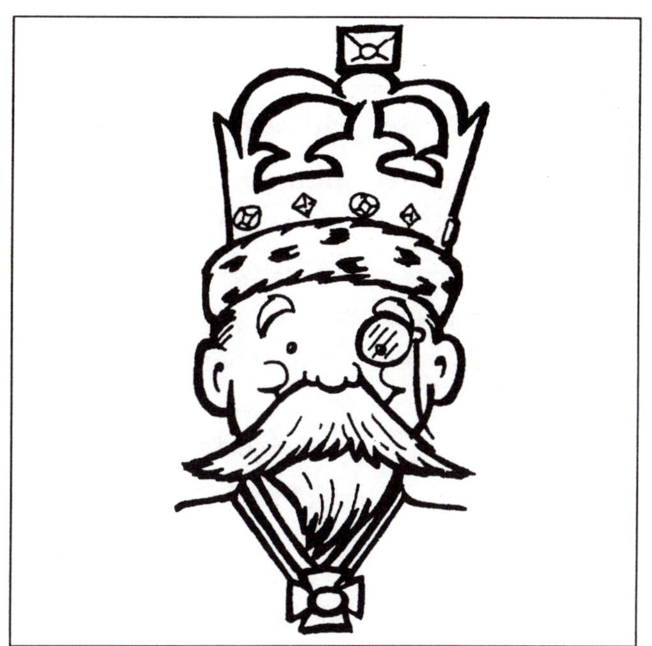

**Target Sound:**
/k/

**Linguistic Level:**
Word/Phrase/Sentence

**Position:**
Initial

## Objective:

To decrease the application of Velar Fronting, the children will produce word-initial /k/ with varying levels of accuracy following the clinician's model or spontaneously.

## Suggestions for Nametags:

In each session, provide a choice between two nametags to elicit productions of the target sound. Suggestions for word-initial /k/ include: *car, cat, coat, cookie, key, king*.

# The King Who Lost His Key

**Target Words:** car, carrot, castle, coat, cookie, country, key, king

**Materials:** initial /k/ illustrations
(e.g., car, carrot, coat, cookie, key, king)
*The King Who Lost His Key* story

**Procedure:** In advance of this activity, duplicate initial /k/ illustrations. Then read the story *The King Who Lost His Key* to the children, bombarding them with initial /k/ words. Use objects or illustrations to depict the target words in the story. Each time the *king* searches for the *key* in a different place and doesn't find it, prompt the children to shout in unison, "NO *KEY!*" When the story is finished, have the children recall the places the *king* searched for his *key*.

**Story:** *The King Who Lost His Key*

Once upon a time there was a *king* who lived in a *castle*. One day he came home from a drive in the *country*. The *king* walked up to the *castle* door. He couldn't find his *key*. The *king* said, "Maybe I left the *key* in my *car*." So the *king* walked back to his *car*. But he couldn't find his *key*. "NO *KEY!*" (encourage everyone to respond in unison). Then the *king* said, "Maybe I left the *key* in my *coat* pocket." So the *king* checked his *coat* pocket. But he couldn't find his *key*. "NO *KEY!*" The *king* said, "Maybe I left the *key* in the *carrot* patch." So the *king* walked to the *carrot* patch. But he couldn't find his *key*. "NO *KEY!*" Then the *king* remembered! He left his *key* in the *cookie* jar at the *castle* door. The *king* ran to the *cookie* jar and found his *key!*

## Cookies or Coca-Cola*

**Target Words:** Coca-Cola, cookie

**Materials:** mini cookies     small cups
Coca-Cola     small plates

**Procedure:** Have the children sit at a small table, ready for snack time. Have one child at a time act as the server and ask the others, "Would you like a *cookie* or *Coca-Cola?*"

## Kiwi or Cookies*

**Target Words:** cookies, kiwi

**Materials:** kiwi fruit     bowl
napkins     small plates
small cookies or small pieces of cookies

**Procedure:** Before the session, cut *kiwi* fruit and place in a bowl. Offer the children a choice of eating *kiwi* or *cookies* for a snack. Have the children take turns serving the food by asking, "Do you want *kiwi* or a *cookie?*" Give small portions of each food item so that the children must use the target words frequently to request more.

## Cake or Carrots*

**Target Words:** cake, carrot

**Materials:** small pieces of cake     carrot sticks
napkins     small plates

**Procedure:** In advance of this activity, prepare *carrot* sticks and *cake*. Offer the children small portions of *cake* and/or *carrot* sticks for a snack. Give each child a turn being the server. Have the child who is the server ask the other children if they want *cake* or a *carrot*.

## Musical /k/ Chairs*

**Target Words:** can, car, cat, cup, king

**Materials:** initial /k/ illustrations (e.g., can, car, cat, cup, king)
heavy stock paper     chairs
cassette player     musical cassette tape

**Procedure:** Duplicate initial /k/ illustrations onto heavy stock paper to form large picture cards. Arrange chairs, one chair per child, in a circle with the backs of the chairs toward the inside of the circle. Place initial /k/ picture cards face down on the chairs. Play music as the children walk around the chairs. Intermittently stop the music. When the music stops, have each child sit on a chair and name the picture on it. Continue to play the game without removing chairs so that each child participates in each round.

(This activity can be modified for use with any target sound or process.)

## Key Keepers

**Target Words:** cake, can, car, cat, coat, cup, key

**Materials:** construction paper
tape
initial /k/ illustrations
   (e.g., cake, can, car, cat, coat, cup)
key illustration or a real key

**Procedure:** Draw a house with a door on construction paper. Create one house for each target word. Cut the doors on the top, bottom, and one side so that they open and close. Tape the houses onto a wall or bulletin board. Duplicate /k/ illustrations and the *key* illustration and cut them out. Place one illustration behind each door. Have the children use a *key* to unlock the doors, but first guess what is inside each by saying *key-can, key-cake,* etc.

(This activity employs the modified paired-stimuli technique and is appropriate only if the children can produce the /k/ correctly in *key*.)

## Captain Cook*

**Target Words:** Captain Cook, kangaroo, kick, kiss

**Materials:** none

**Procedure:** Play a *"Captain Cook"* game (similar to "Simon Says"). Demonstrate the different actions the children can perform (e.g., *kick, kiss,* hop like a *kangaroo*) when they are *Captain Cook.* Give each child a turn being *Captain Cook* and choosing an action (target word) for everyone to perform.

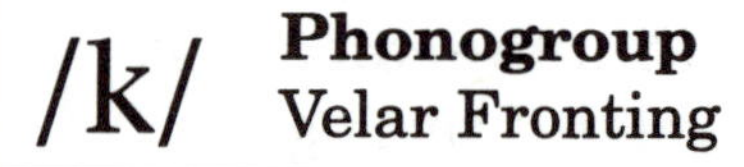



# Who Stole the Cookie?*

**Target Word:** cookie

**Materials:** cookie illustration
cookie jar
markers or crayons
real cookies

**Procedure:** Before the session, duplicate several copies of the *cookie* illustration and color each. Place paper *cookies* in a *cookie* jar or tin. Seat the children in a circle. Have one child (the *Cookie* Monster) leave the circle and cover her or his eyes. Pass the *cookie* jar around the circle. Instruct one child to take a *cookie* out of the jar and hide it (by sitting on it) when given a nonverbal cue from you. Have the *Cookie* Monster return to the circle. Encourage everyone to say, "Who stole the *cookie* from the *cookie* jar?" Direct the *Cookie* Monster to walk around the circle and ask each child "Do you have a *cookie?*" If the child doesn't have one, instruct her or him to say, "No *cookie!*" If the child does have the *cookie,* the response should be "Yes, *cookie!*" This child then becomes the new child to leave the circle and cover his or her eyes. Continue the activity until each child in the circle has at least one paper *cookie.* Then allow the children to cash them in for real *cookies.*

## What's in the Cave?

**Target Words:** candy, car, cave, coat, comb, cup, key

**Materials:** table or chair
blanket
initial /k/ objects
  (e.g., candy, [toy] car, coat, comb, cup, key)
flashlight

**Procedure:** Set up a *cave* in a corner of the room by covering a table or chair with a blanket. Place initial /k/ objects in the *cave*. Turn the lights off in the room. Tell the children what objects are in the *cave*. Have the children take turns going into the *cave* and searching for a specific object with a flashlight. Provide the children with a choice, such as "Do you want to find a *car* or a *comb?*" before they enter the *cave*.

## What's Under the Cup?

**Target Words:** candy, car, comb, cookie, cup, key

**Materials:** initial /k/ objects
    (e.g., candy, [toy] car, comb, cookie, cup, key)
serving tray
cup

**Procedure:** Play a memory game with the children. Place approximately four to six small initial /k/ objects on a tray. Name the items on the tray several times with the children. Have the children close their eyes. Hide one of the objects under the *cup*. Have the children open their eyes and guess what is hidden under the *cup*. Give each child an opportunity to hide an object under the *cup*.

## Cookie Game

**Target Words:** can, car, carrot, cat, cookie, comb, cup, king

**Materials:** game board (See *Appendix H.*)
initial /k/ illustrations
    (e.g., can, car, carrot, cat, comb, cookie, cup, king)
game pieces
two dice

**Procedure:** In advance of the session, make a simple game board containing a variety of initial /k/ illustrations, including illustrations of *cookies*. Also use the *cookie* illustration to create *cookie* tokens (*cookie* cutouts). Have the children take turns rolling the dice and moving their game pieces along the board. As they move along the board, have them name each illustration. If they land on a *cookie*, give them a *cookie* token to be turned in at snack time for a *cookie* or other treat.

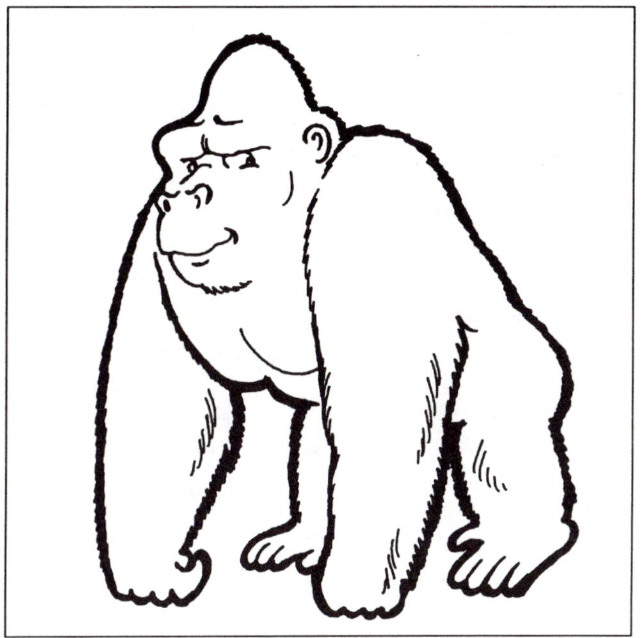

**Target Sound:**
/g/

**Linguistic Level:**
Word/Phrase

**Position:**
Initial

**Objective:**
To decrease the application of Velar Fronting, the children will produce word-initial /g/ with varying levels of accuracy following the clinician's model or spontaneously.

**Suggestions for Nametags:**
In each session, provide a choice between two nametags to elicit productions of the target sound. Suggestions for word-initial /g/ include: *gate, ghost, girl, gorilla, gum.*

## Gabe the Gatekeeper

**Target Words:** Gabe, gate, gatekeeper, gave, Gertie, go, goat, good, goose, Gordon, gorilla, Gus

**Materials:** *Gabe the Gatekeeper* story
illustrations of the goat, goose, and gorilla

**Procedure:** Duplicate illustrations of the animals mentioned in the story. Read the story *Gabe the Gatekeeper* to the children, bombarding them with initial /g/ words. Show illustrations of the animals as the story is read. Afterwards, incorporate target words into a discussion about the animals who enjoyed their baths.

**Story:** *Gabe the Gatekeeper* (by Lynne C. Miller)
*Gabe* was the *gatekeeper* at the zoo. *Gabe* sat by the *gate* and watched the children come and *go*. Early in the morning, *Gabe gave Gus* the *Gorilla* a bath. *Gus* the *Gorilla* loved his bath because it felt so *good*. *Gabe gave Gordon* the *Goat* a bath too. *Gordon* the *Goat* loved his bath because it felt so *good*. *Gabe gave Gertie* the *Goose* a bath. *Gertie* the *Goose* loved her bath, because it felt so *good*. After the baths, *Gabe* returned to sit at the *gate*. *Gabe* loved to watch the children come and *go*.

## Gaston the Goldfish

**Target Words:** Gail, game, Gaston, go, goal, goldfish, good, gorgeous, gosh

**Materials:** *Gaston the Goldfish* story
fish illustration

**Procedure:** Make two copies of the fish illustration to use as *Gaston* and *Gail* from the *Gaston the Goldfish* story. Color them each in a distinct way so that *Gail* can be distinguished from *Gaston*. Emphasize target words as the story is read. Afterwards, have two children act out the events in the story (with assistance from you), producing the target words.

**Story:** *Gaston the Goldfish* (by Lynne C. Miller)
*Gaston* the *Goldfish* lived in a pond. One day there was a new *girl* in *Gaston's* class at school. Her name was *Gail. Gaston gazed* at *Gail.* "*Gosh,* she's *gorgeous,*" he said. *Gaston* went over to *Gail* and said, "Hi, my name is *Gaston.*" *Gail* said, "Hello, *Gaston.* My name is *Gail.*" *Gaston* asked *Gail* if she would like to *go* to the big *game* at the *Goldfish* Bowl on Saturday. *Gaston* loved to *go* to the *Goldfish* Bowl! *Gail* said, "Yes, that sounds like *good* fun." On Saturday, *Gaston* and *Gail* went to the *game.* The *Goldfish* team scored a *goal.* Everyone cheered "*GO, GO, GO* TEAM *GO!*" *Gaston* and *Gail* had a *good* time.

## Gold Guitars*

**Target Words:** gate, ghost, goat, gold, goose, guitar

**Materials:** initial /g/ illustrations (e.g., gate, ghost, goat, goose)
guitar illustration          glue or glue sticks
gold glitter

**Procedure:** Before the session, duplicate several initial /g/ illustrations per child and enlarge and duplicate one illustration of the guitar per child. The initial /g/ illustration should be small in relationship to the guitar. Cut them out. Give each child a *guitar* to decorate with *gold* glitter and small initial /g/ illustrations. Have the children request the *gold* glitter and the illustrations to glue onto their *guitar*. After the children have finished, have them tell each other about their *guitars*.

## Garage or Garden?

**Target Words:** garage, garden, gate, ghost, goat, goose, guitar

**Materials:** initial /g/ illustrations
   (e.g., garage, garden, gate, ghost, goat, goose, guitar)
chalk and chalkboard
tape

**Procedure:** Before this activity, duplicate initial /g/ illustrations. Enlarge and duplicate the *garage* and *garden* illustration and tape them to the chalkboard. Have each child verbally select initial /g/ illustrations and decide whether to put them in the *garage* or in the *garden*. Provide the children with a choice of where to put each picture (e.g., "Do you want to put the *goat* in the *garage* or in the *garden?*"). Instruct them to tape the illustrations in the chosen place. After all the illustrations are posted, recall with the children what they put in the *garage* and in the *garden*.

## /g/ Memory*

**Target Words:** gate/date
gill/dill
go/dough
goo/dew

**Materials:** minimal pairs illustrations (See pages 316–322.)
(e.g., gate/date, gill/dill, go/dough, goo/dew)
glue or glue sticks
index cards

**Procedure:** Before the session, duplicate the minimal pairs illustrations, making two copies of each picture. Glue these to index cards to form a set of cards. Instruct the children to form groups of two to play this memory game. Give each group a set of cards containing two copies for each of two minimal pairs of words (e.g., *gate/date, goo/dew*). Place the eight cards face down on the table. Have one child turn a card over, name it, then turn another card over to try to find the match. Instruct the children to name the cards whether they match or not. If a match is found, allow the child to take another turn. If the cards do not match, direct the other child to take a turn. After each child's production, provide a correct model. If the child produces the word incorrectly, ask for clarification. For example, if the child turns over *gate* but calls it *date,* say, "Did I hear you say *gate* or *date?*" In this way, the child begins to recognize the contrast.

## Ghostly Bingo*

**Target Words:** garage, garden, gate, ghost, goat, goose, gorilla

**Materials:** bingo boards (See *Appendix H.*)
initial /g/ illustrations
  (e.g., garage, garden, gate, goat, goose, gorilla)
cloth grab bag (See *Appendix H.*)
ghost illustration

**Procedure:** Before the session, prepare bingo boards with four to six initial /g/ illustrations on them. Make an identical set of illustrations to use as calling cards and place them in the cloth grab bag. Also, duplicate four to six *ghost* illustrations per child to use as bingo markers. Give each child a bingo board. Have the children take turns being the "caller" by drawing a /g/ card from the bag and naming it for the others. If the picture named is on a child's board, have the child cover it with a picture of a *ghost*. Continue the game until all children have covered all of their illustrations. Have the children name the pictures covered as they remove their *ghosts*.

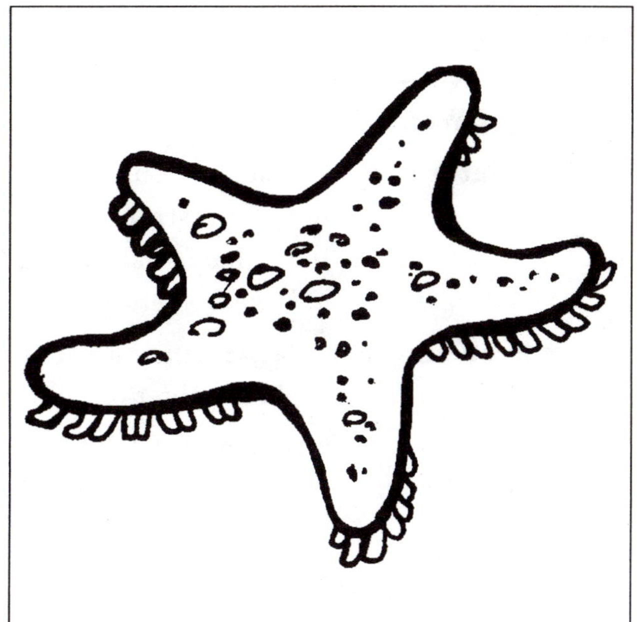

**Target Sound:**
/ʃ/

**Linguistic Level:**
Isolation/Word/
Phrase/Sentence

**Position:**
Isolation/Final

**Objective:**
To decrease the application of Depalatalization, the children will produce word-final /ʃ/ with varying levels of accuracy following the clinician's model or spontaneously.

**Suggestions for Nametags:**
In each session, provide a choice between two nametags to elicit productions of the target sound. Suggestions for word-final /ʃ/ include: *bush, dish, hair-brush, fish, leash, starfish.*

# Tish the Dog

**Target Words:** bush, crash, fish, leash, Nash, splash, Tish, trash

**Materials:** dog illustration
final /ʃ/ illustrations
  (e.g., bush, fish, leash, trash)
*Tish the Dog* story

**Procedure:** Enlarge and duplicate the dog (*Tish*) illustration. Duplicate the final /ʃ/ illustrations. Read the story *Tish the Dog* to the children, bombarding them with final /ʃ/ words. Present the illustrations at important parts of the story. Have the children hang the illustrations on the wall (or set them up along a chalkboard). Emphasize target words and ask questions about the story to elicit productions.

**Story:** *Tish the Dog*
Mr. *Nash* has a dog named *Tish*. *Tish* always had to stay on a *leash* so she wouldn't get into trouble. One day *Tish* was outside without a *leash*. Mr. *Nash* saw *Tish* hiding behind a *bush*. He called, "*Tish, Tish,* come inside!" But *Tish* wouldn't come. Then Mr. *Nash* heard a *crash*. *Tish* knocked over a *trash* can, and was eating *fish!* Mr. *Nash* ran after *Tish*. *Tish* found a puddle. She decided to *splash* in the water. Mr. *Nash* finally caught *Tish* and put on her *leash*.

**Questions:** What is the dog's name? *Tish* or *Nash?*
Where did *Tish* hide? Under a *bush* or in the *trash?*
What did *Tish* knock over? A *trash* can or a *bush?*
What did *Tish* eat? A *fish* or *trash?*
What did Mr. *Nash* finally put on *Tish?* A *leash* or a *fish?*

162

## Crush 'n Mash*

**Target Words:** crush, dish, mash, shhhh

**Materials:** graham crackers
bananas
canned whipped cream
plastic bags that can be sealed
rolling pin
potato masher
dishes

**Procedure:** Prepare a snack with graham crackers, bananas, and whipped cream. Have each child *crush* graham crackers (place graham crackers in a sealed plastic bag and *crush* with a rolling pin) while saying *crush, crush, crush. Mash* bananas (place bananas in a *dish* and *mash* with a potato masher) while saying *mash, mash, mash.* Ask each child if they want to *crush* or *mash* first, thus providing an opportunity to elicit a target word from the child through choices. Direct the children to layer the graham crackers and mashed bananas in the *dish.* Spray on top whipped cream from the can while saying *shhhh.* After all the ingredients have been added, let the children eat the snack.

## Banana Mush*

**Target Words:** fish, mash, mush

**Materials:**

| | |
|---|---|
| bananas | crackers or bread |
| potato mashers or forks | bowls |
| peanut butter | |
| cookie cutter in the shape of a fish | |

**Procedure:** Give each child a banana to *mash* to make banana *mush*. While the children *mash* their bananas, encourage them to say *mash, mash, mash.* Combine the mashed banana with peanut butter and spread on crackers or slices of bread. Cut the bread out in the shape of *fish.* Have the children take turns passing out the *fish,* asking the other children if they want a *fish* to spread their *mush* on.

## Making Slush Puppies

**Target Words:** crush, dish, push, slush, splash, squish

**Materials:**

| | |
|---|---|
| ice cubes | bowls |
| blender | spoons |
| juice concentrate or juice | napkins |

**Procedure:** Make *slush* puppies (the recipe follows) for a snack. Incorporate the target words listed. Encourage the children to chant *crush, crush, crush* as the ice is crushed in a *slush* machine (blender). Give each child the opportunity to ask if they may *push* the *crush* button (on the blender panel) on the *slush* machine.

**Recipe for Slush Puppies:** Place ice cubes in a blender and blend until crushed. Add small amounts of juice or juice concentrate and blend again until desired consistency is reached.

## Fishing Fun

**Target Words:** bush, dish, fish, hairbrush, leash, starfish, wash, wish

**Materials:** final /ʃ/ illustrations
   (e.g., bush, dish, hairbrush, leash, starfish, wash)
fishing pole (See *Appendix H.*)
construction paper
paper clips
bucket or large bowl

**Procedure:** Before the session, duplicate final /ʃ/ illustrations and prepare a fishing pole. Cut *fish* out of construction paper and attach the final /ʃ/ pictures to them with paper clips. Name the pictures on the *fish*, and then place them in a big bowl or bucket. Give each child a turn fishing with the fishing pole. Before fishing, instruct each child to tell which *fish* they *wish* for. When the *fish* is caught, direct the children to name the final /ʃ/ picture attached to the *fish*.

# Trash and Fish Clean Up

**Target Words:** crush, fish, trash

**Materials:** construction paper or wrapping paper
pieces of waste paper, crumpled
bucket or a fish bowl
wastebasket

**Procedure:** Before the session, cut *fish* out of construction paper or wrapping paper. Put *trash* (lightly crumpled paper) and the paper *fish* around the room. Have the children pick up the *trash* and *fish* to clean up the room. Have the children *crush* the *trash* and put it in a *trash* can (wastebasket), and put the *fish* in the *fish* bowl. Encourage the children to talk about what they are looking for, what they have found, and where they want to put it (in the *trash* can or in the *fish* bowl) during this activity.

## Passing Fish

**Target Word:** none (discrimination of /ʃ/ versus /s/)

**Materials:** sponges
medium-size box
fish bowl filled with water

**Procedure:** Before the session, cut *fish* shapes out of sponges. Seat the children on the floor in a line. Place a box of cut-out sponge *fish* at one end of the line and place a *fish* bowl with water in it at the other end. The child next to the box of *fish* takes one out and passes it along to the next child, who passes it to the next until the last child puts it into the *fish* bowl. Produce /ʃ/ in a continuous airstream as the *fish* are passed along. Occasionally shift from producing /ʃ/ to producing a prolonged /s/ without stopping the airstream. Instruct the children to stop passing the *fish* when they hear a change in the sound that is produced.

## Does It Squish?*

**Target Word:** squish

**Materials:** squishable objects
   (e.g., sponge, socks, cotton balls, Nerf ball)
nonsquishable objects
   (e.g., blocks, key, pencil, rock)
feely box (See *Appendix H.*)

**Procedure:** Demonstrate for the children that some of the objects *squish* and some do not *squish*. Place the squishable and nonsquishable objects into the feely box. In turn, have each child reach into the feely box and feel an object. Encourage the child to tell the others in the group whether or not the object squishes by saying, "*Squish*" or "No *squish*."

## Spraying and Washing

**Target Words:** /ʃ/ in isolation, wash

**Materials:** water spray bottles
paper towels

**Procedure:** Give each child a spray bottle filled with water. Have the children clean the furniture in the room. While they spray the furniture, tell the children to produce /ʃ/, /ʃ/, /ʃ/. Then with paper towels, have them wipe up the water while saying *wash, wash, wash.*

## Pushing in a Box*

**Target Words:**  dish, fish, hairbrush, push, trash

**Materials:**  final /ʃ/ illustrations
(e.g., dish, fish, hairbrush, trash)
one sturdy cardboard box, large enough to sit in
cheerleader pom-poms

**Procedure:**  Duplicate four final /ʃ/ illustrations and display them around the room at a child's eye level. Give each child a turn to choose and identify one picture. Have that child sit in a large cardboard box while you and another child *push* him or her to the designated illustration. Have the other children shake cheerleader pom-poms and chant *push, push, push!*

## Wish Grab Bag

**Target Words:**  brush, leash, wish

**Materials:**  dog leashes
dog brushes
cloth grab bag (See *Appendix H.*)
toy dogs

**Procedure:**  Collect dog *leashes* and dog *brushes* and put them in a cloth grab bag. Direct each child to take a turn reaching in the bag while saying "I *wish* for a (*leash* or *brush*)." Then have them either *brush* a toy dog or put a *leash* on it.

## Swish, Swish Go the Fish

**Target Words:**  fish, splash, swish

**Materials:**  sponges
masking tape or blue construction paper
bucket filled with water

**Procedure:**  Cut *fish* out of sponges. Place tape or strips of blue paper on the table as if it were a stream or river. Seat the children around the table. Give each child a *fish* sponge to swim in the stream. Allow each child to take a turn moving the fish-shaped sponge along the stream while saying *swish, swish, swish*. At the end of the river, instruct the children to make their *fish* dive into a pond (a bucket filled with water) while saying *splash, splash, splash*.

## Funny Food for Fishing

**Target Words:**  bush, cash, dish, fish, hairbrush, leash, wash

**Materials:**  chalk and chalkboard          fish bowl (optional)
final /ʃ/ illustrations          paper clips
  (e.g., bush, cash, dish, hairbrush, leash, wash)
fishing poles (See *Appendix H*.)

**Procedure:**  Draw a picture on the chalkboard of *fish* swimming. Duplicate final /ʃ/ illustrations and attach a paper clip to each. Place them on the floor, the table, or in a *fish* bowl. Tell the children that they are going to catch funny food to feed the *fish*. Instruct the children to *fish* for food with fishing poles. As they catch funny food, ask them what they caught by providing choices such as, "Did you catch a *brush* or a *leash*?" or "The *fish* will eat a *dish*, etc."

(This is an appropriate activity for initial /f/ with modification of target words.)

## Cash or Trash

**Target Words:** cash, trash, wish

**Materials:** play money
crumpled paper
cloth grab bag (See *Appendix H.*)
toy cash register
trash can

**Procedure:** Place *cash* (play money) and *trash* (crumpled paper) in a cloth grab bag. Have each child take a turn reaching into the bag, saying if they *wish* for *cash* or *trash*. Elicit a response from the children by asking, "Do you *wish* for *cash* or *trash?*" After they have chosen from the grab bag, have the children state whether they want to put it in the *cash* register or the *trash* can.

## Caring for Baby

**Target Words:** brush, mush, rash

**Materials:** dolls
blankets
bowls and spoons
brushes
small bottles of hand cream or lotion

**Procedure:** Give each child a baby doll to care for. Have each child prepare her or his baby doll for bed. Direct the children to feed the babies *mush,* *brush* the babies' hair, and put cream on their baby's *rash.* To elicit the target words, encourage the children to share and request items from each other.

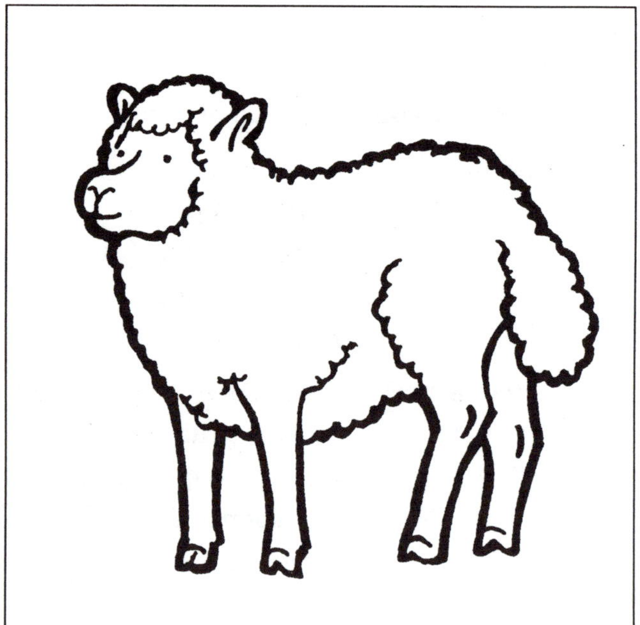

**Target Sound:**
/ʃ/

**Linguistic Level:**
Isolation/Word/Sentence

**Position:**
Isolation/Initial

**Objective:**
To decrease the application of Depalatalization, the children will produce word-initial /ʃ/ with varying levels of accuracy following the clinician's model or spontaneously.

**Suggestions for Nametags:**
In each session, provide a choice between two nametags to elicit productions of the target sound. Suggestions for word-initial /ʃ/ include: *sheep, shell, sheriff, shoe.*

## Shhhh . . . It's Storytime

**Target Word:** /ʃ/ in isolation

**Materials:** any appropriate storybook

**Procedure:** Read a story to the children. While reading, have another person (e.g., another educator) make a noise around the room or while sitting with the group. Tell the children they must quiet the noisy person by saying *shhhh*. Direct the person to be quiet for a brief time and then make noise again, to elicit more productions.

## Shhhh, I'm Sleeping!

**Target Word:** /ʃ/ in isolation

**Materials:** blankets (optional)
pillows (optional)
musical instruments or noisy objects

**Procedure:** Tell all the children, except one, to pretend to be sleeping. (Blankets or pillows can be used to set the mood.) Dim the lights. Instruct the children to be very quiet but, if they hear a noise, to say *shhhh*. Have the child who is not sleeping walk around the room and make noise with musical instruments or noisy objects. Encourage the children to respond by loudly saying *shhhh*. Give each child a turn to make noise.

## Sleeping Baby

**Target Word:** /ʃ/ in isolation

**Materials:** baby doll with eyes that close
doll blanket
cassette tape of common noises
cassette player

**Procedure:** Introduce a sleeping baby doll and explain to the children that they have to be very quiet so that the baby does not wake up. Play the cassette tape of noises. Every time a noise is heard, have the children say *shhhh*.

## Balloon Shaving

**Target Word:** shave

**Materials:** balloons
string
whipped cream
tongue depressors

**Procedure:** Before this activity, blow up several balloons and hang them from the ceiling at a child's eye level. Spread whipped cream on them. Have each child select a balloon to *shave*. Use tongue depressors to *shave* the cream off the balloons and have the children say *shave, shave, shave*.

## Shoot the Basketball

**Target Word:** shoot

**Materials:** basketball hoop (for sponge ball) or trash can
sponge or Nerf basketball

**Procedure:** Set up an indoor basketball hoop. Have the children take turns *shooting* baskets. Have the other children cheer *shoot, shoot, shoot* as each child *shoots* the ball.

## Searching for Ships and Shells

**Target Words:** shell, ship

**Materials:** ship and shell illustrations
chalk and chalkboard
tape

**Procedure:** Before the session, duplicate several *shell* and *ship* illustrations and hide them around the room. Draw a scene of the sea and sand on a chalkboard. Have the children search for *shells* and *ships*. Once the children find the pictures, have them bring the pictures back to you and name what they found. After the search is over, instruct the children to sit on the floor in front of the chalkboard and request a *ship* to put in the sea, or a *shell* to put in the sand. (Affix the illustrations to the chalkboard with small pieces of tape.)

## Dish Search

**Target Words:** sheep, shell, ship, shoe

**Materials:** initial /ʃ/ illustrations
(e.g., sheep, shell, ship, shoe)
dish illustration

**Procedure:** In advance of this session, duplicate initial /ʃ/ illustrations and make several copies of the dish illustration. Hide the /ʃ/ pictures under the illustrations of dishes. Have each child close his or her eyes and choose a dish. Then, instruct each child to lift up the dish and say *dish-sheep, dish-shoe,* etc. (This activity uses the modified sensory-motor technique and is appropriate only if the children can produce the final /ʃ/ correctly in *dish.*)

## Shopping for /ʃ/

**Target Words:** shampoo, shaver, sheets, shell, shirt, shoelaces, shoes, sure

**Materials:** /ʃ/ items
(e.g., shampoo, shaver, sheets, shell, shirt, shoelaces, shoes)
toy cash register
play money

**Procedure:** Before this activity, collect initial /ʃ/ items. Set up a store in the room. Have one child act as the *shopkeeper* and sell the /ʃ/ items to the rest of the children. While *shopping,* have the children ask the *shopkeeper* questions such as, "Do you have any *shoes?*" Instruct the *shopkeeper* to respond by saying *"Sure!"* Direct the *shopkeeper* to name the items as he or she rings up the purchases. Give each child a turn being the *shopkeeper.*

## /ʃ/ **Memory**

**Target Words:** sell/shell, sign/shine, sip/ship, Sue/shoe

**Materials:** minimal pairs illustrations (See pages 316–322.)
(e.g., sell/shell, sign/shine, sip/ship, Sue/shoe)
glue or glue sticks
index cards

**Procedure:** Before the session, duplicate the minimal pairs illustrations, making two copies of each picture. Glue these to index cards to form sets of cards. Instruct the children to form groups of two to play this memory game. Give each group a set of cards containing two copies of each of two minimal pairs of words (e.g., *Sue/shoe, sip/ship*). Place the eight cards face down on the table. Have one child turn a card over, name it, then turn another card over to try to find the match. Instruct the children to name the cards whether they match or not. If a match is found, allow the child to take another turn. If the cards do not match, direct the other child to take a turn. After each child's production, provide a correct model. If the child produces the word incorrectly, ask for clarification. For example, if the child turns over *shoe* and says *Sue*, say, "Did you mean *shoe* or *Sue?*" In this way, the child begins to recognize the contrast.

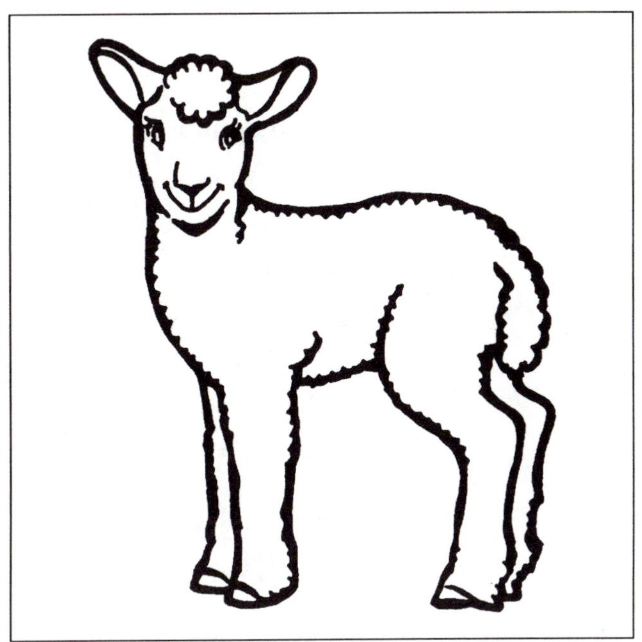

**Target Sound:**
/l/

**Linguistic Level:**
Word/Phrase/Sentence

**Position:**
Initial

## Objective:
To decrease the application of Gliding of Liquids, the children will produce word-initial /l/ with varying levels of accuracy following the clinician's model or spontaneously.

## Suggestions for Nametags:
In each session, provide a choice between two nametags to elicit productions of the target sound. Suggestions for word-initial /l/ include: *ladybug*, *lamb*, *leaf*, *lemon*, *lion*, *log*.

Note: In advance of these activities, make a request to parents, caregivers, and teachers to send stuffed animals or nonbreakable objects representing animals whose names begin with /l/ for use in this section. Collect the stuffed animals over a week's time and label them with the owner's name (a piece of tape on the bottom).

# Lost Animals

**Target Words:** ladybug, lamb, lion, lizard, llama, lobster, lollipop, lost

**Materials:** initial /l/ stuffed animals, toy animals, or illustrations (e.g., ladybug, lamb, lion, lizard, llama, lobster)
*Lost Animals* story

**Procedure:** Duplicate initial /l/ animal illustrations or use the collection of toy or stuffed animals. Read the *Lost Animals* story to the children, bombarding them with initial /l/ words. As each *lost* animal is mentioned, show a stuffed animal or a picture of the animal to the children. Pass it around the circle. Have the children discuss the story, incorporating the target words.

**Story:** *Lost Animals*

*Lots* of animals *lived* on *Lollipop* Farm. One day the *lock* on the gate was broken and all the animals *left* *Lollipop* Farm. They quickly got *lost*. The *llama* got *lost*. The *lion* got *lost*. The *ladybug* got *lost* . . . (fill in with as many /l/ animals as you have). After awhile, the animals were *lonely*. They didn't *like* being *lost*. So they all found their way back to *Lollipop* Farm and *lived* happily ever after.

# Leon and Lisa Go to London

**Target Words:** laces, lamp, leaves, lemon, licorice, lime, lollipop, luggage

**Materials:** illustrations of a girl and a boy (See pages 323–326.)
*Leon and Lisa Go to London* story
initial /l/ items
  (e.g., [shoe]laces, lamps, leaves, lemons, licorice, limes, lollipops)
suitcase

**Procedure:** Duplicate an illustration of a girl (*Lisa*) and a boy (*Leon*). Use the illustrations to add interest to the story. Read the story *Leon and Lisa Go to London* to the children, bombarding them with initial /l/ words. Inform the children that as *Leon* and *Lisa* prepare for a trip, they will pack their *luggage* with *lemons*, *limes*, *laces* (shoelaces), *lollipops*, *licorice*, *lamps*, and *leaves*. While the story is read, have the children take turns placing the /l/ items into the *luggage* (suitcase).

**Story:** *Leon and Lisa Go to London*

*Leon* and *Lisa* are very excited! They are *leaving* on a trip to *London*. Before *leaving*, they packed their *luggage*. *Leon* and *Lisa* packed silly things! *Leon* put *lollipops* and *licorice* in the *luggage*. *Lisa* likes *lemons* and *limes*, so she put them in the *luggage*. *Leon* packed *leaves* and *laces*. *Lisa* took a *lamp*. Finally the *luggage* was packed and they *left* for *London!*

## Lazy Leo

**Target Words:** late, laundry, lazy, leaves, Leo, licorice, lie, lights, likes, lion, litter, lollipops, long, loses, loves, lying

**Materials:** lion illustration
*Lazy Leo* story
initial /l/ items
(e.g., licorice, litter [crumpled paper], lollipops)

**Procedure:** Duplicate the *lion* illustration (*Lazy Leo*). Read the story *Lazy Leo* to the children, bombarding them with initial /l/ words. Show the pictures or real objects representing the target words in the story to the children. Once the story is read, discuss ways in which *Leo* is *lazy*.

**Story:** *Lazy Leo* (by Erin Black)

This is *Leo* the *Lion*. *Leo* is very *lazy*. All *Leo likes* to do is *lie* down and sleep. If he does anything, he never finishes it. *Leo leaves* the *lights* on all the time. He eats only *lollipops* and *licorice*, and then he *leaves litter*. *Leo loses* all his toys. He *lets* the grass grow *long* and never rakes the *leaves*. His *laundry* is dirty and he is always *late* for school. *Lazy Leo* just *loves lying* in bed all day *long*.

## Making Ladybugs

**Target Words:**  ladybug, large, legs, little, lots

**Materials:**  large ladybug illustration (including legs and spots)
glue or glue sticks
construction paper

**Procedure:**  Before the session, duplicate the *large ladybug* illustration, *ladybug legs,* and spots. Cut out the *ladybug, legs,* and spots. Glue the body of the *ladybug* to construction paper. Show the children a *ladybug* already assembled. Have the children then make their *ladybugs* by gluing *large* and *little* spots and *legs* onto the oval body. Give them the opportunity to glue *lots* of *legs* onto the *ladybug*.

## Leapfrogs and Ladybugs

**Target Words:**  ladybug, leapfrog, lily pad, log

**Materials:**  illustrations of a leapfrog, ladybug, lily pad, and log
paper clips
fishing poles (See *Appendix H.*)
glue or glue sticks

**Procedure:**  Duplicate the initial /l/ illustrations and cut them out. Attach a paper clip to the *leapfrog* and *ladybug* pictures. Spread them out on the floor. Have the children catch *leapfrogs* and *ladybugs* with a fishing pole. Then instruct them to glue the *leapfrogs* and *ladybugs* on the cutouts of the *log* or the *lily pad*.

## Lemonade*

**Target Words:** lemon, lemonade, little, (a) lot

**Materials:**

| | |
|---|---|
| lemons | pitcher |
| spoon | cups |
| sugar | juicer |
| knife (for clinician use only) | water |

**Procedure:** Gather together a juicer and the ingredients to make *lemonade* with the children (and possibly their parents). Have the children request the items they need from you or from their parents. After the *lemonade* is made, give the children the opportunity to request a *lot* or a *little* to drink.

## Lemonade or Licorice*

**Target Words:** lemonade, licorice, like, little, long, lot, lunch

**Materials:**

| | |
|---|---|
| lemonade | long and little licorice pieces |
| apron | napkins |
| cups | child-size pitcher |
| bowl (for licorice) | |

**Procedure:** Prepare *lemonade* ahead of time or with the children. Have the children eat a *lunch* together consisting of *lemonade* and *licorice*. Allow the children to take turns being the server (designated by wearing an apron). Tell them to ask the others if they want *licorice* or *lemonade*. If the child responds *licorice*, give him or her a choice of *long* or *little licorice*. If the response is *lemonade*, give the choices of a *little* or a *lot*. Discuss what they *like* the best as the children eat and drink.

## Lemon/Lime Lunch

**Target Words:** large, lemon, like, lime, little, lunch

**Materials:** lemon and lime JELL-O
napkins
tongs or serving spoons
plates
apron

**Procedure:** Prepare firm *lemon* and *lime* JELL-O before this activity. Cut into *little* or *large* pieces. Give the children a turn serving *little* or *large* pieces of *lemon* or *lime* JELL-O to peers. Allow the server to wear the apron. Have the children talk about whether they *like* the *lemon* or *lime* JELL-O better as they eat their *lunch*.

## Logs and Ladybugs*

**Target Words:** ladybug, little, log, long

**Materials:** plastic knives or popsicle sticks
peanut butter
celery
raisins
plates
knife (for clinician use only)

**Procedure:** For a snack, have the children use the plastic knives or popsicle sticks to spread peanut butter on *logs* (celery sticks) and put *ladybugs* (raisins) on top. Then cut the *logs* into *long* and *little* pieces to elicit the target words.

## Lunchtime at the Zoo

**Target Words:** lamb, leaves, lemon, lettuce, limes, lion, lizard, llama, lunch

**Materials:** initial /l/ stuffed animals, toy animals, or illustrations of zoo animals (e.g., lamb, lion, lizard, llama)
berry baskets or laundry baskets
table
real /l/ foods for animals
(e.g., leaves, lemons, lettuce, limes)

**Procedure:** Before the session, duplicate illustrations of initial /l/ zoo animals or use the toy or stuffed animals collected. Put them into berry or *laundry* baskets that are face down (to replicate a cage) on a table. Invite the children to feed the zoo animals their *lunch*. Explain what the animals can eat for *lunch* (e.g., *leaves, lemons, lettuce,* etc.). Provide the children with a choice of which animal to feed and what to feed it.

## Animal Lunch*

**Target Words:** lamb, lemon, lettuce, licorice, like, lime, lion, lizard, llama, lobster, lunch

**Materials:** picnic basket
a variety of initial /l/ foods
   (e.g., lemon, lettuce, licorice, lime)
blanket or tablecloth
initial /l/ stuffed animals, toy animals, or illustrations
   (e.g., lamb, lion, lizard, llama, lobster)

**Procedure:** Before the session, prepare a picnic basket with /l/ foods. Place a tablecloth or blanket on the floor. Invite the children to have a picnic *lunch* with their animal friends. Place the picnic basket with /l/ objects in the center of the tablecloth. Have each child choose an animal and decide what /l/ food the animal would *like* for *lunch*. Provide choices for the child by asking, "Do you want to feed the *lion* or the *lamb?*" or "Would the *lamb like* some *lettuce* or a *lemon?*" Modify your questions according to each child's linguistic level.

# Looking for Lost Animals

**Target Words:** ladybug, lamb, light, like, lion, lizard, llama, lobster, love

**Materials:** initial /l/ stuffed animals, toy animals, or illustrations
(e.g., ladybug, lamb, lion, lizard, llama, lobster)
flashlights

**Procedure:** Duplicate the initial /l/ animal illustrations or use the toy or stuffed animals collected. Hide the stuffed animals, toys, or illustrations around the room. Say that the animals are *lost* and the children need to help the zookeeper find them. Give each child a flashlight and turn the *lights* off. Have the children bring each animal to you and identify it. After all the animals are found, have the children talk about the ones they *like* and the ones they *love*.

## Funny Lunch*

**Target Words:** lamb, laundry, lawn, lemonade, lettuce, licorice, like, lily pad, lips, log, lollipops, lunch, lunch box

**Materials:** initial /l/ illustrations
(e.g., lamb, laundry, lawn, lily pad, lips, log)
initial /l/ items
(e.g., lemonade, lettuce, licorice, lollipops)
child's lunch box
cloth grab bag (See *Appendix H*.)

**Procedure:** Duplicate the initial /l/ illustrations or use real /l/ items. Seat the children in a circle on the floor. Place a child's *lunch box* in the center of the circle. Place objects or illustrations of /l/ words in a cloth grab bag to pass around the circle. Explain to the children that they will choose what they would *like* to eat for *lunch*, and then they will place those illustrations/objects in the *lunch box*. Make illustrations/objects that are both food and nonfood items. Give the children the opportunity to be silly and choose nonfood items as well as food items. Pass the bag of illustrations from child to child. Have each child take a turn picking an object or picture and deciding whether to put it in the *lunch box* or not. Model the target word after the child produces it, and then ask, "Do you want to eat (*lettuce*) for *lunch?*" Review what was put in the *lunch box* after a few children have taken a turn.

(This activity serves as a memory recall task as well as additional sound practice.)

## /l/ Store*

**Target Words:** lace, lamb, leaf, leash, lemon, light, like, lime, lion, lock

**Materials:** toy cash register or scanner
baskets
play money
/l/ items
(e.g., lace, lamb, leaf, leash, lemon, light, lime, lion, lock)

**Procedure:** Set up a department store with the /l/ items placed at various locations around the room. Have a child (storekeeper) stand at each location. Have one other child act as the cashier, and the rest as shoppers. Instruct the shoppers to request the /l/ items from the storekeeper and also to identify the items as they pay the cashier.

## Lily Pads and Logs*

**Target Words:** leader, leap, lily pad, lizard, log

**Materials:** lily pad and log illustrations
green paper
brown paper
lizard illustration

**Procedure:** Duplicate and cut out several *lily pads* (using green paper), *logs* (using brown paper), and *lizards*. Place the *lily pads* and *logs* randomly on the floor. Designate one child as the *leader*. Have the *leader* instruct the other children to *leap* to a *log* or a *lily pad*. After several turns, have the children cover their eyes. Hide a *lizard* under a *log* or a *lily pad*. Make the child who finds the *lizard* the next *leader*.

## Washing Laces or Lambs

**Target Words:**  laces, lamb, laundry, lay, line, little, (a) lot

**Materials:**  clothesline (or string) and clothespins
chairs
plastic toy lambs or lamb illustration
shoelaces
large bucket of water
soap
laundry basket

**Procedure:**  Before the session, string a clothesline between two chairs to be at a child's eye *level*. Gather *laces* (shoelaces) and toy *lambs* (or duplicate the *lamb* illustration, laminate, and cut out). Place a *large* bucket of water in front of the children. Give them a choice of whether to put a *lot* or a *little* soap in it. Have the children identify and wash *laces* (shoelaces) and plastic or laminated *lambs* one by one. Once the *laces* and *lambs* are washed, have the children choose whether to hang them on the *line* or *lay* them in a *laundry* basket.

## Lost Animal Lockup

**Target Words:** ladybug, lamb, lion, lizard, llama, lock, loose

**Materials:** initial /l/ animal illustrations
  (e.g., ladybug, lamb, lion, lizard, llama)
laundry baskets, berry baskets, or any baskets without
  large handles

**Procedure:** Duplicate /l/ animal illustrations. Show the illustrations of several of them. Have the children name the animals. Place the baskets upside down to look like cages. Set the scene by saying that the animals are *loose* and need to be *locked* up in their zoo cages. Have the children take turns choosing animals and *locking* them up in the zoo cages.

## Lucy Lamb

**Target Words:** lamb, large, little, lonely, look, Lucy

**Materials:** lamb illustration

**Procedure:** Before the session, duplicate the *lamb* illustration making several *large* copies and several *little* copies. Hide *large* and *little lambs* around the room. Tell the children that *Lucy Lamb* is very *lonely* because all her *lamb* friends ran away. Enlist the help of all the children to find the runaway *large* and *little lambs*. Have the children call *Lucy* during their search.

## Leaping Lizard

**Target Words:** laundry, lawn, leap, lily pad, lips, lizard, lobster, log

**Materials:** initial /l/ illustrations

(e.g., laundry, lawn, lily pad, lips, lobster, log)

**Procedure:** Before the session, enlarge and duplicate the /l/ illustrations. Spread the pictures out on the floor for the children to *leap* onto. Have the children take turns being the *leaping lizard*. Encourage the other children to chant *leap*, *leap*, *leap* while one child is *leaping*. Have the *lizard* identify the picture he or she will *leap* onto.

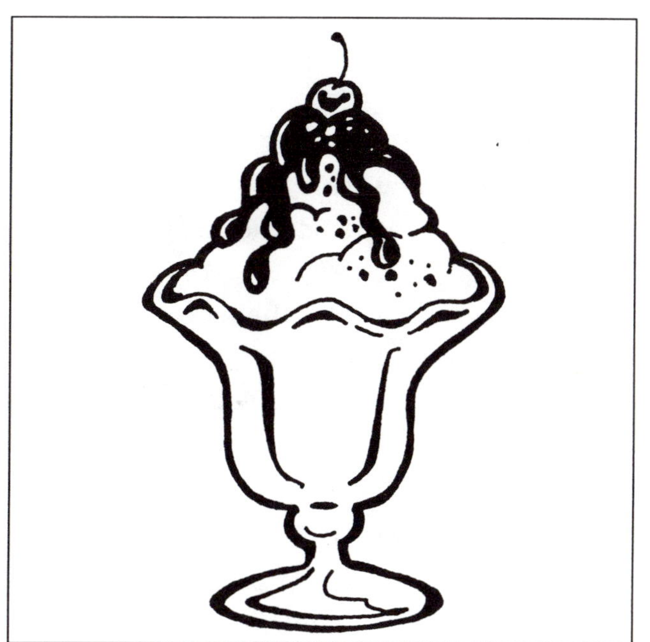

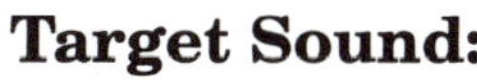

**Target Sound:**
/s/

**Linguistic Level:**
Word/Phrase/Sentence

**Position:**
Initial

## Objective:

To decrease the application of Stopping, the children will produce word-initial /s/ with varying levels of accuracy following the clinician's model or spontaneously.

## Suggestion for Nametags:

In each session, provide a choice between two nametags to elicit productions of the target sound. Suggestions for word-initial /s/ include: *sailboat, seal, seashell, soap, socks, sundae.*

Note: All activities in this section can also be used for Dentalization, Interdentalization, and Lateralization.

## Salt Paint*

**Target Words:** sailboat, salt, sandwich, sea, seal, seashell, sundae

**Materials:** salt
food coloring (several colors)
tray
salt shakers
initial /s/ illustrations
   (e.g., sailboat, sandwich, sea, seal, seashell, sundae)
large sheets of construction paper
glue

**Procedure:** Before the session, make several shakers of various colors of *salt* paint (the recipe follows). Duplicate initial /s/ illustrations and glue several of them on large sheets of construction paper. Give one sheet to each child. Have the children choose the order in which to decorate the illustrations with colored *salt*. Once they have selected a picture, have them put glue on it, then sprinkle *salt* paint on the glue. After the children have finished decorating their picture, have them tell the rest of the group about it. Have different illustrations available to add variety to the discussion.

**Recipe for Salt Paint:** (from Ranya Awwad)
Combine ½ cup salt with ¼ teaspoon of food coloring. Spread out on a tray to dry. Fill a salt shaker with the salt when it is dry.

## By the Sea

**Target Words:** sailboat, sand, sea, seaside, sun

**Materials:** sailboat illustration
yellow construction paper
heavy paper or tag board
glue or glue sticks
sand
blue cellophane or blue construction paper

**Procedure:** Duplicate and cut out the *sailboat* illustration. Cut several circles for the *sun* out of yellow construction paper, at least one per child. Have the children create a *seaside* picture on heavy paper or tag board. Instruct each child to verbally request the items to glue onto their paper. Items include: *sand* (put glue along the bottom of the paper and sprinkle real *sand* on it), the *sea* (blue cellophane or blue construction paper placed above the *sand),* a *sailboat* (placed in the *sea*), and the *sun* (placed in the sky). Elicit target words through providing choices of the items to glue on (e.g., "Do you want to glue the *sea* or the *sun?*"). Have conversations about the illustrations.

# Cereal, Seeds, and Cider*

**Target Words:** cereal, cider, seeds, sip, so

**Materials:** cereal
sunflower seeds
bowls
apple cider
small cups

**Procedure:** Before the session, put *cereal* and sunflower *seeds* in small bowls. Gather apple *cider* and cups. Seat the children around a table. Have each child take a turn being the server. Have the other children ask for either *cereal* or *seeds*. Serve small portions so there are many opportunities for the children to produce the target words. Serve small amounts of *cider* so the children will ask for more. Model "This *cereal* is *so* good!" or "I'm taking a *sip* of *cider*" as the children are eating and drinking.

## Sock Search

**Target Words:** sailboat, sea, seal, search, searchlight, seashell, soap, socks

**Materials:** initial /s/ illustrations
(e.g., sailboat, sea, seal, seashell, soap)
socks
flashlights

**Procedure:** Before the session, duplicate initial /s/ illustrations and put them into *socks*. Hide *socks* around the room before the children come in. Have the children *search* around the room for the *socks* with *searchlights* (flashlights). After the children find all the *socks,* have them return to the circle and name the /s/ illustrations they find in their *socks*.

## Silly Soup*

**Target Words:** salt, sand, silly, sip, soap, socks, soup

**Materials:** initial /s/ items
(e.g., salt, sand, soap, socks)
serving tray
large pot
large spoon

**Procedure:** Make a *silly soup* out of common objects that begin with /s/. Introduce each item by saying its name slowly and clearly. Then place the item on a tray. Have the children take turns selecting and naming an item, then have them put it into the *soup* using a large *soup* pot and large spoon to stir. Let the children pretend to *sip* the *soup*.

## Sending Postcards

**Target Words:** sack, saddle, sailboat, Sally, sandwich, seal, send, Sid, soap, sundae

**Materials:** initial /s/ illustrations
(e.g., saddle, sailboat, sandwich, seal, soap, sundae)
tape
envelopes
illustrations of a boy and a girl (See pages 323–326.)
two toy mailboxes
(or shoeboxes with a mail slot cut on top)
cloth grab bag (See *Appendix H.*)

**Procedure:** Duplicate initial /s/ illustrations and tape them onto envelopes. Also duplicate an illustration of a boy (*Sid*) and a girl (*Sally*). Place two toy mailboxes near the children. Tape the drawing of *Sid* on one mailbox, and the drawing of *Sally* on the other. Have the children pick an envelope from a mail *sack* (a cloth grab bag) and identify the picture taped to it. Then instruct them to decide whether to *send* (mail) it to *Sally* or to *Sid*. Allow them to place the envelope in the appropriate mailbox.

## Searching the Sea

**Target Words:** saddle, sailboat, sea, seal, search, seashell, sign, soap

**Materials:** initial /s/ illustrations
(e.g., saddle, sailboat, seal, seashell, sign, soap)
sailor hats (paper)

**Procedure:** Duplicate and hide initial /s/ illustrations around the room before the session. Tell the children that they are *sailors* and need to find some things that are lost at *sea*. Instruct the children to put on *sailor* hats and *search* for things in the *sea* (room).

# Silly Salad*

**Target Words:** saddle, sailboat, salad, sandwich, seashell, sign, silly

**Materials:** initial /s/ illustrations
  (e.g., saddle, sailboat, sandwich, seashell, sign)
large salad bowl
salad tongs

**Procedure:** Before the session, duplicate initial /s/ illustrations. Seat the children in a *circle* with a large *salad* bowl in the *center*. Explain that they will make *silly salad*. Have the children choose illustrations to toss into the *salad* using *salad* tongs. As a picture is selected, provide an obvious foil (e.g., "James picked a coat," to which the children respond, "No, *soap!*"). After a few items are tossed, have the children recall what is in the *silly salad*.

(The modified sensory-motor approach can also be used in this activity by combining the word *toss* with initial /s/ target words as in *toss-soap, toss-sign,* etc.)

## Wash with Soap

**Target Words:** circle, sailboat, soapy, socks, sun

**Materials:** chalk and chalkboard
bucket of soapy water
sponges

**Procedure:** Draw several *socks, sailboats, suns,* and *circles* on the chalkboard and prepare a bucket of *soapy* water. Have the children work in pairs. Have one child ask the other, "Do you want to wash a *circle* or a *sun?*" Have the other child make the choice, then dip his or her sponge in the *soapy* water and wash the selected picture. Incorporate foils in this activity. For example, say, "You're doing a great job washing those pajamas." Expect the child to respond with, "No, *socks!*" If the child does not notice the error, call attention to it by saying, e.g., "Did I say pajamas? I meant *socks.*"

## Sam Says*

**Target Words:** circle, Sam, saw, sip, sit, soup

**Materials:** none

**Procedure:** Select one child to be the leader. Give the child a choice between two actions (e.g., *sit* or *saw)* to have the other children perform. Have the child say, *"Sam says (sit)."* Give each child a turn being *Sam.* Choices for actions are *saw* (pretend to cut wood), *sit* (*sit* down on the floor), *circle* (make a *circle* in the air with one hand), and *sip soup* (pretend to *sip* from a cup). Modify as needed according to the children's linguistic abilities.

## /s/ Memory

**Target Words:** tail/sail, tea/sea, toe/sew

**Materials:** minimal pairs illustrations (See pages 316–322.)
(e.g., tail/sail, tea/sea, toe/sew)
glue or glue stick
index cards

**Procedure:** Before the session, duplicate the minimal pairs illustrations, making at least two copies of each picture. Glue
these to index cards to form sets of cards. Instruct the
children to form groups of two to play this memory
game. Give each group a set of cards containing two
cards for each of two minimal pairs of words (e.g.,
*tea/sea, toe/sew*). Place the eight cards face down on the
table. Have one child turn a card over, name it, then
turn another card over to try to find the match. Instruct
the children to name the cards whether they match or
not. If a child finds a match, allow that child to take
another turn. If the cards do not match, direct the other
child to take a turn. After each child's production,
provide a correct model. If the child produces the word
incorrectly, ask for clarification. For example, if the
child turns over *sail* but calls it *tail,* say, "Did I hear you
say *sail* or *tail?*" In this way, the child begins to
recognize the contrast.

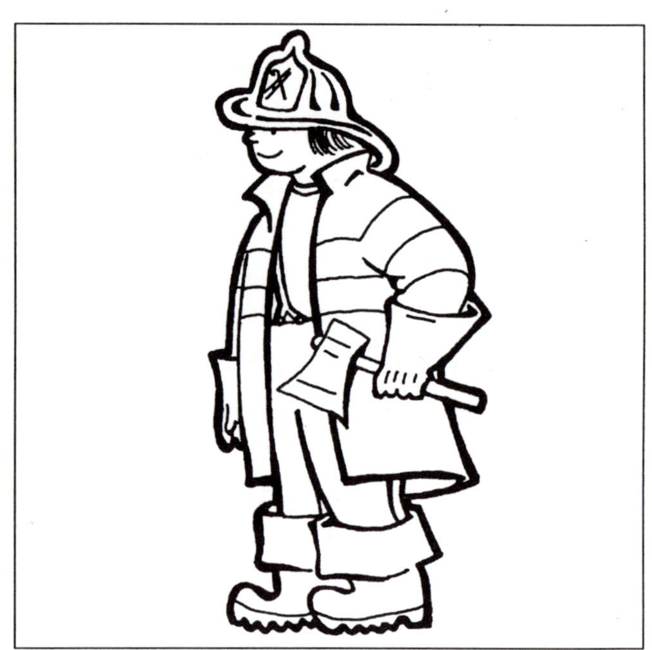

**Target Sound:**
/f/

**Linguistic Level:**
Word/Phrase/Sentence

**Position:**
Initial

**Objective:**
To decrease the application of Stopping, the children will produce word-initial /f/ with varying levels of accuracy following the clinician's model or spontaneously.

**Suggestions for Nametags:**
In each session, provide a choice between two nametags to elicit productions of the target sound. Suggestions for word-initial /f/ include: *firefighter, fish, foot, football, fork.*

## Farm on Fire!

**Target Words:** farm, farmer, father, fenced, fire, firefighter, fire truck, five, Phil

**Materials:** initial /f/ illustrations
(e.g., fence, fire, firefighter, fire truck)
*Farm on Fire!* story

**Procedure:** Duplicate illustrations depicting target words. Read the story *Farm on Fire!,* bombarding the children with initial /f/ words. Present the pictures that illustrate parts of the story. Emphasize target words and ask questions about the story to elicit target productions.

**Story:** *Farm on Fire!*

Once upon a time there was a *farmer* named *Phil. Phil* had *five* animals on his *farm*. He kept them in a *fenced* yard. One day *Phil found* a *fire* on his *farm*. He quickly took all the *farm* animals out of the *fenced* yard. Then he called his *father* who was a *firefighter*. *Phil's father* came right away with his *fire truck*. *Phil's father* put out the *fire*. The *five* animals came back to the *farm*.

## Fish or Fudge*

**Target Words:** fish, fudge

**Materials:** goldfish crackers
small pieces of fudge
napkins
serving tray
small plates

**Procedure:** Before the session, purchase goldfish crackers and *fudge*. Give the children a choice of eating *fish* crackers or small pieces of *fudge*. Have the children take turns serving the snack and offering each other a choice between *fish* or *fudge*.

## Musical Feet*

**Target Words:** fence, fish, football, footprint, fork, found

**Materials:** brown construction paper
initial /f/ illustrations (e.g., fence, fish, football, fork)
tape
cassette tape player
musical cassette tape

**Procedure:** Trace *footprints* on brown construction paper, cut them out, and tape an initial /f/ picture to the bottom of each. Place the *footprints* on the floor to form a winding path around the room. Tell the children to *follow* the *footprints* as the music is played. Stop the music intermittently. When the music stops, have the children turn over the *footprint* they are closest to and tell the rest of the group which picture they have *found*.

# Feeding Funny Philip

**Target Words:**  fan, feed, fire truck, fish, football, footprints, funny, Philip

**Materials:**  initial /f/ illustrations
(e.g., fan, fire truck, fish, football, footprints)
illustration of a boy's face (See page 327.)
tape
tag board
small paper bag

**Procedure:**  Duplicate initial /f/ illustrations. Enlarge and duplicate the illustration of the boy's *face* (*Philip*). Tape it to tag board and then cut the mouth out. Attach a small paper bag to the back of the poster, below the mouth, to catch the *food* illustrations. Give the children an opportunity to take turns *feeding funny Philip* by placing silly *food* illustrations (e.g., *football, fire truck,* etc.) in his mouth. Have one child choose a *food* picture for another child, by requesting, for example, *"Feed Philip a football."* Model correct productions and provide some obvious foils (e.g., "Philip ate a bird!", to which the children respond, "No, *fish!*").

## Is It Fuzzy?*

**Target Words:** feel, find, fuzzy

**Materials:** fuzzy objects
(e.g., slippers, stuffed animals)
nonfuzzy objects
(e.g., cup, rock)
feely box (See *Appendix H.*)

**Procedure:** Collect objects that are *fuzzy* and objects that are not *fuzzy*. Have the children collect objects from around the room or request them to bring items from home. Place all objects in a *feely* box. Have the children take turns *feeling* an object in the box (without looking) and then telling if it *feels fuzzy* or not *fuzzy*. Before the child reaches into the box, ask if he or she wants to *find* something *fuzzy* or not *fuzzy*. Let the rest of the children assist in making the choice (e.g., *"Find* something that is *fuzzy"*). Children can ask each other, "How does it *feel?"*

## Go Fish*

**Target Words:** fairy, fan, fence, fire, fish, football, footprints, fork

**Materials:** initial /f/ illustrations

(e.g., fairy, fan, fence, fire, fish, football, footprints, fork)

heavy stock paper

**Procedure:** Create several decks of cards for this activity (one deck per pair of children). Duplicate initial /f/ illustrations onto heavy stock paper. Make two copies of each illustration for each deck. Cut illustrations apart forming cards. For each group of two children, deal each child *four* cards. Have each child in the group hold the cards so the other player can't see them. Place additional cards in a pile on the table. Have one child ask the other for a card (e.g., "Do you have *fence?*"). If the other child has the card, guide him or her to respond with "Yes, I have *fence,*" and then give the card to the child who asked. If the other child doesn't have the card requested, then instruct him or her to respond with "No *fence.* GO *FISH!*" and take a card from the pile on the table. Continue the activity until all the children have matching pairs. Modify responses to single words if necessary.

(This activity works best if another adult is available to assist.)

# Firefighter Bingo*

**Target Words:** fairy, fence, fire, firefighter, fire truck, football, footprints

**Materials:** bingo boards (See *Appendix H.*)
initial /f/ illustrations
 (e.g., fairy, fence, fire, fire truck, football, footprints)
cloth grab bag (See *Appendix H.*)
firefighter illustration

**Procedure:** Before the session, prepare bingo boards with four to six initial /f/ illustrations on them. Make an identical set of illustrations to use as calling cards and place them in the cloth bag. Also duplicate four to six *firefighter* illustrations per child to use as bingo markers. Give each child a bingo board. Have the children take turns being the "caller" by drawing an /f/ calling card from the bag and naming it for the others. If the picture named is on a child's board, instruct him or her to cover it with a picture of a *firefighter*. Continue the game until all children have covered all of their illustrations.

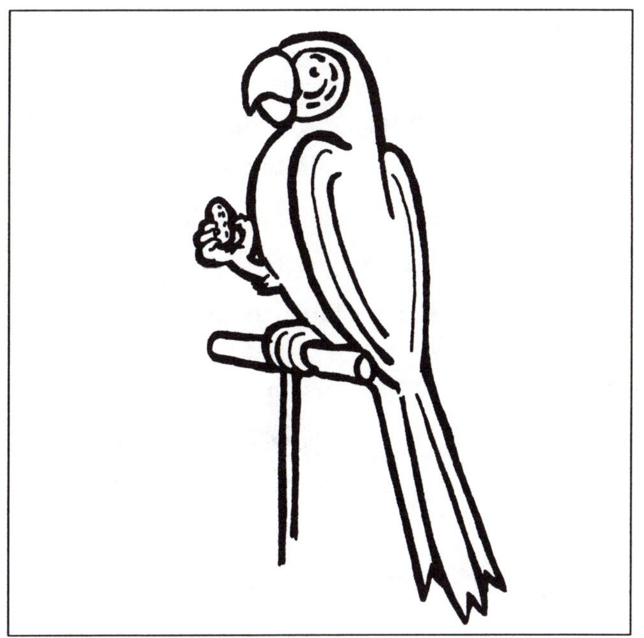

**Target Sound:**
/p/

**Linguistic Level:**
Word/Phrase/Sentence

**Position:**
Initial

**Objective:**
To decrease the application of Initial Voicing, the children will produce word-initial /p/ with varying levels of accuracy following the clinician's model or spontaneously.

**Suggestions for Nametags:**
In each session, provide a choice between two nametags to elicit productions of the target sound. Suggestions for word-initial /p/ include: *panda, parrot, pear, penguin, pickle, pig.*

## Picnic in the Park

**Target Words:** Pam, panda, park, parrot, Patty, pen, penguin, Penny, Peter, picnic, pig, pool

**Materials:** initial /p/ illustrations (e.g., panda, parrot, penguin, pig)
*Picnic in the Park* story

**Procedure:** Duplicate several /p/ illustrations depicting target words in the story. Read the story *Picnic in the Park* to the children, bombarding them with initial /p/ words. Show the illustrations to the children as the story is read. Afterwards, discuss the story, eliciting target words.

**Story:** *Picnic in the Park*

Many animals lived in a *pen*. The animals were *Peter* the *Pig*, *Penny* the *Parrot*, *Patty* the *Penguin*, and *Pam* the *Panda*. One day they wanted to go on a *picnic*. They couldn't decide where to go. *Peter* the *Pig* said, "Let's have a *picnic* at the *park!*" *Penny* the *Parrot* said, "Let's have a *picnic* at the *pool!*" *Pam* the *Panda* said, "I want to go to the *park.*" *Patty* the *Penguin* said, "No, I want to go to the *pool!*" Finally, *Penny* the *Parrot* had a good idea. *Penny* said, "Let's go to the *park* for our *picnic*. THEN let's go to the *pool.*" That's what they did, and they had a wonderful time at their *picnic* AND at the *pool!*

# A Picnic Lunch*

**Target Words:**   pancakes, pear, pickle, picnic, pie, pizza, popcorn

**Materials:**   initial /p/ food illustrations
    (e.g., pancakes, pear, pickle, pie, pizza, popcorn)
newspapers or magazines (optional)
tablecloth
picnic basket
glue or glue sticks
paper plates

**Procedure:**   Duplicate several copies of initial /p/ food illustrations or cut photographs from newspapers or magazines. Prepare to have a *picnic.* Spread out a tablecloth on the floor. Place a *picnic* basket in the center of the tablecloth. Put *pictures* of foods whose names begin with /p/ inside the *picnic* basket. In turn, allow the children to select a *picture* from the basket and identify what they will eat. Before each child selects a *picture,* provide a choice of what they might *pick* from the basket (e.g., "Do you want a *pickle* or *pizza?*"). After all the initial /p/ *pictures* are selected, have the children glue their *pictures* onto their *paper* plates.

## Popcorn and Pickles*

**Target Words:** pickle, pig, popcorn

**Materials:** pickle and pig illustrations
popcorn (illustration or real)
glue or glue sticks

**Procedure:** Enlarge and duplicate the *pig* illustration, preparing one per child. Also duplicate several illustrations of the *pickle* and cut them out. *Pop* the *popcorn* in advance of this activity (or duplicate several *popcorn* illustrations). Give each child a *picture* of the large *pig*. Model choices for the children (e.g., "Do you want *popcorn* or a *pickle?*"). After modeling, have the children take turns asking each other if they want *popcorn* or a *pickle* to glue onto the *pig*. Give each child several opportunities to produce the target words until the *pig* is covered with *popcorn* and *pickles*.

## Play-doh Creations*

**Target Words:** pancake, pea, pickle, pie, pizza, potato

**Materials:** Play-doh

**Procedure:** Have the children make a variety of initial /p/ foods (e.g., *pancakes, peas, pickles, pie, pizza, potatoes)* out of Play-doh. Model target words and engage the children in conversation to elicit productions.

## Pig or Panda Puzzle

**Target Words:** panda, piece, pig, puzzle

**Materials:** pig and panda illustrations
glue or glue sticks
construction paper

**Procedure:** Enlarge and duplicate the illustration of the *pig* and the *panda*. Make two copies of each per child. Glue one of each onto construction paper and cut to form *puzzle pieces*. Trace the *puzzle pieces* onto one of the remaining illustrations of a *pig* or a *panda* to form the *piece* outlines. Show the children large illustrations of a *pig* and a *panda* with outlines of *puzzle pieces* on them. Have each child complete both a *pig* and a *panda puzzle*. Give the children choices by asking, "Which *puzzle piece* do you want—one for the *pig* or one for the *panda?*" After responding with a target word, have the child glue the *piece* on the appropriate *puzzle*.

## Pink and Purple Paint

**Target Words:** paint, parrot, pear, pie, pig, pink, pizza, pond, purple

**Materials:** initial /p/ illustrations
  (e.g., paint, parrot, pear, pie, pig, pizza, pond)
large sheets of construction paper
glue or glue sticks
pink and purple paint
paintbrushes

**Procedure:** Duplicate /p/ illustrations. Give each child a large *piece* of *paper*. Have each child choose which *picture* to glue onto their *paper*. Then have them choose to *paint* each *picture* *pink* or *purple*. In turn, the children can offer each other choices of illustrations to glue onto their *papers*.

## Peeling Peanuts

**Target Words:** pan, peanuts, pot

**Materials:** peanuts in a shell
cooking pot
baking pan

**Procedure:** Seat the children around a table. Pass out *peanuts* to be *peeled* (shelled) by the children. Direct the children to *peel* the *peanuts* and *put* the shells in either the *pot* or the *pan*. After the sorting task is completed, have everyone eat the *peanuts*. *Peas* in the shell can be used in place of or in addition to the *peanuts*.

## Pop, Pop, Pop!

**Target Word:** pop, popcorn

**Materials:** popcorn
hot air popper
large bowl
napkins

**Procedure:** Make *popcorn* in a hot air *popper*. Have the children shout *pop, pop, pop!* as the *popcorn* is *popping*. Then allow the children to eat the *popcorn*. Have the children talk about the *popping* sound and the delicious *popcorn*.

## Peaches or Pears*

**Target Words:** peach, pear

**Materials:** fresh or canned peaches and pears (sliced)
small plates or bowls
napkins
spoons (or forks)

**Procedure:** Offer the children a choice of sliced *peaches* or *pears* for a snack. Give each child an opportunity to be the server. Have the server ask the others if they would like a *peach* or a *pear*.

## Peanuts and Popcorn Here!*

**Target Words:** peanut, pink, popcorn

**Materials:** peanuts in a bowl
popcorn in a bowl
serving tray
pitcher of pink lemonade
small cups
napkins

**Procedure:** Provide the children with the choice of eating *peanuts* or *popcorn* for a snack. Put the food items on a tray and have the children take turns asking each other if they want *peanuts* or *popcorn*. Serve *pink* lemonade as part of the snack.

# Feed the Penguin or the Pig

**Target Words:** pancakes, pear, penguin, pickles, pie, pig, pizza, popcorn

**Materials:** penguin and pig illustrations
initial /p/ food illustrations (or empty food containers)
  (e.g., pancakes, pear, pickle, pie, pizza, popcorn)
basket
tape

**Procedure:** Enlarge and duplicate the illustrations of the *penguin* and *pig* and mount them onto the chalkboard or wall. Also duplicate initial /p/ food pictures or use real food. Explain to the children that the *penguin* and the *pig* are hungry and would like to be fed. Show the children a basket of initial /p/ food. Provide models of each target item, then have the children verbally select what to feed the animals. Allow them to pretend to feed the animals. If the items are illustrations, tape them to the animals.

## Spin for Circles

**Target Words:**  pea/bee, pear/bear, pen/Ben, pie/bye

**Materials:**  minimal pairs illustrations (See pages 316–322.)
   (e.g., pea/bee, pear/bear, pen/Ben, pie/bye)
construction paper
spinner board (See *Appendix H.*)

**Procedure:**  Duplicate the minimal pairs illustrations, making two copies of each. Cut large circles out of construction paper and attach a picture illustrating one member of a minimal pair (e.g., *pea* or *bee)* to each. Place these on the floor near each other. Mount identical illustrations on the spinner board. Have the children take turns spinning and instructing the others to "put your hand on *pea*" or "put your foot on *bee*," until both hands and feet are placed on illustrations. Pass the spinner to another child.

(This activity can be played on a "Twister" board game if available.)

## Bunny Hop

**Target Words:** paint, pants, parrot, pie, pig, pond

**Materials:** initial /p/ illustrations
  (e.g., paint, pants, parrot, pie, pig, pond)
construction paper
carrot
toy bunny (optional)

**Procedure:** Prepare for this activity by duplicating /p/ illustrations and cutting a bunny ear headband out of construction paper. Place initial /p/ illustrations face-up on the floor. In turn, instruct one child to act as the bunny (by wearing the bunny ears headband and holding a carrot) and hop from *picture* to *picture*. Have the others say *hop-pie, hop-pig*, etc. as the bunny hops. Ask the bunny what *picture* he or she is going to hop to.

This activity can also be done by placing initial /p/ illustrations face-up on the table. Have the children make a toy bunny hop from *picture* to *picture* while saying *hop-pie, hop-pig*, etc. The second word is the *picture* that the bunny hops to.

In this modified sensory-motor technique, word pairs (e.g., *hop-pie)* are produced to sound like one word, without pausing between them. This technique is appropriate only if /p/ is correctly produced in word-final position.

## Pin the Pants on Peter or Pam

**Target Words:** Pam, pants, Peter, pin

**Materials:** illustrations of a boy and a girl (See pages 323–326.)
pants illustration
blindfold
tape

**Procedure:** Enlarge and duplicate the illustrations of a boy (*Peter*) and a girl (*Pam*). Also duplicate and cut out the illustration of a *pair* of *pants*. Mount the picture of *Peter* and *Pam* on the board or wall. Give each child an opportunity to *pin pants* on either *Peter* or *Pam*. Put a blindfold on the child and provide a *picture* of *pants* with tape on the back. Spin the child around slowly and have him or her attempt to place the *pants* as close to where they belong as possible. Give the children the opportunity to make choices for each other.

# Pink and Purple Postcards

**Target Words:** parrot, penguin, pink, postcard, purple

**Materials:** two toy mailboxes (or shoeboxes)
penguin and parrot illustrations
glue or glue stick
index cards
pink and purple markers (or crayons)

**Procedure:** Obtain two toy mailboxes or create them by cutting slots in the tops of shoeboxes. Duplicate the *penguin* and *parrot* illustrations. Glue the *picture* of the *parrot* on one mailbox and the *picture* of the *penguin* on the other. Invite the children to decorate *postcards* (index cards) with *pink* or *purple* markers (or crayons) which will be mailed to the *parrot* or the *penguin*. Offer a choice of markers as well as a choice of who to mail the *postcards* to. If the children know the *pink* and *purple* color names, provide foils when offering them the markers (e.g., "Here's the green marker," to which the children respond, "No *pink!*").

## Shopping for /p/*

**Target Words:** pancakes, pear, pickle, pie, pizza, popcorn

**Materials:** initial /p/ illustrations of grocery items
(e.g., pancakes, pear, pickle, pie, pizza, popcorn)
empty containers of initial /p/ grocery items
(e.g., pancakes, pears, pickles, pie, pizza, popcorn)
bags or grocery baskets

**Procedure:** In advance of this activity, duplicate initial /p/ food illustrations. Then set up a grocery store by placing /p/ food items around the room. Divide the children into two groups—store clerks and shoppers. Have the shoppers pick two *pictures* depicting the foods they want to buy. Have the children shop for their designated items. Place the items just out of reach of the shoppers, so they must request them from the store clerks (e.g., "*Popcorn please!*", "Can I have a *pear?*"). Have the store clerks give the shoppers choices, for example, "Do you want *pizza* or *pie?*" After a few turns, have the store clerks and shoppers change roles. Modify requests based on the linguistic abilities of the children.

## No Peeking!*

**Target Words:**  paintbrush, pencil, penny, pillow, pinecone

**Materials:**  feely box (See *Appendix H.*)
initial /p/ objects
(e.g., paintbrush, pencil, penny, pillow, pinecone)

**Procedure:**  Provide the children with a feely box filled with objects beginning with /p/. Allow the children to reach into the box with their eyes closed (no *peeking!*), feel an object, and guess what it is. Before the children reach into the box, identify all the objects so the children know what choices are available. Also provide models and choices of the target words such as, "Do you want to feel a *penny* or a *pinecone?*" before each child reaches into the box.

## /p/ Memory*

**Target Words:** bear/pear, bee/pea, bunch/punch, bye/pie

**Materials:** minimal pairs illustrations (See pages 316–322.)
(e.g., bear/pear, bee/pea, bunch/punch, bye/pie)
glue or glue sticks
index cards

**Procedure:** Before the session, duplicate the minimal pairs illustrations, making at least two copies of each picture. Glue these to index cards to form sets of cards. Instruct the children to form groups of two to play this memory game. Give each group a set of cards containing two cards for each word of two minimal pairs (e.g., *bee/pea, bunch/punch*). Place the eight cards face down on the table. Have one child turn a card over, name it, then turn another card over to try to find the match. Instruct the child to name the cards whether they match or not. If a match is found, allow that child to take another turn. If the cards do not match, direct the other child to take a turn. After each child's production, provide a correct model. If the child produces the word incorrectly, ask for clarification. For example, if the child turns over *pear* but calls it *bear*, say, "Did you mean *pear* or *bear?*" In this way, the child becomes aware of the contrast.

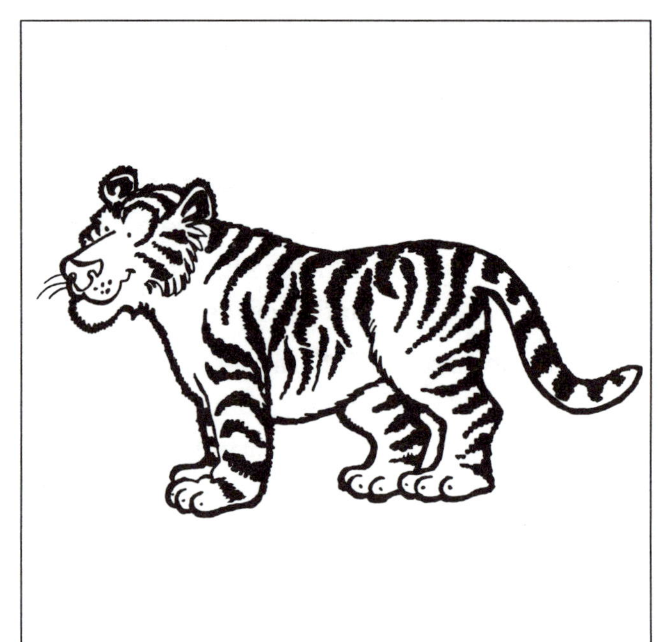

**Target Sound:**
/t/

**Linguistic Level:**
Word/Phrase/Sentence

**Position:**
Initial

**Objective:**
To decrease the application of Initial Voicing, the children will produce word-initial /t/ with varying levels of accuracy following the clinician's model or spontaneously.

**Suggestions for Nametags:**
In each session, provide a choice between two nametags to elicit productions of the target sound. Suggestions for word-initial /t/ include: *teddy bear, telephone, tiger, turkey, turtle.*

# Tony Lost His Tail

**Target Words**:  tail, take, teddy bear, tiger, toad, Tony, turkey, turtle

**Materials**:  initial /t/ animal illustrations
(e.g., teddy bear, tiger, toad, turkey, turtle)
popsicle sticks
tape
*Tony Lost His Tail* story

**Procedure**:  Before the session, duplicate and cut out the illustrations of the *teddy bear, tiger, toad, turkey,* and *turtle,* so that there will be at least one character per child. Cut off the tiger's *tail* and *tape* it to the feathers of the *turkey.* Mount the illustrations on popsicle sticks. Keep the *tiger* yourself, and have each child select one of the other characters. Read the story *Tony Lost His Tail.* As each character is mentioned, instruct the child who has that picture to hold it up and say, "No, I did not take your *tail!* or just "No *tail!*"

**Story**:  *Tony Lost His Tail* (by Caren Leamon)

*Tony* the *Tiger* was sad because he lost his *tail.* (Hold up the tiger without the tail.) *Tony* decided to ask his friends for help. First he asked the *toad,* "*Toad,* did you take my *tail?*" The *toad* answered, "No, I did not *take* your *tail.*" (Have the child who has the *toad* character hold it up and say, "No, I did not take your *tail!*" or simply "No *tail!*") Next *Tony* asked his friend the *teddy bear,* "Did you *take* my *tail?*" The *teddy bear* replied, "No, I did not take your *tail.*" (Instruct the child who has the *teddy bear* character to hold it up and repeat the sentence or just say, "No *tail!*")

*(continued)*

*Tony Lost His Tail—Continued*

Very soon, *Tony* the *Tiger* saw a *turtle*. He asked, *"Turtle,* did you take my *tail?"* The *turtle* answered, "No, I did not *take* your *tail!"* (or "No *tail!"*). (Direct the child holding the *turtle* character to respond.) Finally, *Tony* saw his friend the *turkey*. *Tony* asked, "Did you *take* my *tail?"* The *turkey* answered, "No, I did not *take* your *tail!"* (or "No *tail!"*). (Have the child holding the *turkey* character respond.)

Just then, *Tony* saw his *tail tucked* in the *turkey's* feathers. *Tony* said, "This *time* you really *teased* me! You *took* my *tail!"* So, *Tony took* back his *tail*. He was very happy to have his beautiful *tail!*

## Tea Party

**Target Words:** table, tart, tea, teacups, teapot, tin

**Materials:** table

teapot (or pitcher)

small teacups

iced tea

cookie tin

poptarts

**Procedure:** Arrange the *table* for a *tea* party. Use a *teapot* and *teacups*. Fill the *teapot* with weak iced *tea*. Fill a cookie *tin* with small pieces of *tarts* (poptarts). Have the children *take turns* asking each other if they would like *tea* or a *tart*.

## Taste Test

**Target Words:** taffy, Tang, tart, taste, tea, tent, toast, tongue, tuna

**Materials:** initial /t/ food items

(e.g., taffy, Tang, poptart, tea, toast, tuna fish)

table

napkins

small cups

plates

tent (optional)

**Procedure:** Gather initial /t/ foods and arrange them on a *table*. Have the children identify the foods and *taste* them. Provide choices of what to *taste* next, such as "*Toast* or *tuna?*" Talk about *tasting* with your *tongue*. Have children ask each other what they want to *taste*. The *taste test* could also be done in a *tent* if available.

## Tossed Salad*

**Target Words:** tape, teddy bear, tie, toothbrush, toss, towel, toy, T-shirt

**Materials:** initial /t/ items
(e.g., tape, teddy bear, tie, toothbrush, towel, toy, T-shirt)
large bowl
salad tongs
table
cookie tin

**Procedure:** Gather initial /t/ items, a large bowl and salad *tongs*. Place some items on a *table* and some in a *tin* (cookie tin). Explain to the children that they will pretend to make a *tossed* salad with the items. Have each child select an item from the *table* or *tin* and place it in the salad bowl. Use *tongs* to *toss* the items *together*. As each item is placed in the bowl, say *toss, toss, toss*. Provide choices of initial /t/ objects to put in the bowl such as a *T-shirt* or *tape*.

## /t/ Store*

**Target Words:** tape, tea, ten, tissue, tool, towel, toy, T-shirt, two

**Materials:** initial /t/ items
(e.g., tape, tea, tissue, tools, T-shirts, towels, toys)
stickers for price tags
toy cash register
pretend money
small shopping baskets

**Procedure:** Arrange the room to look like a store with initial /t/ items in various places. Price each item to be *two* or *ten* cents. Assign each child a role to play (such as shopper, cashier, or storekeeper). Recreate a shopping trip by acting out each role. Place the items for purchase just beyond reach of the shoppers, so they must ask the storekeeper for the items they wish to purchase. Have the storekeeper provide the shoppers with a choice of items to purchase and have the cashier name the items as the shoppers go through the checkout. Give each child an opportunity to play each role.

## Tennis Toss

**Target Words:** teddy bear, tennis ball, tiger, toss, turtle

**Materials:** teddy bear, tiger, and turtle illustrations
tape
large grocery bags or laundry baskets
tennis ball

**Procedure:** Duplicate and enlarge the *teddy bear, tiger,* and *turtle* illustrations. *Tape* one of each to the front of a large grocery bag or laundry basket. Have the children stand a designated distance from the pictures and verbally choose which one to *toss* a *tennis ball* to. As one child is *tossing,* encourage the other children to shout *toss, toss, toss!*

## Minimal Pairs Musical /t/ Chairs*

**Target Words:** ten/den, tie/die, time/dime, toe/dough

**Materials:** minimal pairs illustrations (See pages 316–322.)
(e.g., ten/den, tie/die, time/dime, toe/dough)
glue or glue stick
index cards
chairs
cassette player
musical cassette tape

**Procedure:** Before the session, duplicate the minimal pairs illustrations and glue them onto index cards. Arrange one chair per child in a circle, with the backs of the chairs toward the inside of the circle. Place the two cards of each of the minimal pairs (e.g., *tie/die*) face down on each chair. (Use only two or three pairs per game.) Play music as the children walk around the chairs. Stop the music intermittently. When the music stops, have each child sit on a chair and name the pair of pictures on it. Provide a correct model immediately after the child's production. Place emphasis on the initial sounds of the words to highlight the minimal pairs contrast. Continue to play the game without removing chairs so that each child participates in each round.

## The Teacher Says*

**Target Words:** talk, tea, teacher, telephone, tickle, tiptoe, tummy, turn

**Materials:** none

**Procedure:** Introduce a modified version of "Simon Says," calling the game "The *Teacher* Says." Demonstrate each action that the *teacher* can do: *tiptoe* (stand on your *toes*), *talk* on the *telephone* (hold a pretend *telephone* to your ear), *tickle* your *tummy* (*tickle* your abdomen), or pour *tea* (pouring action with pretend *teapot* and cup). Have the children produce the target words as they take *turns* being the *teacher*. As each child is selected, say "( _____'s) *turn!*" Have the children chorally repeat the target words as they perform the action (e.g., *tickle, tickle, tickle*).

Bankson, N.W., and Bernthal, J.E. (1990). *Bankson-Bernthal test of phonology.* Chicago, IL: Riverside Press.

Camarata, S. (1993). The application of naturalistic conversation training to speech production in children with speech disabilities. *Journal of Applied Behavior Analysis, 26,* 173–182.

Chabon, S., and Prelock, P. (1991). *Meta magic: A metalinguistic approach to the training of closed syllables.* Tucson, AZ: Communication Skill Builders.

Compton, A.J. (1970). Generative studies of children's phonological disorders. *Journal of Speech and Hearing Disorders, 35,* 315–339.

Compton, A.J. (1975). Generative studies of children's phonological disorders: A strategy of therapy. In S. Singh (Ed.), *Measurements in hearing, speech, and language* (pp. 55–90). Baltimore, MD: University Park Press.

Compton, A.J. (1976). Generative studies of children's phonological disorders: Clinical ramifications. In D.M. Morehead and A.E. Morehead (Eds.), *Normal and deficient child language: Selected readings* (pp. 61–96). Baltimore, MD: University Park Press.

Compton, A.J., and Hutton, J.S. (1978). *Compton-Hutton phonological assessment.* San Francisco, CA: Carousel House.

Comras, R. (1974). Tartamudez o espasmofemia funcional. Relato y aportes conceptuales. *Revista Cubana de Pediatria, 46,* 595–605.

Conture, E.G. (1990). *Stuttering* (2nd ed.). Englewood Cliffs, NJ: Prentice-Hall.

Conture, E.G., Louko, L.J., and Edwards, M.L. (1993). Simultaneously treating stuttering and disordered phonology in children: Experimental treatment, preliminary findings. *American Journal of Speech-Language Pathology, 2,* 72–81.

Edwards, M.L. (1979). *Patterns and processes in fricative acquisition: Longitudinal evidence from six English-learning children.* Unpublished doctoral dissertation, Stanford University, Stanford, CA.

Edwards, M.L. (1992). In support of phonological processes. *Language, Speech, and Hearing Services in Schools, 23,* 233–240.

Edwards, M.L. (in press). Phonological process analysis. In K. Pollock (Ed.), *Children's phonology disorders.* Rockville Pike, MD: American Speech-Language-Hearing Association.

Edwards, M.L., and Bernhardt, B.H. (1973). *Phonological analyses of the speech of four children with language disorders.* Unpublished manuscripts, Stanford University, Institute for Childhood Aphasia, Stanford, CA.

Edwards, M.L., and Kelman-Maziuk, M. (1993, November). *Enhancing phonological remediation with preschool-aged children: Parental involvement.* Paper presented at the Annual Convention of the American Speech-Language-Hearing Association, Anaheim, CA.

Edwards, M.L., Kelman-Maziuk, M., and Louko, L. (1991, November). *Preschool phonology groups: Maximizing remediation efficiency.* Paper presented at the annual convention of the American Speech-Language-Hearing Association, Atlanta, GA.

Edwards, M.L., and Shriberg, L.D. (1983). *Phonology: Applications in communicative disorders.* San Diego, CA: College-Hill Press.

Eiserman, W., Weber, C., and McCoun, M. (1992). Two alternative program models for serving speech-disordered preschoolers: A second year follow-up. *Journal of Communication Disorders, 25,* 77–106.

Elbert, M., Rockman, B., and Saltzman, D. (1980). *Contrasts: The use of minimal pairs in articulation training.* Austin, TX: Exceptional Resources.

Gierut, J. (1989). Maximal opposition approach to phonological treatment. *Journal of Speech and Hearing Disorders, 54,* 9–19.

Gierut, J. (1990). Differential learning of phonological oppositions. *Journal of Speech and Hearing Research, 33,* 540–549.

Goldman, R., and Fristoe, M. (1986). *Goldman-Fristoe test of articulation.* Circle Pines, MD: American Guidance Service.

Grunwell, P. (1982). *Clinical phonology.* Rockville, MD: Aspen Systems.

Grunwell, P. (1985). *Phonological assessment of child speech* (PACS). San Diego, CA: College-Hill Press.

Grunwell, P. (1987). *Clinical phonology* (2nd ed.). Baltimore, MD: Williams and Wilkins.

Hodson, B.W. (1980). *The assessment of phonological processes*. Danville, IL: Interstate Printers and Publishers.

Hodson, B.W. (1985). *Computer analysis of phonological processes* [Computer program]. Stonington, IL: PhonoComp.

Hodson, B.W. (1986). *Assessment of phonological processes-revised (APP-R)*. Danville, IL: Interstate Printers and Publishers.

Hodson, B.W., and Paden, E.P. (1981). Phonological processes which characterize unintelligible and intelligible speech in early childhood. *Journal of Speech and Hearing Disorders, 46*, 369–373.

Hodson, B.W., and Paden, E.P. (1983). *Targeting intelligible speech*. San Diego, CA: College-Hill Press.

Hodson, B.W., and Paden, E.P. (1991). *Targeting intelligible speech* (2nd ed.). Austin, TX: PRO-ED.

Hoffman, P., Norris, J., and Monjure, J. (1990). Comparison of process targeting and whole language treatments for phonologically delayed preschool children. *Language, Speech, and Hearing Services in Schools, 21*, 102–109.

Ingram, D. (1973). *Phonological analysis of a child*. Unpublished paper. Also in (1976), *Glossa, 10*, 1–27.

Ingram, D. (1974). Phonological rules in young children. *Journal of Child Language, 1*, 49–64.

Ingram, D. (1976). *Phonological disability in children*. New York: American Elsevier.

Ingram, D. (1981). *Procedures for the phonological analysis of children's language*. Baltimore, MD: University Park Press.

Ingram, D. (1989). *Phonological disability in children* (2nd ed.). San Diego, CA: Singular Publishing Group.

Jenkins, R., and Bowen, L. (1994). Facilitating development of preliterate children's phonological abilities. *Topics in Language Disorders, 14,* 26–39.

Khan, L.M., and Lewis, N.P. (1986). *Khan-Lewis phonological analysis (KLPA).* Circle Pines, MN: American Guidance Service.

Kiernan, K.L., and Zentz, B.W. (1987). *Contrastive word pairs.* Baltimore, MD: K.Z. Associates.

Long, S., and Fey, M. (1988). *Computerized profiling* [Computer program]. Ithaca, NY: Department of Speech Pathology and Audiology, Ithaca College.

Lorentz, J.P. (1974). A deviant phonological system of English. *Papers and Reports on Child Language Development*, Linguistics Department, Stanford University, *8,* 55–64.

Lorentz, J.P. (1976). An analysis of some deviant phonological rules of English. In D.M. Morehead and A.E. Morehead (Eds.), *Normal and deficient child language: Selected readings* (pp. 29–59). Baltimore, MD: University Park Press.

Martin, M., and Ausberger, C. (1981). *Frequent error pairs.* Tucson, AZ: Communication Skill Builders.

McDonald, E. (1964). *Articulation testing and treatment: A sensory-motor approach.* Pittsburgh, PA: Stanwix House.

McReynolds, L.V., and Bennett, S. (1972). Distinctive feature generalization in articulation training. *Journal of Speech and Hearing Disorders, 37,* 462–470.

McReynolds, L.V., and Engmann, D. (1975). *Distinctive feature analysis of misarticulations.* Baltimore, MD: University Park Press.

McReynolds, L.V., and Huston, K. (1971). A distinctive feature analysis of children's misarticulations. *Journal of Speech and Hearing Disorders, 36,* 156–166.

Monahan, D. (1984). *Remediation of common phonological processes*. Tigard, OR: C.C. Publications.Oller, D.K. (1973). Regularities in abnormal child phonology. *Journal of Speech and Hearing Disorders, 38*, 36–47.

Oller, D.K. (1990). *Logical international phonetic programs (LIPP)* [Computer program]. Miami, FL: Intelligent Hearing Systems.

Perrone, V. (1989). *Working papers—Reflections on teachers, schools, communities*. New York: Teacher's College Press.

Ruscello, D.M., Cartwright, L.R., Haines, K.B., and Schuster, L.I. (1993). The use of different service delivery models for children with phonological disorders. *Journal of Communication Disorders, 26*, 193–203.

Shriberg, L.D. (1986). *PEPPER: Programs to examine phonetic and phonologic evaluation records* [Computer program]. Hillsdale, NJ: Lawrence Erlbaum.

Shriberg, L.D., and Kwiatkowski, J. (1980). *Natural process analysis (NPA): A procedure for phonological analysis of continuous speech samples*. New York: John Wiley & Sons.

Shriberg, L.D., and Kwiatkowski, J. (1982). Phonological disorders III: A procedure for assessing severity of involvement. *Journal of Speech and Hearing Disorders, 47*, 256–270.

Stampe, D. (1969). The acquisition of phonetic representation. In R.T. Binnick, A. Davison, G. Green, and J. Morgan (Eds.), *Papers from the Fifth Regional Meeting of the Chicago Linguistic Society* (pp. 443–454). Chicago, IL: Chicago Linguistic Society.

Tyler, A.A., Edwards, M.L., and Saxman, J.H. (1987). Clinical application of two phonologically based treatment procedures. *Journal of Speech and Hearing Disorders, 52*, 393–409.

Weiner, F. (1979). *Phonological process analysis*. Baltimore, MD: University Park Press.

Weiner, F. (1981). Treatment of phonological disability using the method of meaningful minimal contrast: Two case studies. *Journal of Speech and Hearing Disorders, 46*, 97–103.

Weiner, F. (1982). *Process analysis: Version 2.0* [Computer program]. State College, PA: Parrot Software.

Weston, A.J., and Irwin, J.V. (1971). Use of paired-stimuli in modification of articulation. *Perceptual and Motor Skills, 32*, 947–957.

Wolk, L., Conture, E.G., and Edwards, M.L. (1990). Comorbidity of stuttering and disordered phonology in young children. *The South African Journal of Communication Disorders, 37*, 15–20.

Wolk, L., Edwards, M.L., and Conture, E.G. (1993). Co-existence of stuttering and disordered phonology in young children. *Journal of Speech and Hearing Research, 36*, 906–917.

Wolk, L., Edwards, M.L., and Louko, L.J. (1990, April). *Phonological remediation: Maximizing efficiency through the use of groups*. Miniseminar presented at the Annual Convention of the New York State Speech-Language-Hearing Association, Kiamesha Lake, NY.

Young, E.C. (1981). *Language approach to open syllables*. Tucson, AZ: Communication Skill Builders.

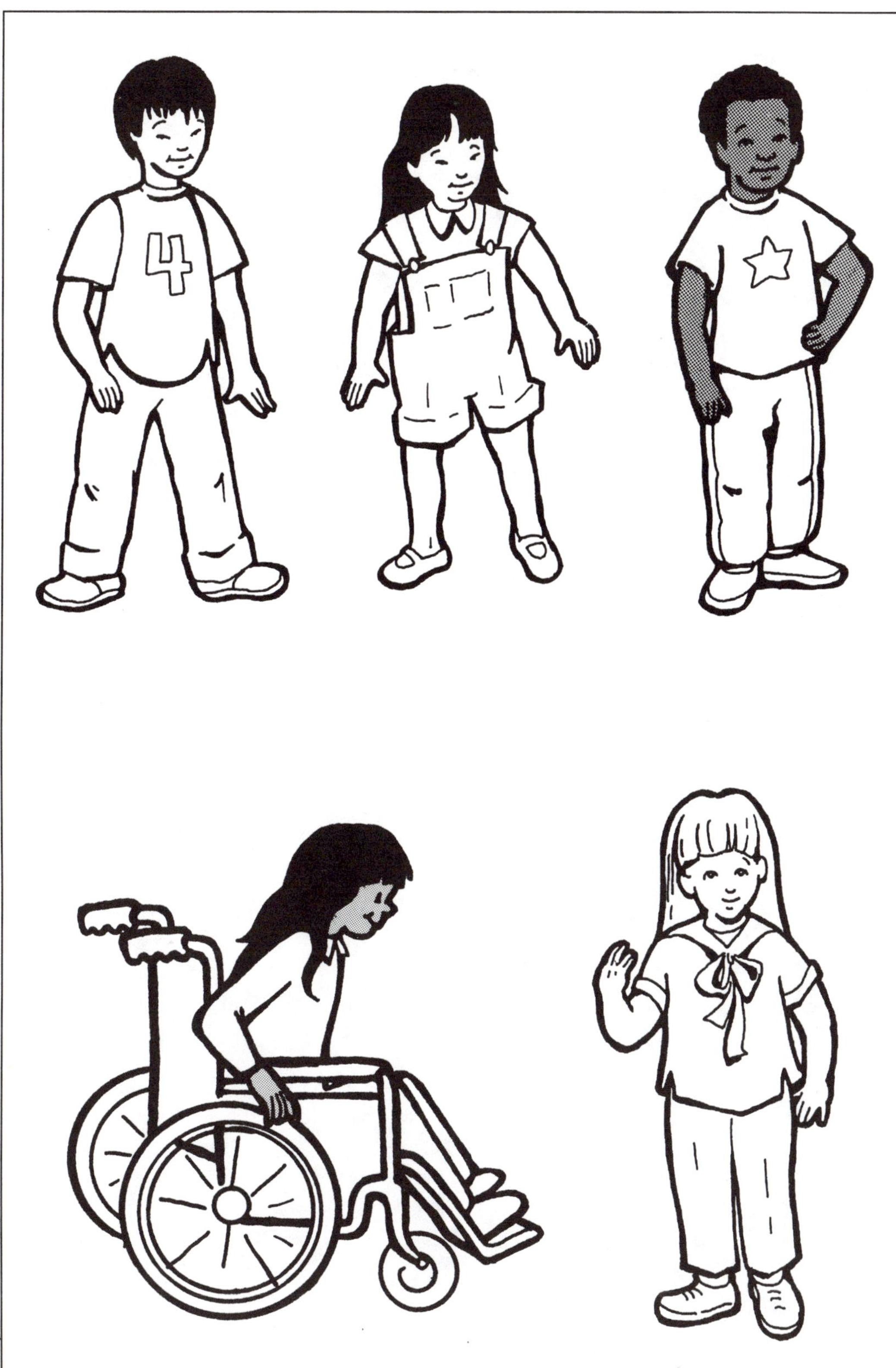

A *phonological process* is a systematic sound change that affects a class of sounds (such as velars or fricatives) or a sound sequence (such as /s/ + stop clusters) (Edwards and Shriberg, 1983). Processes are organized here according to syllable structure changes, assimilation processes, changes in place, manner, and voicing, etc. Note that various clinical phonologists may organize processes differently. In addition, terms and definitions may differ somewhat.

## Syllable Structure Changes

1. *Weak Syllable Deletion (WSD)*—An *unstressed* (i.e., weak) syllable is deleted. Children may exhibit WSD up to age 3:6 for three-syllable words and up to age 4–4:6 for longer words.*

   *banana* [ˈnænə]          *television* [ˈtɛˌvɪzən]          *butterfly* [ˈbʌˌfaɪ]

2. *Final Consonant Deletion* (FCD)—Word-final consonants are deleted. Most words are produced with final consonants by age 3:0, though they may not be correct.

   *dog* [dɔ]          *cat* [kæ]          *fish* [fɪ]

3. *Reduplication* (R)—An entire syllable (or part of a syllable) is repeated. (An early process used extensively by some children; used rarely by others.)

   *pudding* [ˈpʊpʊ]          *water* [ˈwɔwɔ]          *blanket* [ˈbɑbɑ]

4. *Cluster Reduction* (CR)—A sequence of two or more consonants in one syllable (i.e., a cluster) is simplified, usually by deletion of the *marked* (i.e., the more difficult) element. This process may occur up to about age 3:0 in normal development, and may be common in severe disorders.

   a. */s/ Cluster Reduction*—Usually the /s/ is deleted, especially in initial clusters.

      *spoon* [pun]          *snow* [noʊ]          *mask* [mæk]

---

*Ages for process suppression throughout this section are based on data from a variety of sources, including Hodson and Paden (1981), Grunwell (1982, 1987), and Ingram (1976, 1989). In some cases, developmental information is not available; therefore, ages of suppression are not given for all processes.

b. *Nasal Cluster Reduction*—Either element may be deleted; this sometimes depends on the voicing of the following obstruent (i.e., fricative, affricate, or stop).

*sink* [sik]          *lamp* [læp]          *sand* [sæn]

c. *Liquid Cluster Reduction*—The liquid is usually deleted. This is an early stage in children's attempts to produce clusters.

*clown* [kaʊn]          *green* [gin]          *belt* [bɛt]

5. *Epenthesis* (E)—A segment is inserted, usually between two elements of a cluster. This is considered to be a late stage in children's attempts to produce clusters.

*green* [gᵊrin]          *frog* [fᵁwɔg]          *blue* [bᵊlu]

6. *Coalescence* (CO)—Features from two adjacent segments or syllables combine (*Segment* or *Syllable Coalescence*). (Examples may be put under Cluster Reduction and Weak Syllable Deletion.)

| *Segment Coalescence* | | *Syllable Coalescence* | |
|---|---|---|---|
| *swing* [fiŋ] | *snow* [n̥oʊ] | *garage* [gɑʒ] | *balloon* [bun] |

7. *Metathesis (M)*—Two consonant elements are reversed or reordered; this is usually not consistent.

mask [mæks]          *basket* [ˈbæksɪt]          *blue* [bul]

## Assimilation Processes

In *assimilation* processes, one sound is influenced by another and becomes similar (or identical) to it. Assimilation may be complete or partial, progressive or regressive. In *progressive* (i.e., forward) assimilation, an early sound in a word affects a later sound, while in *regressive* (i.e., backward) assimilation, a later sound affects an earlier sound.

1. *Velar Assimilation* (VA)—A sound becomes a velar due to the influence of a nearby velar (i.e., /k, g, ŋ/). This process is very common in early acquisition and may persist until the age of about 2:6.

| *Complete Progressive* | *Complete Regressive* | *Partial Regressive* |
|---|---|---|
| *cat* [kæk] | *doggie* [ˈgɔgi] | *snake* [ŋek] |

2. *Labial Assimilation* (LA)—A sound becomes a labial due to the influence of a nearby labial. This process is noted in severe phonological disorders, as well as early normal development.

| *Partial Progressive* | *Complete Regressive* | *Partial Regressive* |
|---|---|---|
| *bait* [bep] | *table* [ˈbebu] | *swim* [fwɪm] |

## Voicing Changes

1. *Initial (Prevocalic) Voicing* (IV/PV)—Voiceless obstruents (i.e., fricatives, affricates, and stops) are voiced in initial position (or preceding a vowel). This may persist in normal acquisition until the age of about 2:8 or 3:0.

| *top* [dɑp] | *cow* [gaʊ] | *pig* [bɪg] |
|---|---|---|

2. *Final Devoicing* (FD)—Word-final obstruents are devoiced. This process may be exhibited even by four-year-olds (Hodson and Paden, 1981).

| *pig* [pɪk] | *bed* [bɛt] | *nose* [nos] |
|---|---|---|

## Changes in Place of Articulation

1. *Fronting of Velars* (VF)—Velars /k, g, ŋ/ are replaced by alveolars [t, d, n]. This process is typically suppressed by about 3:0 and is common in disordered phonology.

| *go* [do] | *wing* [wɪn] | *cookie* [ˈtuti] |
|---|---|---|

2. *Depalatalization or Palatal Fronting* (PF)—Palatals /ʃ, ʒ, tʃ, dʒ/ are replaced by alveolars. This process may be exhibited even by four-year-olds (Hodson and Paden, 1981).

| *show* [so] | *juice* [dzus] | *watch* [wɑts] |
|---|---|---|

3. *Labialization* (LB)—Front (nonlabial) sounds are replaced by labials.

| *mouth* [maʊf] | *brother* [ˈbrʌvɚ] | *see* [fi] |
|---|---|---|

245

4. *Alveolarization* (AL)—Front (nonalveolar) sounds are replaced by alveolars.

*thumb* [sʌm]          *leaf* [wis]          *mother* [ˈmʌzɚ]

## Changes in Manner of Articulation

1. *Stopping* (ST)—Fricatives/affricates are replaced by stops. This process begins to disappear by age 2:6–3:0 for most sounds, but persists for some fricatives (e.g., /ð, v/). Sometimes broken down into "early" and "late" Stopping.

   *fall* [pɔl]      *see* [ti]      *this* [dɪs]      *vest* [bɛst]      *chair* [teɚ]

2. *Gliding of Fricatives* (GF)—Fricatives are replaced by glides. This process is not as common as Stopping (Edwards, 1979).

   *food* [wud]          *vase* [wes]          *shoe* [ju]

3. *Gliding of Liquids* (GL)—Liquids are replaced by glides. This process may persist up to age 4:0 for /l/, and even longer for /r/.

   *light* [jaɪt]          *clown* [kwaʊn]          *pillow* [ˈpɪjo]
   *run* [wʌn]          *green* [gwin]          *very* [ˈvɛwi]

4. *Vocalization* (V)—Syllabic or postvocalic liquids are replaced by vowels. This process may be exhibited past age 4:0, even for /l/.

   *bell* [bɛʊ]          *milk* [mɪʊk]          *whistle* [ˈwɪso]
   *bird* [buəd]          *car* [kaʊ]          *under* [ˈʌndə]

5. *Affrication* (AF)—Fricatives are replaced by affricates (any stop + fricative combination).

   *shoe* [tʃu]          *bus* [bʌts]          *fish* [pfɪʃ]

6. *Deaffrication* (DA)—Affricates /tʃ, dʒ/ are replaced by fricatives (e.g., /tʃ→ʃ, dʒ→ʒ/).

   *chin* [ʃɪn]          *juice* [ʒus]          *page* [peʒ]

## Vowel Changes

Vowels are generally acquired early; vowel errors are rare in normal development. Vowels may be lowered, diphthongized, reduced to [ə], etc. If many vowel errors occur, try to find patterns (e.g., neutralization to [ʌ]), as in the following examples.

*bed* [bʌd]          *mad* [mʌd]          *cat* [kʌt]          *bird* [bʌd]

## Some Atypical Sound Changes

1. *Initial Consonant Deletion* (ICD)—Word-initial consonants are deleted. This is normal only for /h/ in early acquisition, is common in severe disorders, and rare for stops.

   *hot* [at]          *toy* [ɔɪ]          *shoe* [u]

2. *Atypical Cluster Reduction* (ACR)—The unmarked (i.e., easier) element of a cluster is deleted.

   *stop* [sɔp]          *snow* [soʊ]          *tree* [wi]          *glue* [lu]

3. *Glottal Replacement* (GR)—Consonant sounds are replaced by a glottal stop ([ʔ]), usually in intervocalic or final position. (Normal for /t, d/ in some dialects.)

   *chicken* [ˈtʃɪʔɪn]          *money* [ˈmʌʔi]          *tub* [tʌʔ]

4. *Velarization / Backing to Velars* (BK)—Front sounds, especially alveolars, are replaced by velars. This may include front fricatives, as in *zoo*→[gu].

   *tea* [ki]          *dough* [go]          *zoo* [gu]          *feather* [ˈfɛgə]

5. *Lateralization* (LAT)—Fricatives (generally sibilants) are produced with lateral emission or are replaced by a lateral fricative [ɬ].

   *sip* [ɬɪp]          *she* [ɬi]          *fish* [fɪɬ]

6. *Neutralization* (N)—One sound is used in place of several different adult sounds, so that adult phonemic contrasts are *neutralized* or merged.

Neutralization of initial fricatives to [j] is demonstrated in the following examples.

*see* [ji]          *thumb* [jʌm]          *ship* [jɪp]          *fish* [jɪs]

## Interacting Processes

Processes *interact* when two or more processes affect the same sound or have some influence on one another (Edwards, 1992). These may be termed *constituent processes* (Stampe, 1969). If the processes have to apply in a certain sequence, they are said to be *ordered*.

1. *Constituent Processes*

    a. *car* [dar]          k→d/#_V  (place, voicing)
    Velar Fronting + Prevocalic Voicing
    (k→t→d or k→g→d)

    b. *bridge* [bɪʃ]          dʒ→ʃ/_# (manner, voicing)
    Deaffrication + Final Devoicing
    (dʒ→ʒ→ʃ or dʒ→tʃ→ʃ)

2. *Ordered Processes*

    a. *pan* [mæ]*          Order:  (1) Regressive Nasal Assimilation (RNA)
                                   (2) Final Consonant Deletion (FCD)

    Derivation:          If FCD *preceded* RNA, /pæn/ would be produced as [pæ]. In this case, RNA could not apply *after* deletion of the final nasal.

    Child's Underlying Form (CUF) /pæn/
    (1) RNA /mæn/
    (2) FCD /mæ/
    Child's Surface Form (CSF) [mæ]

* This example is taken from Shriberg and Kwiatkowski's (1980) *Natural Process Analysis* (NPA). The *NPA* is one of the few published procedures in which the issue of process ordering is discussed.

b. *sweet* [pit]        Order: (1) Segment Coalescence (CO) (sw→f)

(2) Stopping (ST) (f→p)

Derivation:        *sweet*

CUF                        /swit/

(1) CO                     /fit/

(2) ST                     /pit/

CSF                        [pit]

In these phonological rules, the correct adult sound is to the left of the arrow, and the child's produced sound is to the right of the arrow. The *arrow* means is replaced by or becomes. The phonetic context in which the change takes place is shown to the right of the slash. The number sign (#) represents a word boundary, and a capital V represents any vowel. So /#_V means "in word-initial position preceding a vowel."

The CSF is the *Child's Surface Form,* or the form produced by the child and transcribed phonetically by the clinician. It is written in square brackets. The CUF is the *Child's Underlying Form*, or underlying representation. This is the "mentally stored" form of the word on which the phonological processes operate. In the approach taken here, the CUF is assumed to be basically equivalent to the broad (phonemic) adult form (after Stampe, 1969). So, even though the child says [pit] for sweet, the CUF is assumed to be /swit/. The CUF is written in slashes. The *derivation* shows all the steps between the CUF and the CSF.

# Nonstandardized Phonological Analysis

## What to Include

A nonstandardized phonological analysis should include the following:

1. A *phonological process analysis* containing a list of the child's major processes (with a brief description of each), sounds and positions affected, and frequency (%) of occurrence.

2. A *phonetic inventory analysis,* resulting in a list of the sounds used by the child in each position, including those used only as substitutes; also a list of absent sounds (i.e., those not used at all).

3. A rough measure of *phonological severity*, such as Shriberg and Kwiatkowski's (1982) percentage of consonants correct (PCC).

4. *Stimulability testing,* especially for sounds missing from the child's phonetic inventory.

5. Any other types of analyses that seem particularly relevant for the child being assessed, such as an analysis of preferred syllable or word shapes (e.g., CV), or the child's use of contrasts or "idiosyncratic rules" (e.g., the first consonant in a word is produced further forward in the mouth than the second consonant).

## Sampling and Transcription

The following steps describe the procedure for obtaining and transcribing a sample for phonological analysis:

1. Obtain a sample of 50–100 different words representing all of the consonant sounds of English in a variety of positions and phonetic contexts, as well as numerous consonant clusters. Also try to sample a variety of phonological processes (e.g., 20–30). (See the list of processes in *Appendix A.*)

2. Try to elecit spontaneous (i.e., non-imitated) productions, for example, by means of object- or picture-naming tasks. (A published articulation test or combination of such tests may be used.) When necessary, elicit delayed

imitations. That is, give the child the name of the object or picture, and then say something about it before asking the child to supply the label.

3. Try to obtain a sample of conversational speech for comparative purposes. In your analysis, do not combine words from conversational speech with words elicited in a more structured way, as the two types of productions may differ.

4. Tape record the sample under the best conditions possible, and use a combination of "live" transcription and transcription from the tape; use the tapes to verify the live transcriptions.

5. Phonetically transcribe each word completely, and transcribe distortions as accurately as possible. Make up symbols if necessary.

6. To streamline the transcription process, write out the broad adult transcriptions of test words ahead of time and then modify them to show the child's productions, as in Hodson (1980, 1986).

*Example:*  $/\overset{g}{\cancel{d}}\mathfrak{o}\cancel{g}/$

In this example, a line is drawn through the initial /d/ of the word *dog* to show that it was produced incorrectly. The substituted sound /g/ is written above the /d/. The line drawn through the final /g/ indicates that it was deleted.

7. To facilitate phonological analysis, use the same page for both phonetic transcription and process coding.

## Guidelines for Phonological Process Analysis

After obtaining and transcribing the child's language sample, the following guidelines are suggested for coding the analysis. (For additional information, see Edwards [in press].)

1. Beside each phonetically transcribed word, write the "substitution rules" for all the sound errors that are evident.

   *Example:* If *fan* is said as [bæ], write b/f (initial) or write f→b/#__ and n→ø/__#. (The ø symbol represents deletion.)

2. For each substitution rule, note the process(es) that would account for it. In phonological rules, the adult sound is written to the left of the arrow, which means *is replaced by* or *becomes*. The child's produced form is to the right of the arrow. The ø signifies deletion and __# indicates word-final position (i.e., preceding a word boundary, #).

   *Example:* ʃ→ø/__# in *push* is accounted for by Final Consonant Deletion (FCD). This rule ʃ→ø/__# means /ʃ/ is deleted (ø) at the end of the word.

3. Begin analyzing with the "easiest" words (i.e., those in which there is just one error that can be accounted for in only one way) as in the preceding FCD example.

4. For "complex substitutions" such a f→b/#__, all relevant processes are coded, in this case Stopping (f→p) plus Initial Voicing (p→b), as in [bæ] for *fan*.

5. If a sound error can be accounted for in more than one way, withhold judgment and look at similar words before making a decision.

   *Example*: [t] for /k/ in *kite* could be due to either Alveolar Assimilation (AA) or Velar Fronting (VF). Look at the production of /k/ in words like *key* or *cape* where assimilation could *not* be a factor.

6. Note any cases in which one process has to precede another to give the correct output. (See the discussion of ordered processes in *Appendix A, pages 248–249* .)

   *Example:* In [taɪ] for *kite*, Alveolar Assimilation (AA) must *precede* Final Consonant Deletion (FCD), or *kite* would be produced as [kaɪ].

7. After all "easy" items have been accounted for (i.e., those that can be coded in only one way), use the processes you have found, along with what you know about typical errors, to deal with any "problem" items or ambiguous errors.

8. Words that cannot be accounted for can be listed as "leftovers" or "isolated examples." For instance, these may be words that simply do not fit with

the child's current phonological system for any number of possible reasons, as in [ˈbabi] for *blanket*.

9. If there are just a few examples of a possible process, try to elicit additional examples. Otherwise, list the error under the heading of "leftovers" or "isolated errors."

   *Example:* If /ʃ/ is replaced by [w] between two vowels only in the word *dishes*, elicit more words with intervocalic fricatives to check for other examples of gliding of fricatives in that position.

10. The analysis procedure can be streamlined if process coding forms are made up ahead of time. For example, list test words down the left-hand side and processes across the top, as in Hodson (1980, 1986) and Khan and Lewis (1986).

11. On the coding form, write symbols in the appropriate spaces to show the sounds and positions affected by each process.

    *Example*: If f→b /#__ in *fish*, write I /f/ in the space under Stopping and across from the test word *fish*.

12. For each process, divide the number of actual occurrences by the number of possible occurrences to determine the frequency (percent) of occurrence.

    *Example*: If 3 out of 4 words with initial /s/ clusters undergo Cluster Reduction, the % occurrence of /s/ CR is 75%.

13. Make a list of the child's *major processes* (i.e., those that have a frequency of occurrence of at least 40%). Write a brief description of each, using information from the coding forms (regarding sounds and positions affected).

    *Example:* Final Consonant Deletion—Word-final consonants (except nasals) are deleted in 50% of all possible cases.

14. Star (*) the processes that are particularly significant for the child being assessed (e.g., processes that are unusual, apply very frequently, or contribute greatly to unintelligibility).

# Review of Selected Published Assessment Procedures

1. *Assessment of Phonological Processes-Revised* (APP-R) (Hodson, 1986)

   a. Includes 50 target words (rather than the 55 included in Hodson's 1980 procedure).

   b. Assesses about 30 error patterns, compared to 42 assessed in the earlier version (Hodson, 1980).

   c. Includes illustrations for 23 of the 50 assessment words (for objects which may be difficult to find).

   d. Has been "simplified substantially" from the 1980 version, according to Hodson (1986).

   e. Can be administered in 15–20 minutes and scored in 30 minutes.

   f. Contains extensive information about Hodson's "cycles" approach to phonological remediation, as well as a case study of a "profoundly unintelligible" five-year-old child.

   g. Includes a preschool phonology screening instrument, as well as a new multisyllabic screening protocol used to identify problem areas in phonology for school-age children. (Illustrations of the 12 multisyllabic screening protocol words are included.)

   h. Scoring keys are included in an appendix.

   i. Percentage of occurrence scores are computed for the basic processes, such as Consonant Sequence Reduction, and class deficiencies, such as Velar Deviations.

   j. A Phonological Deviancy Score can be computed by using the average of the percentage-of-occurrence scores and adding age compensatory points.

   k. Severity interval categories (from mild to profound) can be derived from the phonological deviancy score.

2. *Khan-Lewis Phonological Analysis* (KLPA) (Khan and Lewis, 1986)

   a. Designed to accompany the *Goldman-Fristoe Test of Articulation* (Goldman and Fristoe, 1986).

   b. Consists of 44 single words.

   c. Takes 15–40 minutes to complete the analysis.

   d. Identifies both specific phoneme errors and "simplification patterns."

   e. Assesses 12 developmental (i.e., normal) phonological processes, as well as 3 "nondevelopmental" processes.

   f. Takes process blocking into account.

   g. Color-coded form facilitates finding position-specific patterns.

   h. Space is provided on a single form to transcribe productions, record sound changes, and code processes.

   i. Includes norms for ages 2:0–5:11; also useful for older children.

   j. Derived scores include an *index of overall phonological process usage*, a *speech simplification rating*, and an *age equivalent* score.

   k. Includes a phonetic inventory analysis for each position.

   l. Includes 10 case studies and guidelines for remediation.

# Process Summary

Date: _______________

| **Process:** | Names | | | |
|---|---|---|---|---|
|  |  |  |  |  |
|  |  |  |  |  |
|  |  |  |  |  |
|  |  |  |  |  |
|  |  |  |  |  |
|  |  |  |  |  |
|  |  |  |  |  |

## Sample Parent Letter

Date: ___*3/15*___

Dear Parents,

This week in our phonology group we are working on the *sh* sound at the end of words. Here are some activities you can enjoy with your child at home:

1. Make *Banana Mush*—a favorite! Take one ripe banana and *mash* it with a fork or potato masher, while saying "Let's *mash*. *Mash, mash, mash!*" Take turns mashing. Add a spoonful of peanut butter and continue to *mash*. Spread on bread or crackers. Delicious!

2. Read the attached story, *Tish the Dog,* to your child at home. Remember to read slowly and emphasize the words that have the *sh* sound in them. These words are in italics for you.

Happy Mashing!

Sincerely,

*Margot Kelman*
Speech-Language Pathologist

## Sample Parent Letter

Date: _____*9/22*_____

Dear Parents,

This week we are working on the *sm* sound in our phonology group. You can help your child with this sound by doing the following activities at home:

1. Go from room to room in your house (particularly the kitchen and bathroom) and talk about items that *smell* or do not *smell*. Emphasize the target word *smell* rather than the name of the item. Find one item in your house that *smells* and one that does not *smell*. Have your child bring them to the phonology group on Thursday.

2. Play "Go Fish" with the *sm* cards sent home.

3. Remember to emphasize modeling the *sm* sound and choices. Praise your child for participating in the activity rather than commenting on the correct or incorrect productions.

Enjoy!

Sincerely,

*Margot Kelman*
___________________________
Speech-Language Pathologist

Activities that lend themselves to parental involvement are listed below. Throughout the activity section of this manual, those that are most appropriate for involving parents have an asterisk (*) after the activity title. Involving parents whenever feasible in any of the activities is suggested. Sending *Phonogroup* stories home to be read to the child is another option for involving parents. The stories provide additional opportunities to bombard the child with a specific sound or cluster and to encourage production of the target words.

## Art Activities

- *Snowperson Art*—page 46
- *Space Spaghetti*—page 53
- *Swimming or Swinging Swan*—page 67
- *Trucks with /tr/ Cargo*—page 95
- *Train Art*—page 97
- *Bright and Brown Bracelets*—page 105
- *Glitter Gloves*—page 134
- *Glitter T-Shirts*—page 136
- *Gold Guitars*—page 158
- *Salt Paint*—page 196
- *A Picnic Lunch*—page 213
- *Play-doh Creations*—page 214

## Snack Activities

- *Peanut Butter Stickies*—page 37
- *Sticks and Stones Stew*—page 38
- */st/ Jigglers*—page 38
- *Sweetheart Snack*—page 68
- *Swirl Snack*—page 69
- *Small Pudding Pies*—page 77
- *Dragon and Droopy Snack*—page 88
- *Trix or Trolls*—page 98
- *Treats and Tropical Drink*—page 99
- *Blue and Black Snack*—page 123
- *Blueberry Blizzards*—page 124
- *Cookies or Coca-Cola*—page 149
- *Kiwi or Cookies*—page 149

- *Cake or Carrots*—page 150
- *Crush 'n Mash*—page 163
- *Banana Mush*—page 164
- *Lemonade*—page 184
- *Lemonade or Licorice*—page 184
- *Logs and Ladybugs*—page 185
- *Cereal, Seeds, and Cider*—page 198
- *Fish or Fudge*—page 206
- *Popcorn and Pickles*—page 214
- *Peaches or Pears*—page 217
- *Peanuts and Popcorn Here!*—page 217

## Songs

Modified versions of familiar childhood songs:

- London *Bridge* is *breaking* down . . . *Bridge, Bridge, Broken*—page 106
- We are *floating,* we are *floating, Float, float, float* . . .—page 130

## Movement

- *Musical Stepping Stones*—page 39
- *Store*—pages 40, 113, 190, 224, 231
- *Activity Stations*—pages 41, 90, 109, 128
- *Star Says*—page 43
- *Start / Stop*—page 43
- *Spin and Pin*—page 61
- *Spot Toss*—page 61
- *Musical Smoke and Smiles*—page 79
- *Show and Smell*—page 80
- *Musical Smiles*—page 81
- *Skip, Skate, and Score*—page 84
- *Skip / Skate to My Lou*—page 85
- *Drip, Drip, Dragon*—page 91
- *Human Train*—page 101
- *Musical Bricks*—page 110
- *Hiding in Grass*—page 115

## Games

# Tally Sheet

Date: _________________________     Process: _________________________________

Target Sound/Cluster: _______________________________

| Training Words | Names | | | | | |
|---|---|---|---|---|---|---|
| | | | | | | |
| | | | | | | |
| | | | | | | |
| | | | | | | |
| | | | | | | |
| | | | | | | |
| | | | | | | |
| | | | | | | |
| | | | | | | |
| | | | | | | |
| | | | | | | |
| | | | | | | |
| | | | | | | |
| | | | | | | |
| | | | | | | |
| | | | | | | |
| | | | | | | |
| | | | | | | |
| | | | | | | |
| | | | | | | |
| | | | | | | |
| | | | | | | |
| | | | | | | |
| | | | | | | |
| | | | | | | |

# Session Log

Date: _______________

| Process: | Names | | | |
|---|---|---|---|---|
| | | | | |
| Sound: | % | % | % | % |
| Position: | C/T | C/T | C/T | C/T |
| Level: | o.p. | o.p. | o.p. | o.p. |

| Process: | Names | | | |
|---|---|---|---|---|
| | | | | |
| Sound: | % | % | % | % |
| Position: | C/T | C/T | C/T | C/T |
| Level: | o.p. | o.p. | o.p. | o.p. |

% = level of accuracy (C ÷ T x 100)        C/T = # of correct productions /# of total productions
o.p. = other production(s) (not correct)

The purpose of probing is to assess the degree to which a child has generalized beyond what has been taught. Therefore, words used for probing should be different from those used in remediation sessions. If words included on these probe lists are incorporated in training, they should not be used as probe words.

## /s/ Cluster Reduction

| **Initial** /sp/ | **Initial** /str/ | **Initial** /st/ | **Initial** /sk/ |
|---|---|---|---|
| spaceship | straight | stair | scarecrow |
| spaghetti | stranger | stand | skate |
| spider | strawberry | stapler | skeleton |
| spider web | street | star | ski |
| spill | string | steak | skip |
| spin | string bean | sticky | skirt |
| sponge | stroller | stocking | skunk |
| spooky | strong | stomach | sky |
| spoon | | stop | |
| sports | | story | |
| spy | | stove | |
| | | student | |

| **Initial** /sn/ | **Initial** /sl/ | **Initial** /sm/ |
|---|---|---|
| snack | sled | smash |
| snail | sleep | smell |
| snake | sleeve | smile |
| sneakers | sleigh | smiling |
| snow | slide | smoke |
| snowball | slippers | smoky |
| snowsuit | slow | |

## Liquid Cluster Reduction

| **Initial** /br/ | **Initial** /tr/ | **Initial** /dr/ | **Initial** /kr/ |
|---|---|---|---|
| bracelet | tractor | dragon | crab |
| braces | traffic | draw | cracker |
| braid | train | dream | crate |
| bread | trap | dress | crawl |
| brick | trash | drink | crayon |
| bride | tray | driving | cream cheese |
| bridge | treasure | drum | crib |
| broom | tree | dryer | cross |
| brother | trick | drying | crosswalk |
| brownie | tricycle | | crumb |
| brush | troll | | crush |
| | truck | | crutches |
| | trumpet | | cry |
| | trunk | | |

| **Initial** /fr/ | **Initial** /pl/ | **Initial** /bl/ | **Initial** /kl/ |
|---|---|---|---|
| frame | placemat | black | clam |
| freezer | plane | blackboard | clap |
| french fries | planet | blanket | clean |
| friend | plant | blastoff | climb |
| frog | plate | blink | clock |
| frosting | playground | blizzard | close |
| Frosty | plow | blocks | closet |
| fruit | plug | bloodhound | clothes |
| | plum | blow | clown |
| | Pluto | blue | |
| | | blueberry | |
| | | bluebird | |
| | | blue jeans | |

## Liquid Cluster Reduction

### Initial /fl/

flag
flame
flashlight
flat
flip
float
floor
flower
flying

### Initial /gl/

glass
glasses
glitter
glove
glue

### Initial /sl/

sled
sleep
sleeping bag
slide
slinky
slippers
slow

## Velar Fronting

| **Initial /k/** | **Medial /k/** | **Final /k/** |
|---|---|---|
| cabbage | blackbird | birthday cake |
| caboose | blanket | black |
| cactus | bookstore | book |
| cage | chicken | candlestick |
| calendar | chocolate | crosswalk |
| can | cookie | cupcake |
| car | rocket | duck |
| carrot | sneakers | rake |
| cat | vacuum | rock |
| caterpillar | | steak |
| cave | | truck |
| coffee | | |
| cookie | | |
| corn | | |
| cowboy/cowgirl | | |
| cup | | |
| kissing | | |
| kite | | |
| kitten | | |

| **Initial /g/** | **Medial /g/** | **Final /g/** |
|---|---|---|
| garage | alligator | bag |
| garden | doghouse | bug |
| gas station | dragon | frog |
| gate | fingernail | hot dog |
| ghost | kangaroo | log |
| girl | magnet | plug |
| gold | pigpen | rug |
| goldfish | spaghetti | sleeping bag |
| gorilla | sugar | |
| guitar | tiger | |
| gum | wagon | |

## Depalatalization

| **Initial /ʃ/** | **Medial /ʃ/** | **Final /ʃ/** |
| --- | --- | --- |
| shadow | bookshelf | ash |
| shampoo | dishes | bush |
| shark | fishing | crush |
| shave | flashlight | flush |
| sheep | horseshoe | goldfish |
| sheet | lotion | hairbrush |
| shelf | machine | leash |
| shell | mushroom | licorice |
| sheriff | ocean | mouthwash |
| ship | sunshine | nail polish |
| shirt | tissue | paintbrush |
| shoe | washcloth | push |
| shoelace | | radish |
| shovel | | rash |
| shower | | relish |
| sugar | | smash |
| | | splash |
| | | starfish |
| | | toothbrush |
| | | trash |

## Depalatalization

### Initial /tʃ/

chair
chalk
cheek
cheer
Cheerios
cheese
cherry
chest
chew
chicken
child
chimney
chimp
chin
chipmunk
chocolate chips
chop
chopsticks

### Medial /tʃ/

branches
chocolate chips
corn chips
crutches
French fries
ketchup
kitchen
lunch box
matches
picture
teacher

### Final /tʃ/

beach
bench
branch
catch
couch
lunch
match
peach
punch
sandwich
scratch
watch
witch

### Initial /dʒ/

giant
giraffe
jacket
jar
jeans
JELL-O
jet
juice
jump rope

### Medial /dʒ/

pages
pajamas
refrigerator
vegetable

### Final /dʒ/

bandage
bridge
cabbage
cage
carriage
cottage
fudge
garage
orange
page
sponge

## Gliding of Liquids*

### Initial /l/

| | |
|---|---|
| ladder | lettuce |
| lady | light |
| lake | lion |
| lamb | lipstick |
| lamp | lizard |
| lawn mower | lock |
| leaf | log |
| leash | lotion |
| legs | lunch |
| lemon | |

### Medial /l/

balloon
color
dollar
elephant
jelly
pillow
sailor
telephone

### Final /l/

ball
bell
bowl
bull
drill
nail
pool
shell
smile
tail
whale
wheel

### Initial /r/

| | |
|---|---|
| rabbit | ribbon |
| raccoon | rice |
| radio | robot |
| rain | rock |
| rainbow | rocket |
| raisin | roof |
| rake | rope |
| rash | rose |
| rattle | Rudolph |
| read | rug |
| red | run |

### Medial /r/

arrow
berry
carrot
cherry
earring
garage
giraffe
married
orange
parachute
parrot
squirrel
strawberry

### Final /r/

bear
door
ear
hair
mirror
pear
reindeer
square
store

*/r/ words are included to assess generalization from trained liquid /l/ to untrained /r/.

**Stopping**

### Initial /f/

| | |
|---|---|
| fan | fire truck |
| feather | first |
| fence | fish |
| fight | five |
| fin | foot |
| finger | fork |
| fire | |

### Medial /f/

breakfast
coffee
elephant
laughing
sofa
telephone
traffic

### Final /f/

cough
giraffe
handkerchief
knife
leaf
sheriff

### Initial /v/

vacuum
valentine
van
vanilla
vase
vegetable
violin
vitamin

### Medial /v/

driving
Grover
heavy
shaving
shovel
silver

### Final /v/

drive
five
glove
olive
wave

### Initial /θ/

Thanksgiving
thank you
thermometer
thorn
thumb
thunder

### Medial /θ/

bathtub
birthday
toothbrush

### Final /θ/

mouth
path
teeth
washcloth
wreath

271

## Stopping

### Initial /ð/

that
there
these
they
this

### Medial /ð/

breathing
brother
father
feather
mother

### Initial /s/

sail
sailboat
scissors
sink
sister
soap
sofa
sunburn

### Medial /s/

bicycle
eraser
glasses
ice cream
kissing
police officer
sister

### Final /s/

bus
caboose
circus
glass
juice
kiss
lettuce
octopus
vase

### Initial /z/

xylophone
zebra
zero
zipper
zoo

### Medial /z/

buzzing
daisy
frozen
magazine
scissors

### Final /z/

berries
cookies
glasses
knees
rose
scissors

## Initial Voicing

### Initial /p/

paint
peach
pear
peas
pie
pig
pipe
police
pool

### Initial /t/

table
tail
tea
teeth
ten
tennis ball
tie
toast
toaster
toilet
tomato
tongue
toolbox
toothbrush
toothpaste
tuna fish
turkey
two

### Initial /k/

cabbage
caboose
cactus
cage
calendar
can
car
carrot
cat
caterpillar
cave
coffee
cookie
corn
cowboy/cowgirl
cup
kissing
kite
kitten

The following materials are required on occasion in *Phonogroup* activities. Often these materials are readily available in preschool programs. However, in the event that they are not accessible, instructions for creating them are included here for the convenience of the speech-language clinician.

## Fishing Pole

**Materials:** dowel rod
magnet
fishing line or string

**Procedure:** Create a fishing pole by attaching a short fishing line or string to the end of a dowel rod. Drill a hole in the end of the dowel rod to tie the fishing line to or tape the line to the pole with duct tape. Tie or tape a magnet to the opposite end of the fishing line or string.

## Cloth Grab Bag

**Materials:** pillow case or laundry bag

**Procedure:** Use cloth bags as grab bags to avoid noisy paper or plastic bags that make it difficult to hear the children's productions.

## Bingo Board

**Materials:** bingo board grid (See page 276.)  glue or glue stick
illustration to be used as marker  heavy stock paper
four to six illustrations of the target sound

**Procedure:** Duplicate the bingo board onto heavy stock paper. Duplicate the target sound illustrations (reduce to 90 percent to fit the bingo board spaces), making at least two copies of each. Glue illustrations to the bingo board spaces. Vary bingo boards from one another by at least one picture. Use any picture twice on one bingo board and also add free spaces if desired. Create the bingo calling cards using the remaining illustrations, making certain that one of each illustration is included. Create the bingo markers by using the illustration cited to be the marker in the individual bingo activities. Reduce and duplicate onto heavy stock paper at least six markers per child.

## Spinner Board

**Materials:** spinner pattern (See pages 278–279).  glue or glue stick
spinner arrow  brass fastener
heavy stock paper or tag board
illustrations of target sound

**Procedure:** Duplicate the spinner pattern and arrow onto heavy stock paper. Color and laminate them. Attach the arrow with a brass fastener to the center of the spinner. Duplicate the target sound illustrations and glue them to the spinner sections. (As another alternative, purchase a spinner from a learning store or borrow one from an existing game, such as "Twister.")

## Feely Box

**Materials:** five-gallon bucket, coffee can, or large box
old sweat pants or sweatshirt with elastic cuffs or an old sock
duct tape or staples

**Procedure:** Remove the elastic cuffs from a pair of old sweatpants or a sweatshirt, or cut the toe end off an old sock, leaving enough room to attach the cuff end to the container. Attach to the bucket, can, or box with duct tape or staples, making sure the cuff's end is centered so that students can use the cuff to put their hands into the container.

## Game Board

**Materials:** game board pattern (See page 277.)
11 x 17" paper
glue
illustrations of target sound
tag board

**Procedure:** Enlarge at 130 percent and duplicate the game board pattern onto 11 x 17" paper. Glue the pattern to tag board. Color it if desired. Reduce to 50 percent, then duplicate the target sound illustrations, cut them out, and attach them to the game board. Laminate the game board for durability.

Phonogroup Bingo Board
Phonogroup

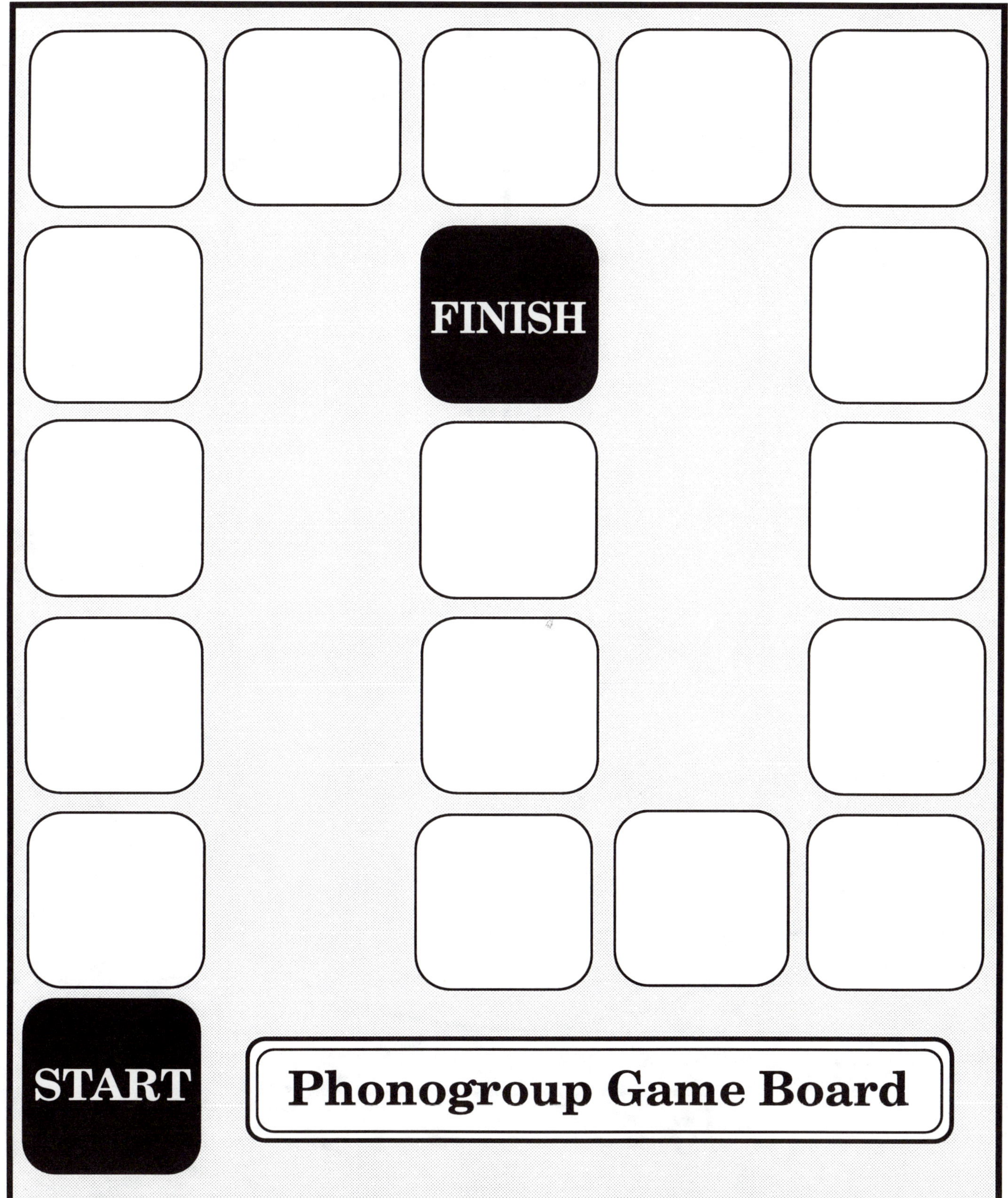
FINISH
START
Phonogroup Game Board

**Spinner Pattern**

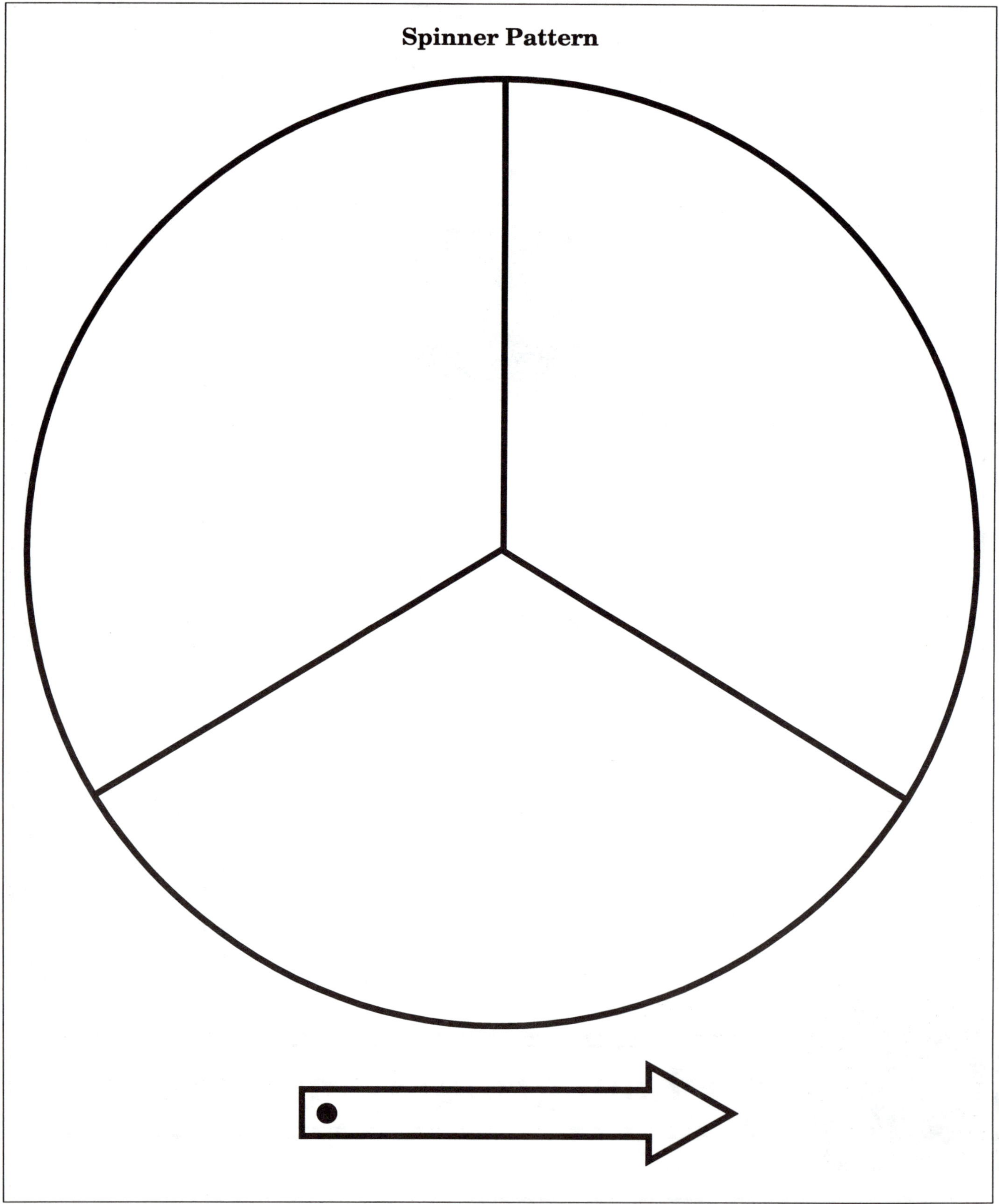

## Spinner Pattern

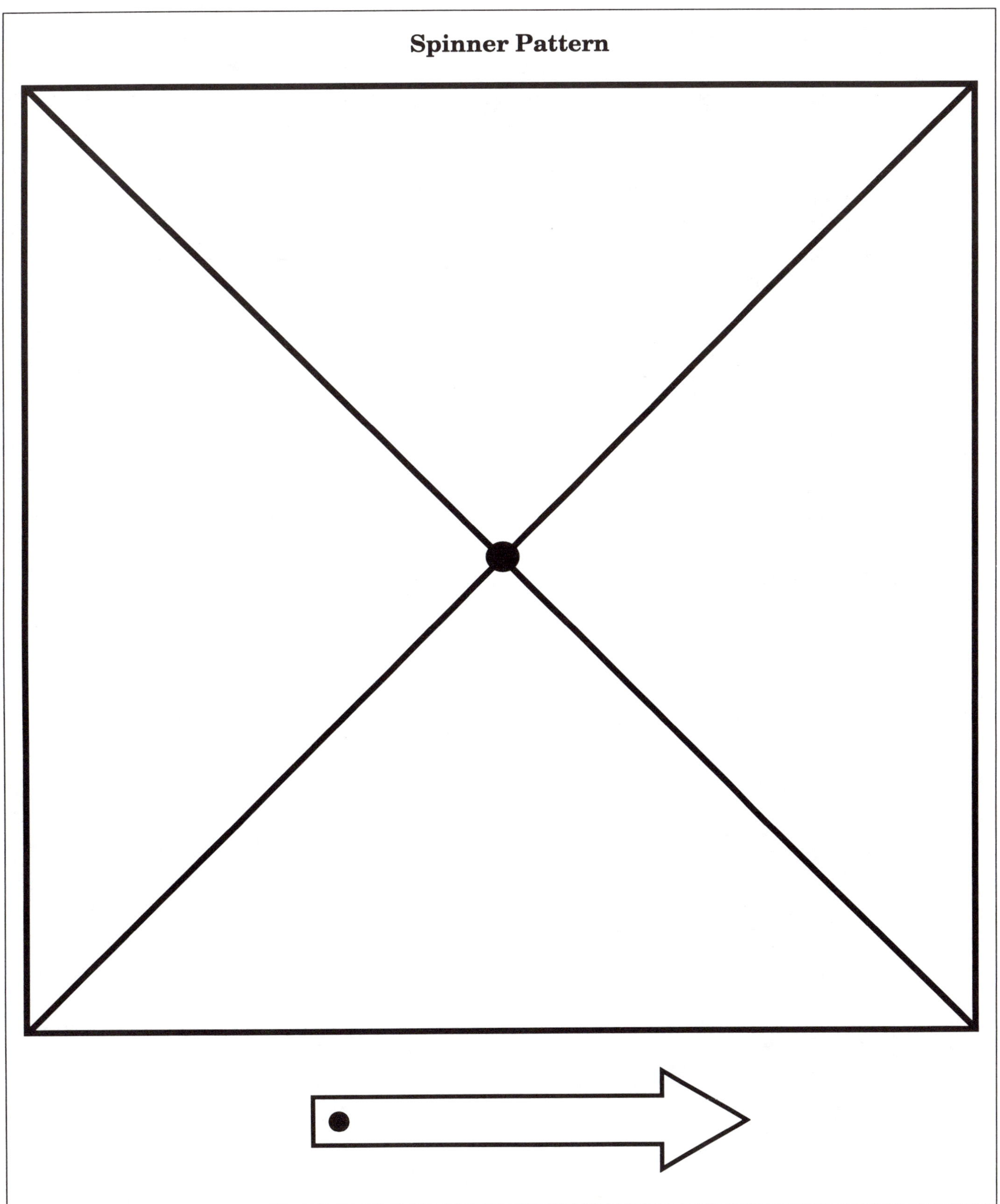

Following is a list of the illustrations included in *Phonogroup*. Illustrations are organized by process, then by target sound, and then in alphabetical order (when possible). The actual illustrations begin on page 285; they may be enlarged or reduced as applicable to the activity. In addition, illustrations of seven children (three boys and four girls) and two dogs are included on pages 322–326. A variety of names can be used for these children and dogs as appropriate for particular target sounds and processes. Also included are a large face of a boy and a girl on pages 327–328. Minimal pairs illustrations are listed on page 284 and then arranged alphabetically on pages 316–322.

## /s/ **Cluster Reduction**

| /st/ | /sn/ | /sp/ |
|---|---|---|
| stairs | snail | spider |
| star | snake | spook |
| starfish | snowperson | spoon |
| steak | | |
| Sticky Bear | | |
| stinky bug | | |
| stove | | |

| /sw/ | /sm/ | /sk/ |
|---|---|---|
| Swami Bear | smoke | scarecrow |
| swamp | smile | scarf |
| swan | | school bus |
| sweatband | | skates |
| sweater | | skeleton |
| sweatshirt | | skirt |
| sweat shorts | | skunk |
| sweat socks | | |
| swim fins | | |
| swim mask | | |
| swimmies | | |
| swimsuit | | |
| swim trunks | | |
| swing | | |

## Liquid Cluster Reduction

### /dr/

dragon
dress
drill
drum

### /tr/

tractor
train
trash can
tree
tricycle
trout
truck
trumpet

### /br/

bread
bricks
bridge
broom
brush

### /gr/

grapes
grass
grasshopper
grizzly bear
groundhog

### /bl/

black cat
black pants
blue jeans

### /fl/

flower

### /gl/

glasses
gloves
glowworm

### /kl/

clam
clock
clouds
clover
clown

### /pl/

plane
plant
plate
plow

## Velar Fronting

### /k/

cake
can
car
carrot
cat
coat
comb
cookie
cup
key
king

### /g/

garage
garden
gate
ghost
goat
goose
gorilla
guitar

## Depalatalization

### /ʃ/ (Final)

bush
cash
dish
fish
hairbrush
leash
starfish
trash
wash

### /ʃ/ (Initial)

sheep
shell
ship
shoe

## Gliding of Liquids

### /l/

ladybug
lamb
laundry
lawn
leapfrog
lily pad
lion
lips
lizard
llama
lobster
log

## Stopping

### /s/

saddle
sailboat
sandwich
sea
seal
seashell
sign
soap
sundae

### /f/

fairy
fan
fence
fire
firefighter
fire truck
fish
football
footprints
fork

## Initial Voicing

| /p/ | /t/ |
|---|---|
| paint | teddy bear |
| pancakes | tiger |
| panda | toad |
| pants | turkey |
| parrot | turtle |
| pear | |
| penguin | |
| pickle | |
| pie | |
| pig | |
| pizza | |
| pond | |
| popcorn | |

## Minimal Pairs Illustrations

| | | |
|---|---|---|
| bear (pear) | pea (bee) | tail (sail) |
| bee (pea) | pear (bear) | tea (sea) |
| Ben (pen) | pen (Ben) | ten (den) |
| bunch (punch) | pie (bye) | tie (die) |
| bye (pie) | punch (bunch) | time (dime) |
| | | toe (sew, dough) |
| date (gate) | sail (tail) | |
| den (ten) | sea (tea) | |
| dew (goo) | sell (shell) | |
| die (tie) | sew (toe) | |
| dill (gill) | shell (sell) | |
| dime (time) | shine (sign) | |
| dough (toe, go) | ship (sip) | |
| | shoe (Sue) | |
| gate (date) | sign (shine) | |
| gill (dill) | sip (ship) | |
| go (dough) | Sue (shoe) | |
| goo (dew) | | |

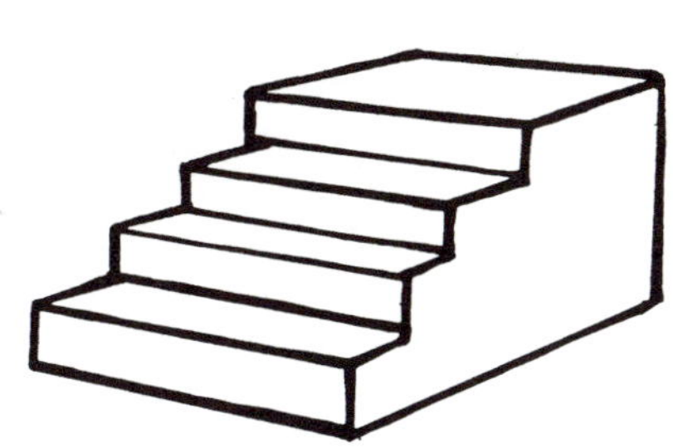

**stairs**

*© 1994 Thinking Publications—Phonogroup*

**star**

*© 1994 Thinking Publications—Phonogroup*

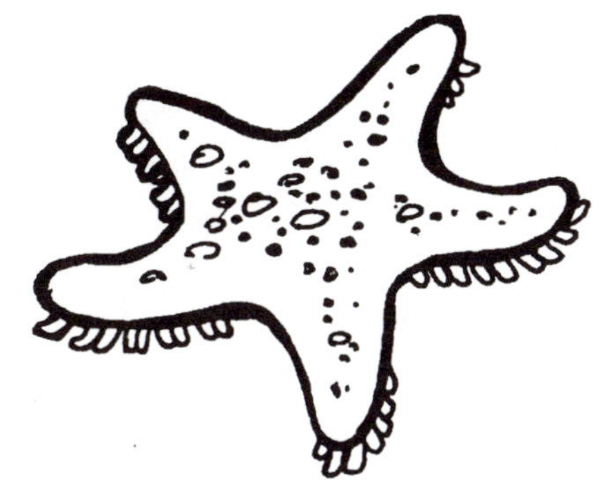

**starfish**

*© 1994 Thinking Publications—Phonogroup*

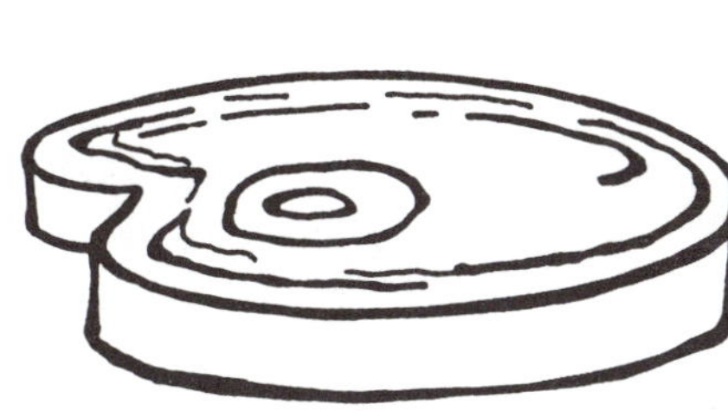

**steak**

*© 1994 Thinking Publications—Phonogroup*

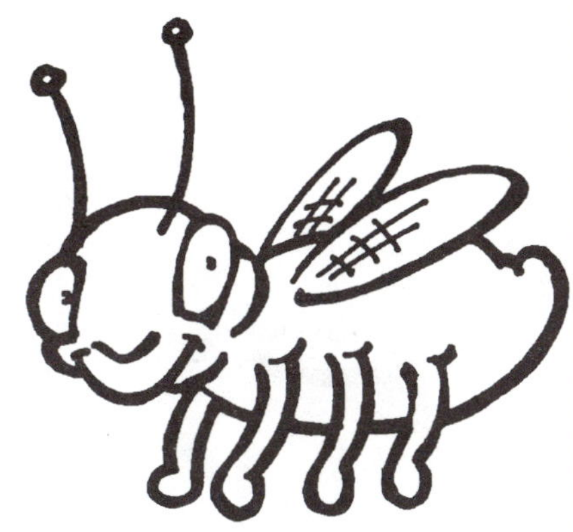

**stinky bug**

*© 1994 Thinking Publications—Phonogroup*

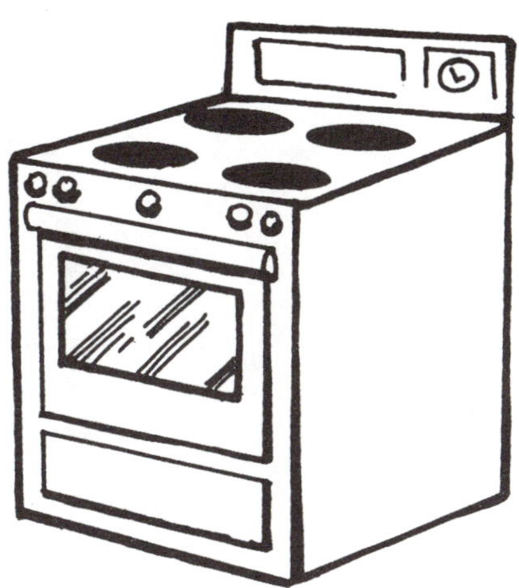

**stove**

*© 1994 Thinking Publications—Phonogroup*

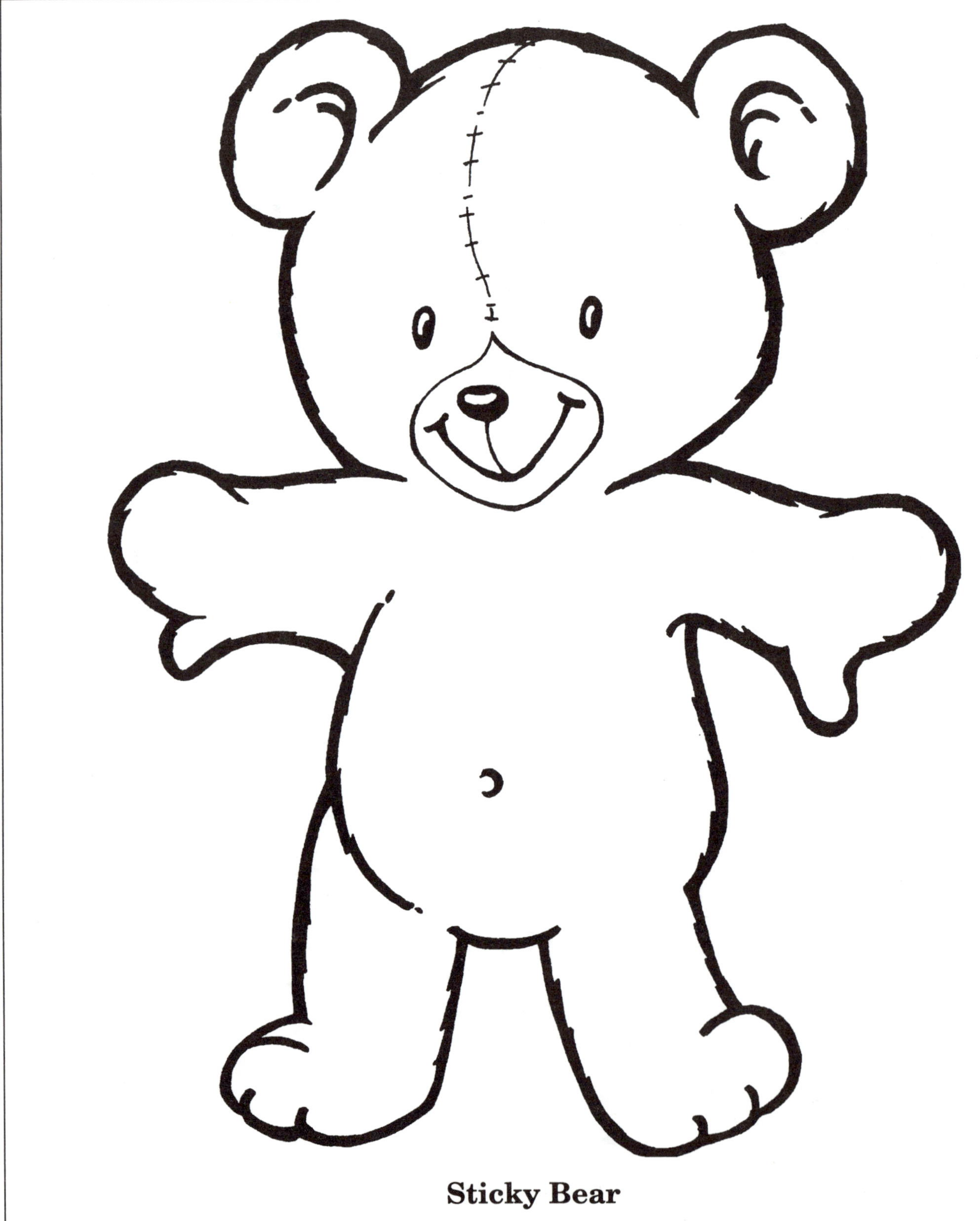

**Sticky Bear**

*© 1994 Thinking Publications—Phonogroup*

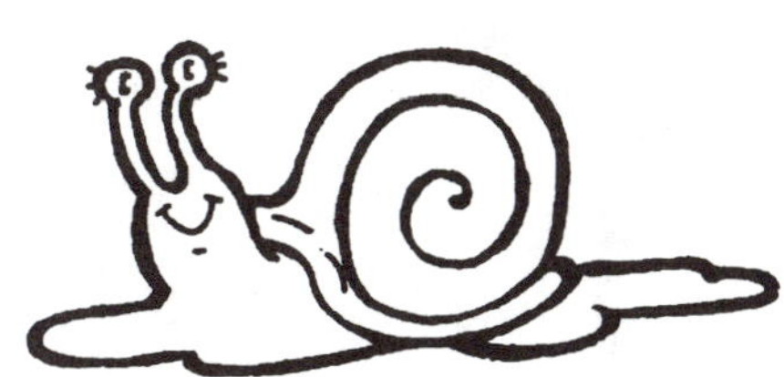

**snail**



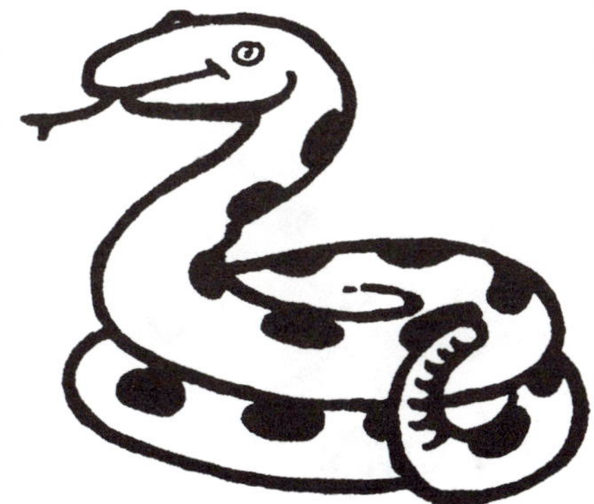

**snake**



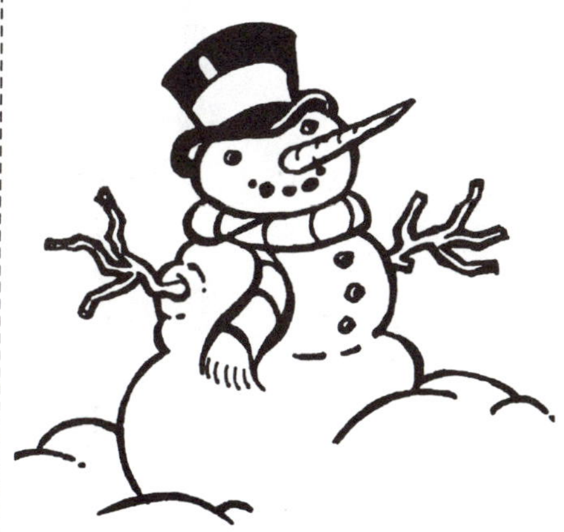

**snowperson**



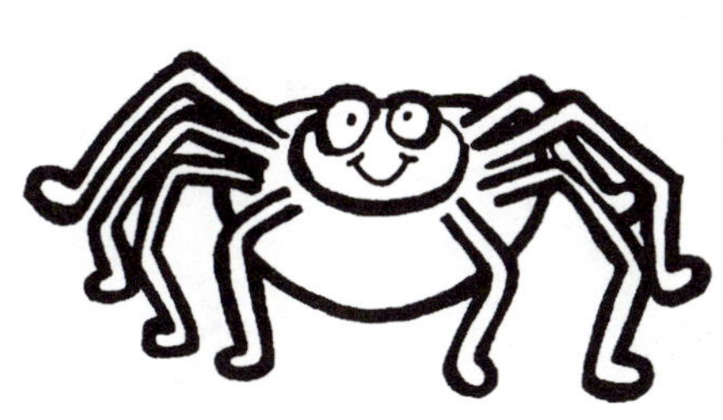

**spider**



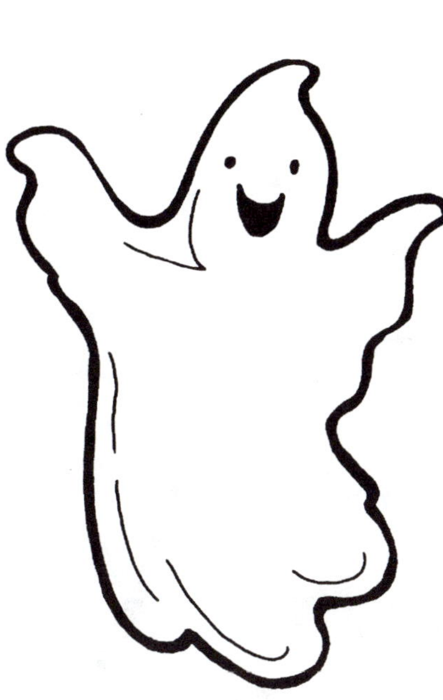
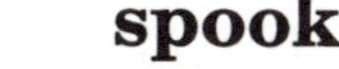

**spook**



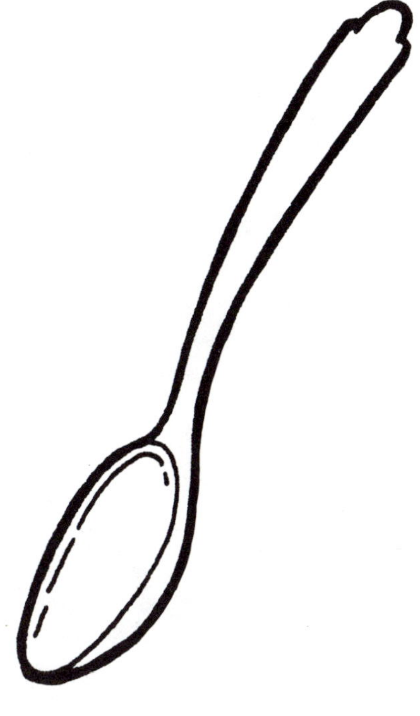

**spoon**

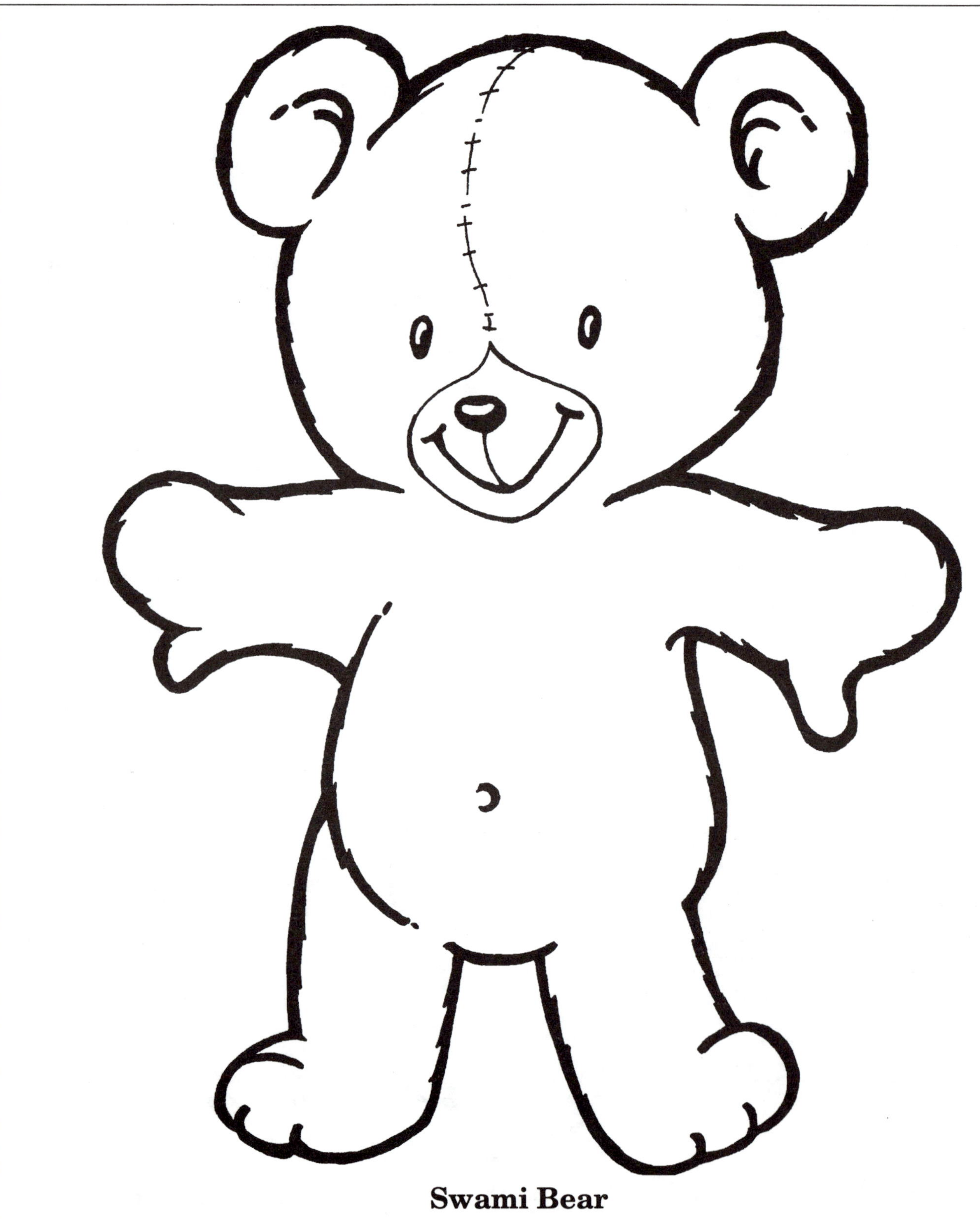

**Swami Bear**

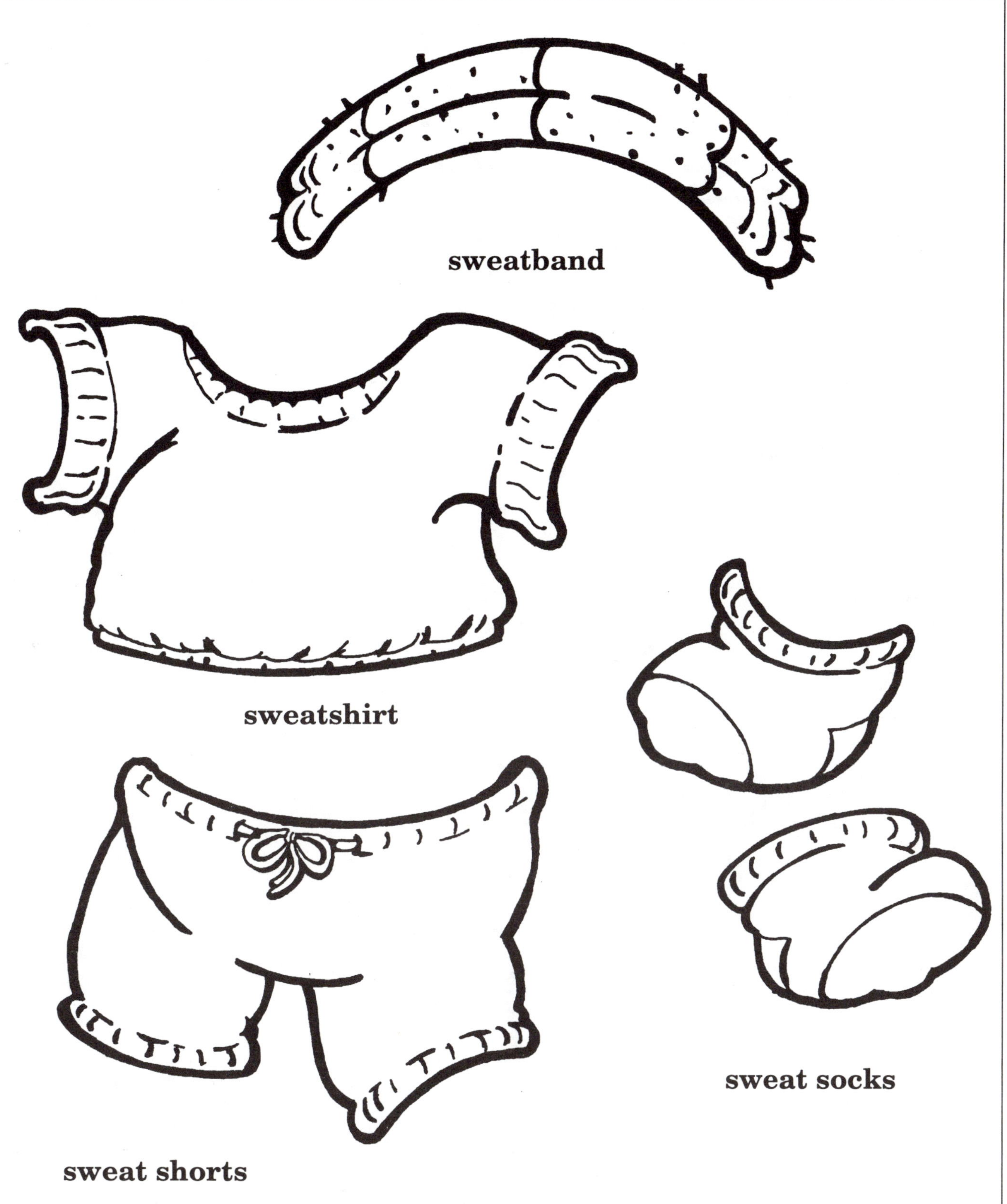

sweatband
sweatshirt
sweat shorts
sweat socks

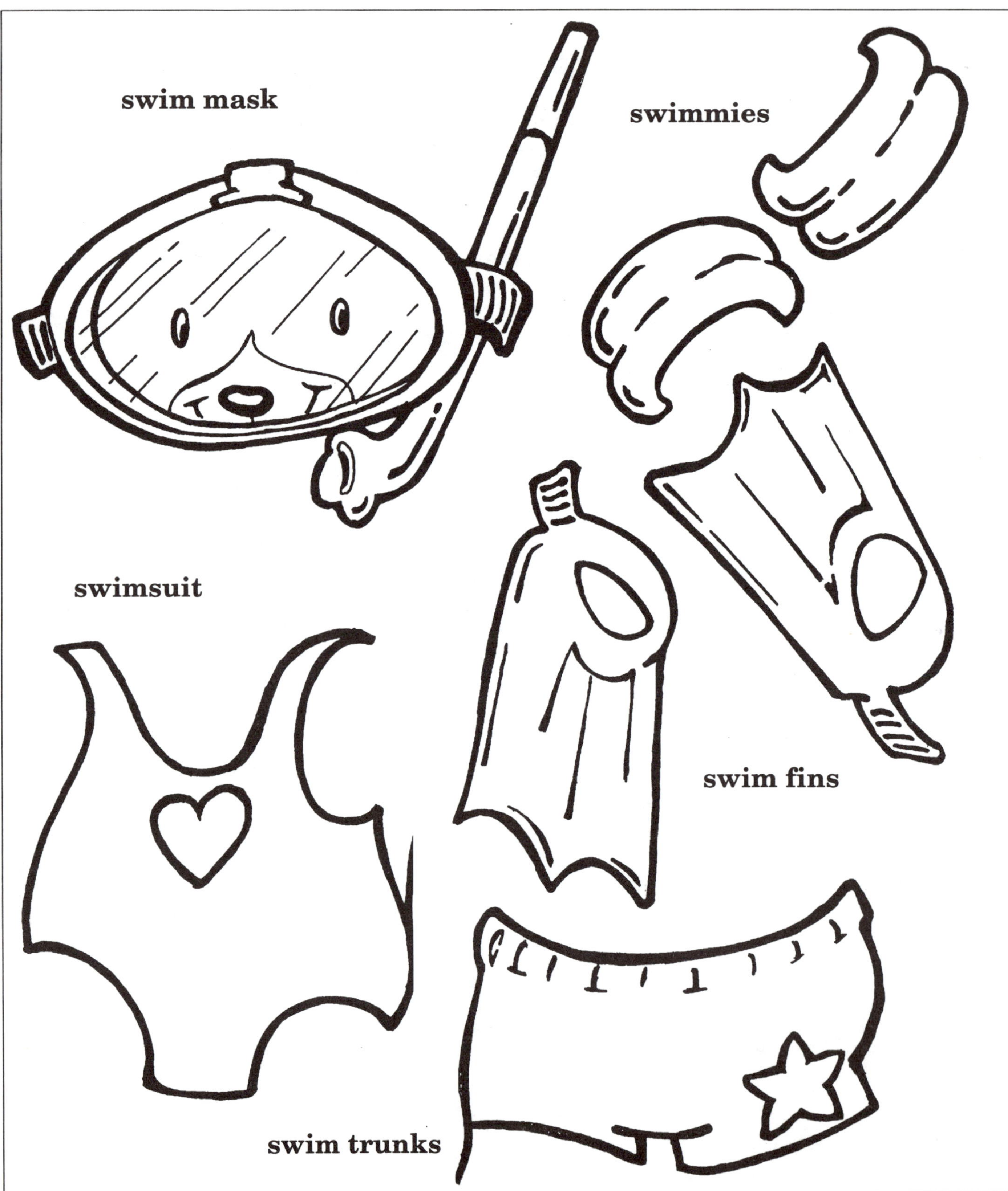


swim mask
swimmies
swimsuit
swim fins
swim trunks

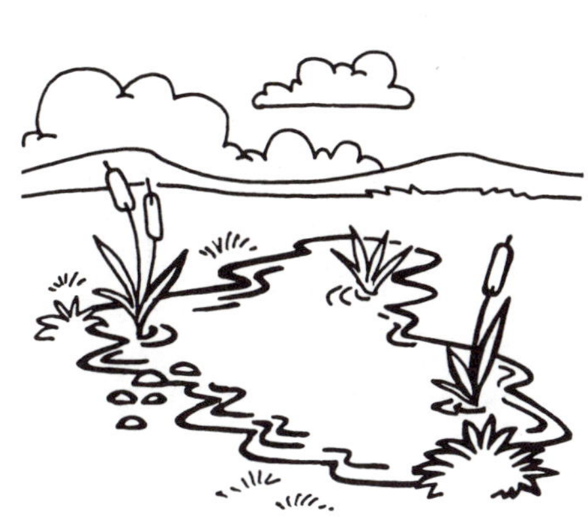

**swamp**

© 1994 Thinking Publications—Phonogroup

**swan**

© 1994 Thinking Publications—Phonogroup

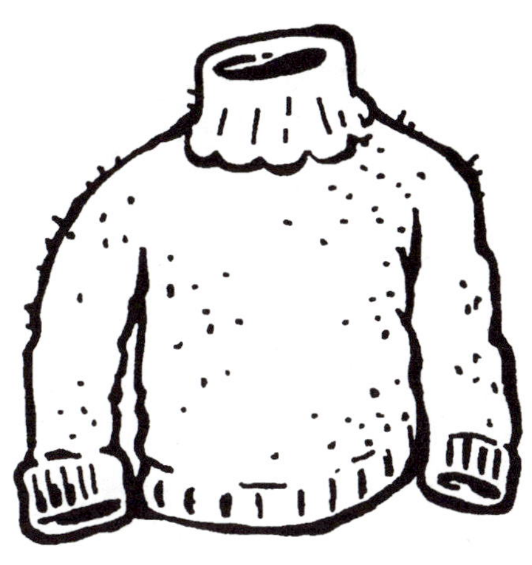

**sweater**

© 1994 Thinking Publications—Phonogroup

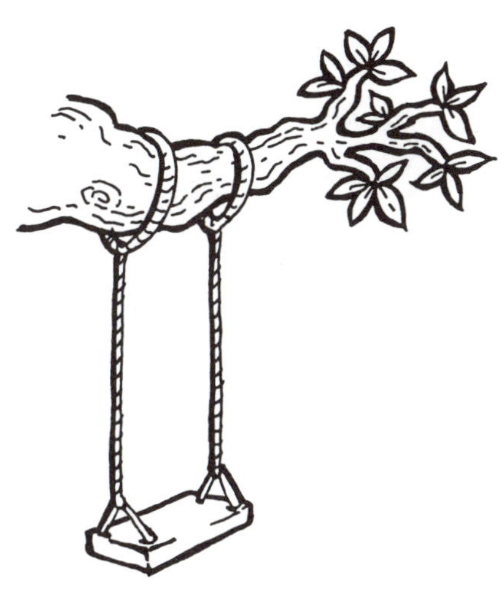

**swing**

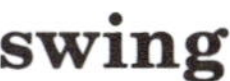

© 1994 Thinking Publications—Phonogroup

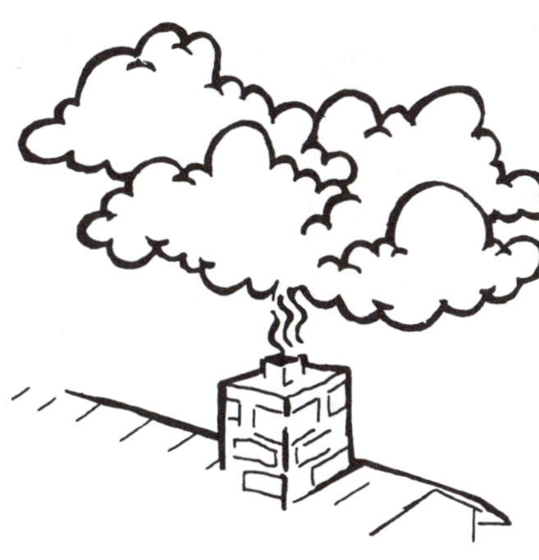

**smoke**

© 1994 Thinking Publications—Phonogroup

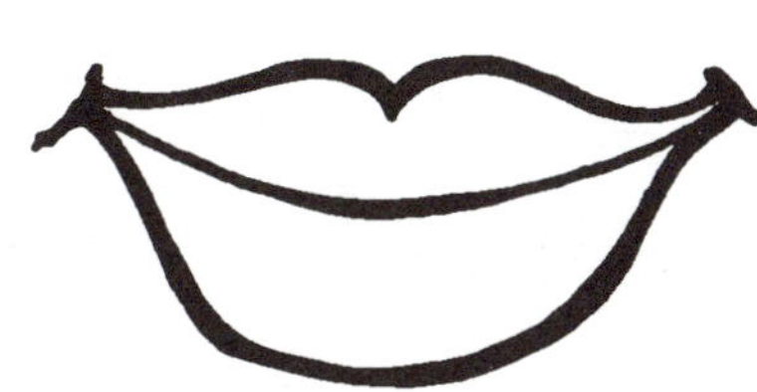

**smile**

© 1994 Thinking Publications—Phonogroup

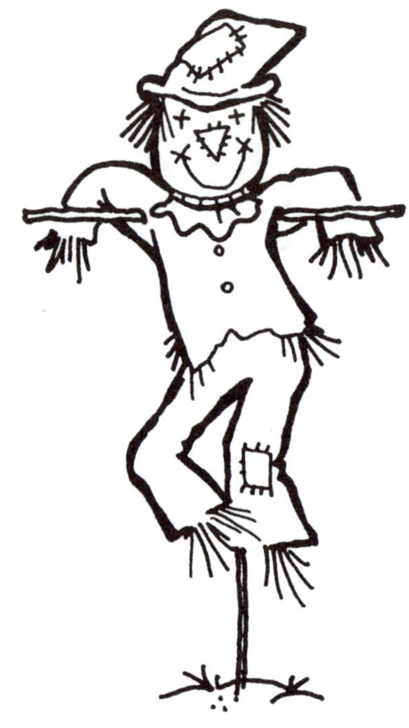
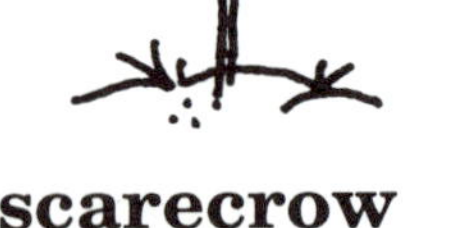

**scarecrow**

*© 1994 Thinking Publications—Phonogroup*

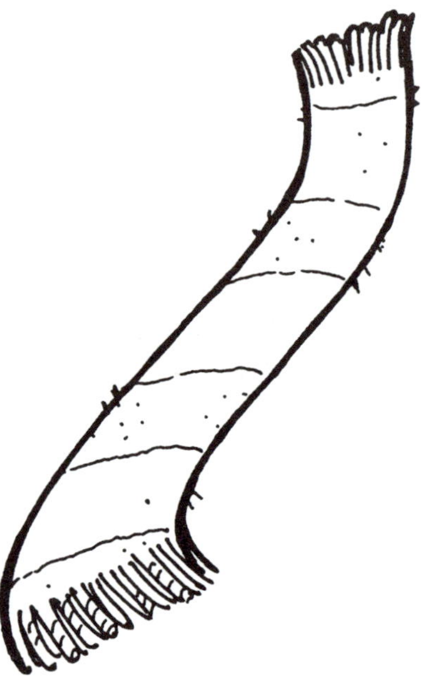

**scarf**

*© 1994 Thinking Publications—Phonogroup*

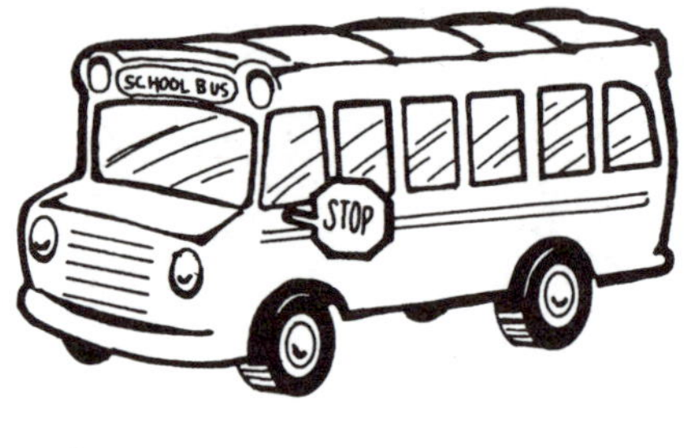

**school bus**

*© 1994 Thinking Publications—Phonogroup*

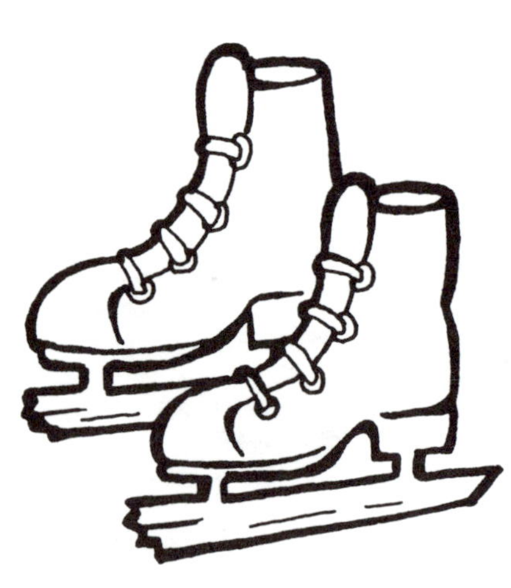

**skates**

*© 1994 Thinking Publications—Phonogroup*

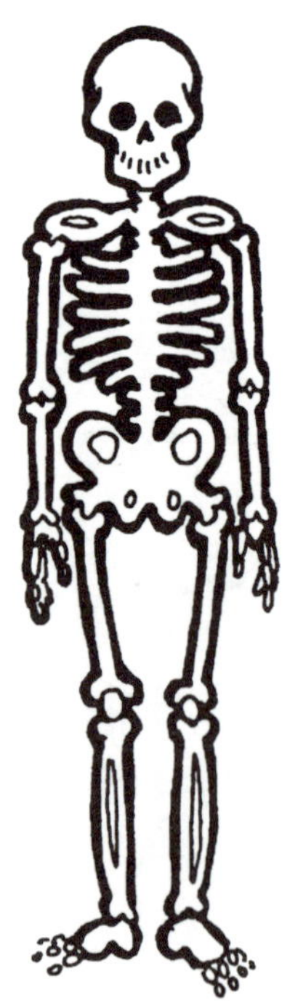

**skeleton**

*© 1994 Thinking Publications—Phonogroup*

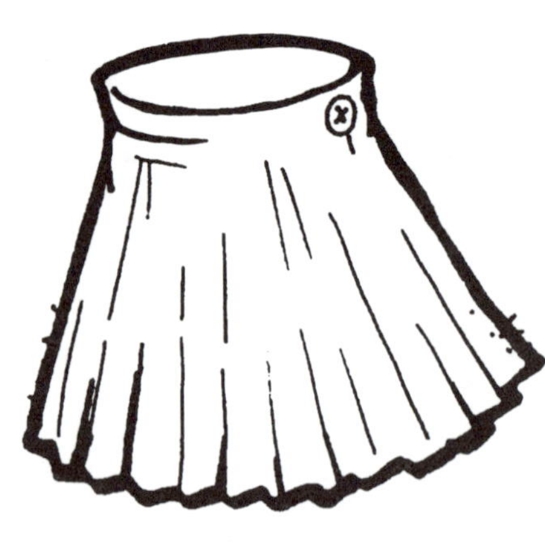

**skirt**

*© 1994 Thinking Publications—Phonogroup*

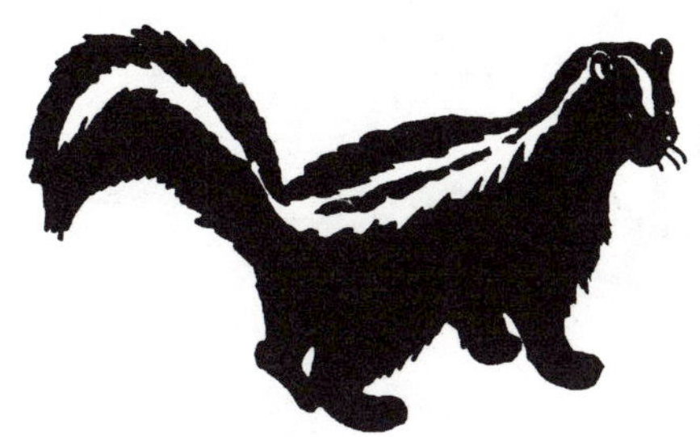

**skunk**



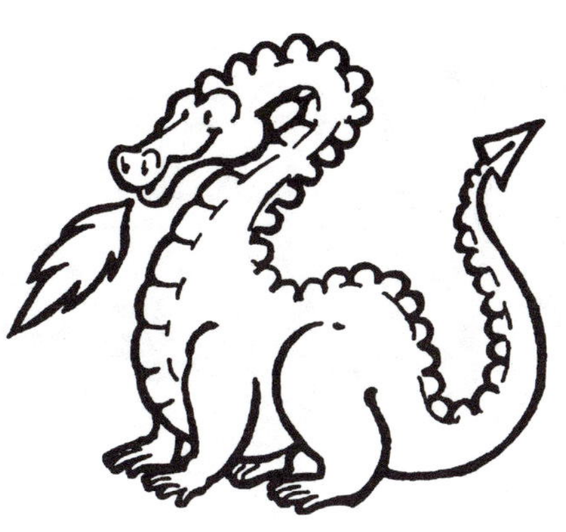

**dragon**



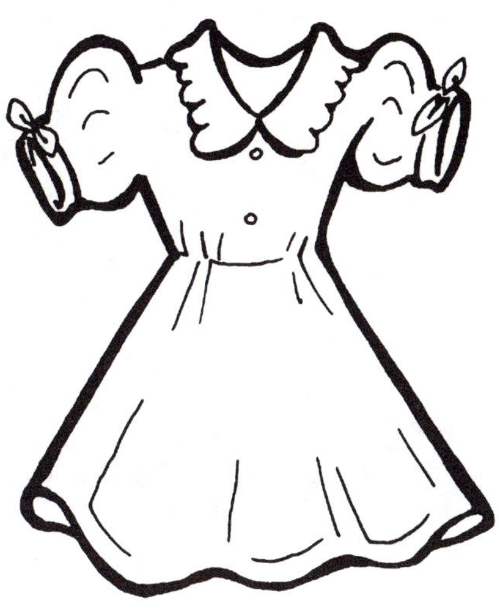

**dress**



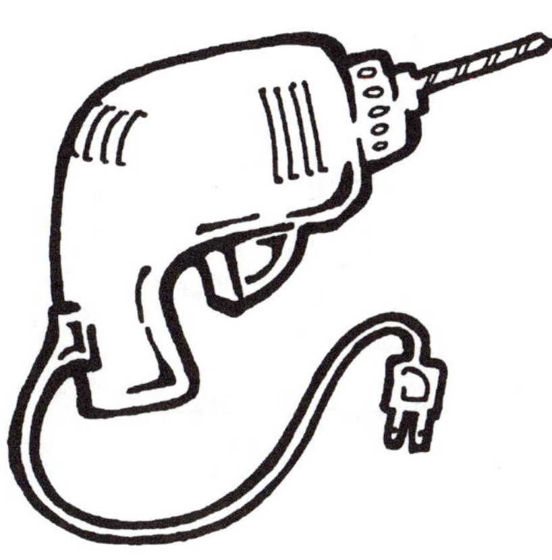

**drill**



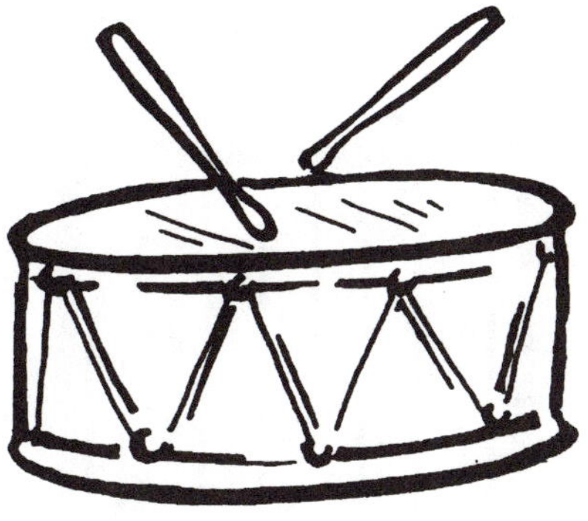

**drum**



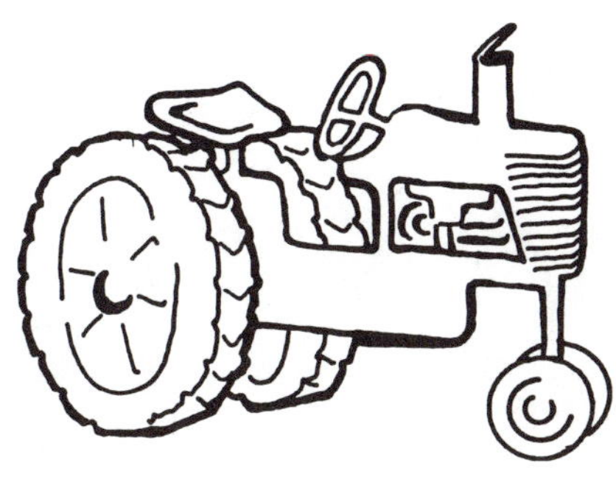

**tractor**

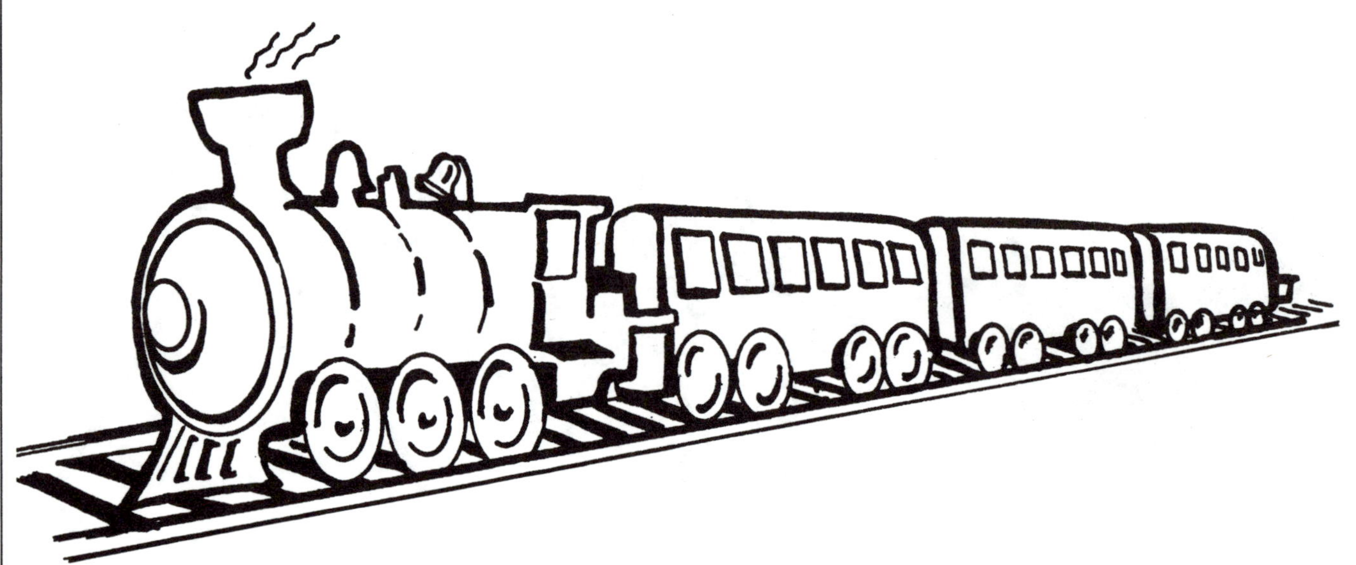

**train**

© 1994 Thinking Publications—Phonogroup

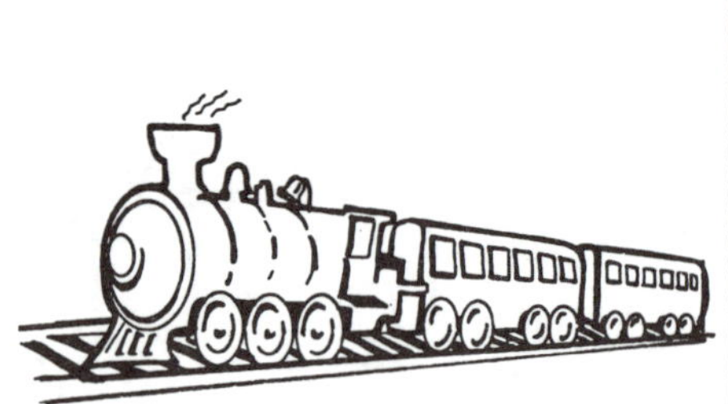

**train**

© 1994 Thinking Publications—Phonogroup

**trash can**

© 1994 Thinking Publications—Phonogroup

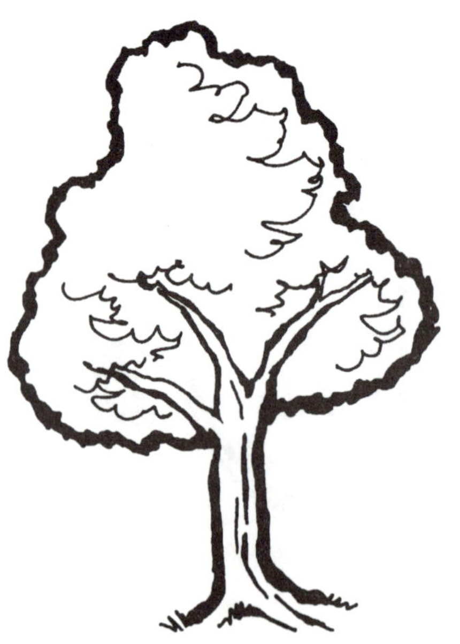

**tree**

© 1994 Thinking Publications—Phonogroup



© 1994 Thinking Publications. Duplication permitted for educational use only.

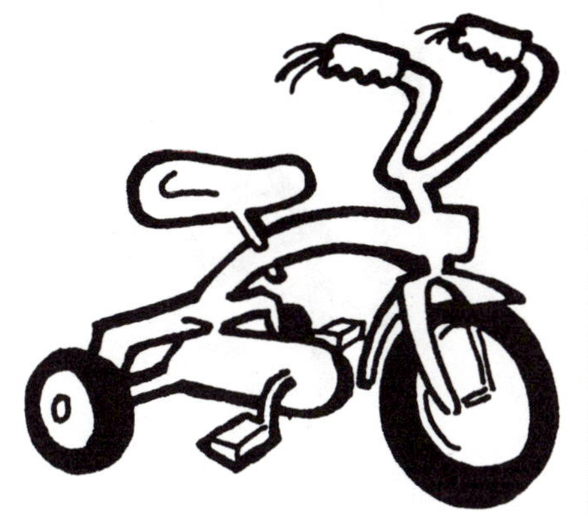

**tricycle**

*© 1994 Thinking Publications—Phonogroup*

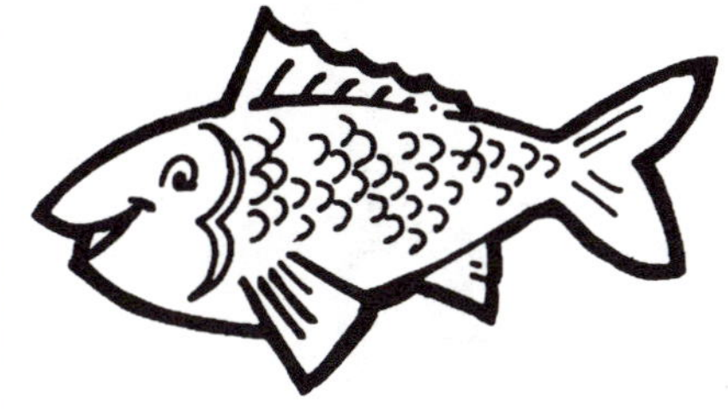

**trout**

*© 1994 Thinking Publications—Phonogroup*

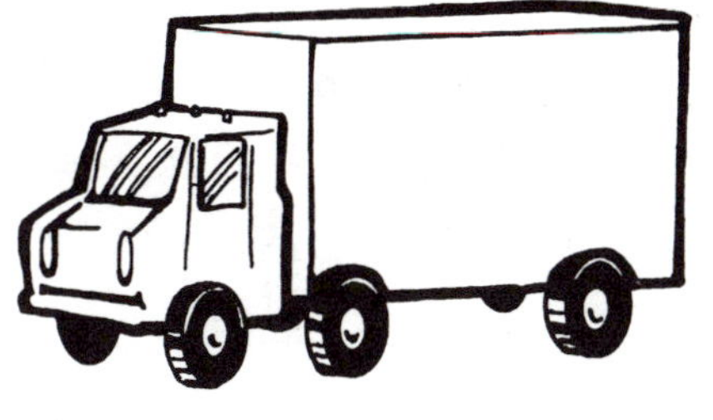

**truck**

*© 1994 Thinking Publications—Phonogroup*

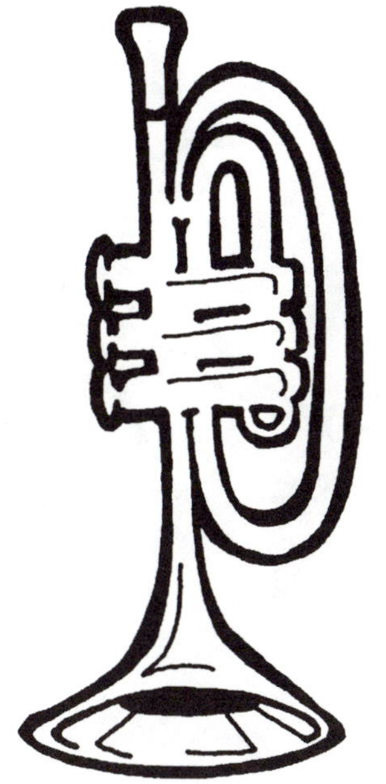

**trumpet**

*© 1994 Thinking Publications—Phonogroup*

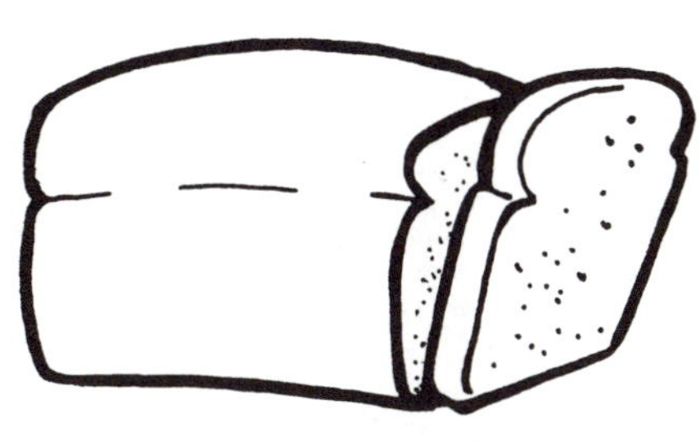

**bread**

*© 1994 Thinking Publications—Phonogroup*

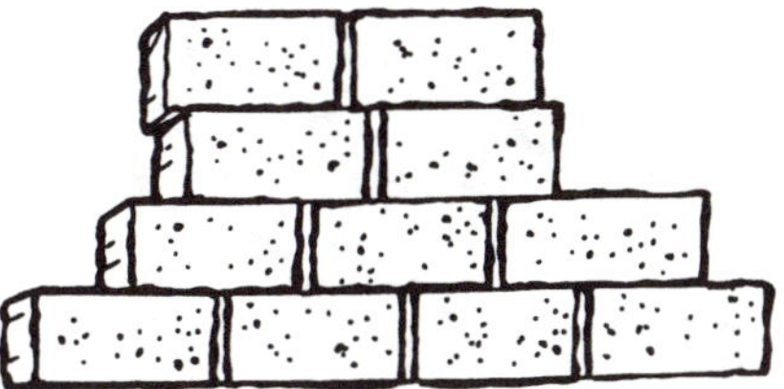

**bricks**

*© 1994 Thinking Publications—Phonogroup*

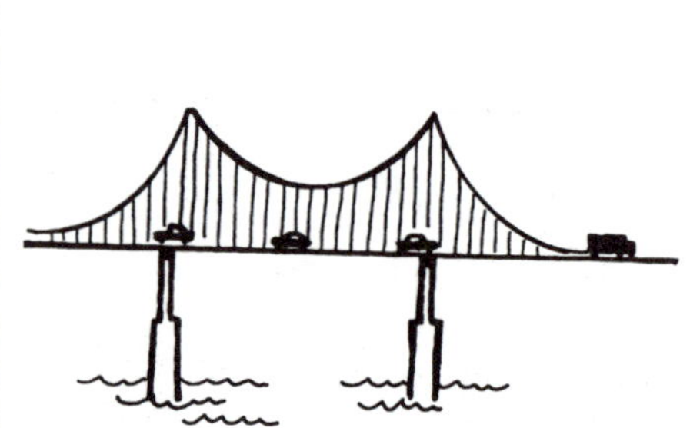

**bridge**



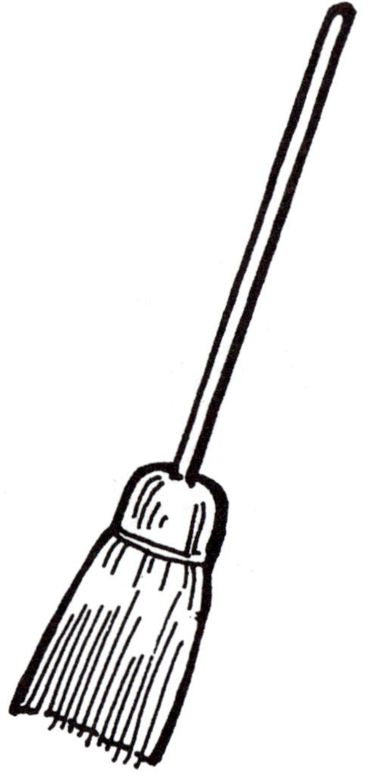

**broom**



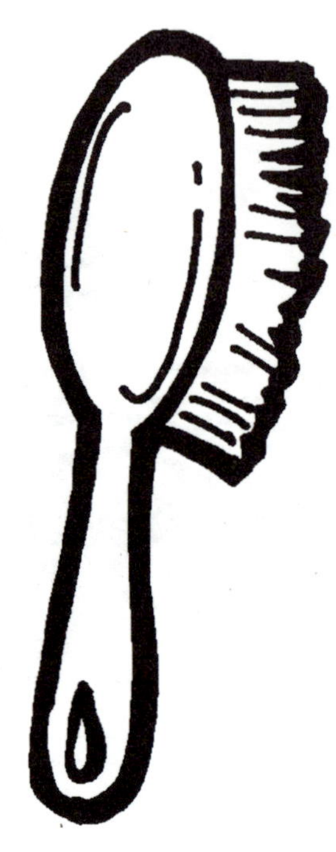

**brush**



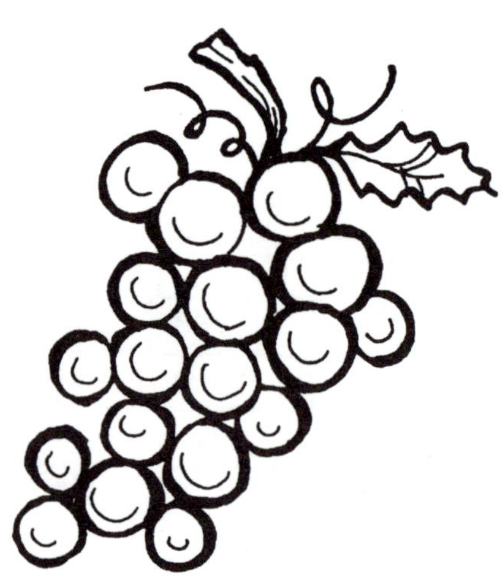

**grapes**



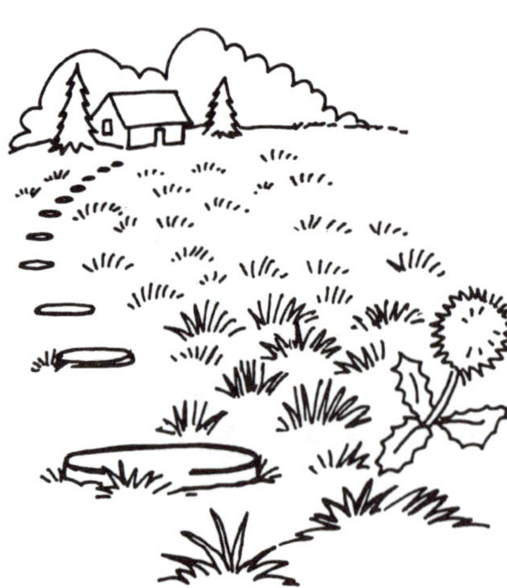

**grass**



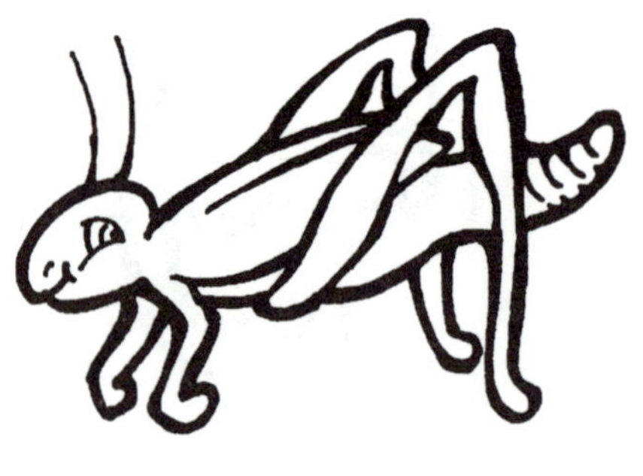

**grasshopper**

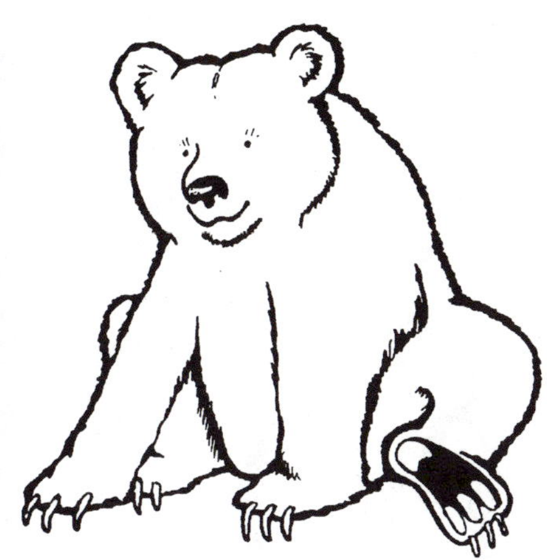

**grizzly bear**
*© 1994 Thinking Publications—Phonogroup*

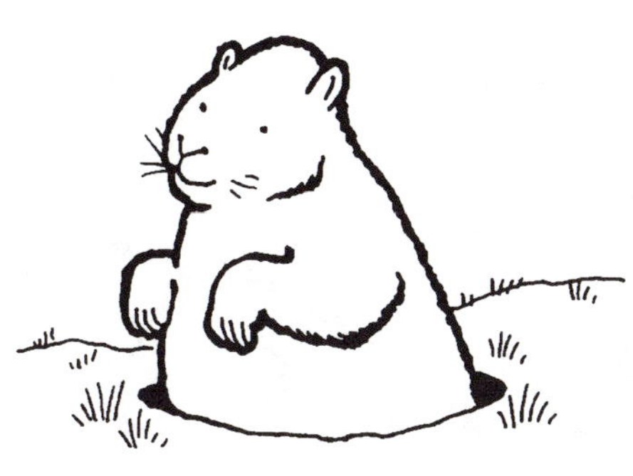

**groundhog**
*© 1994 Thinking Publications—Phonogroup*

**black cat**
*© 1994 Thinking Publications—Phonogroup*

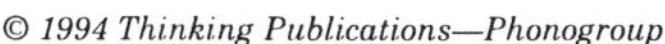

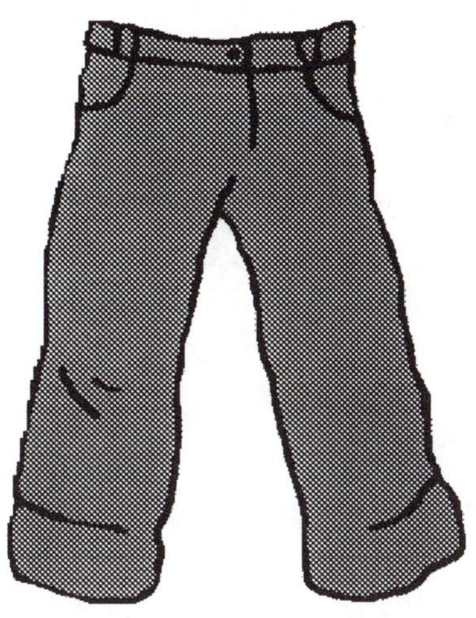

**black pants**
*© 1994 Thinking Publications—Phonogroup*

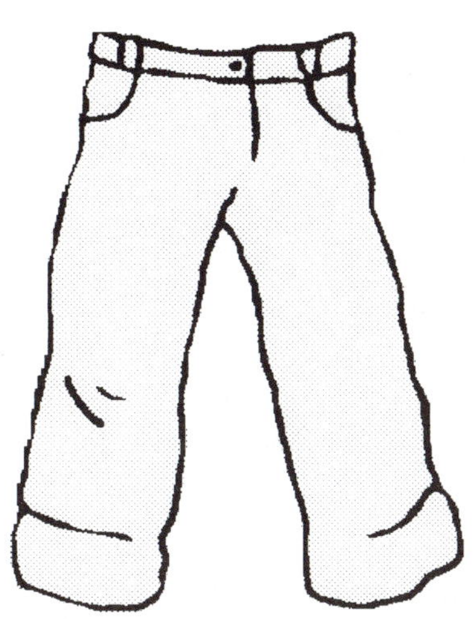

**blue jeans**
*© 1994 Thinking Publications—Phonogroup*

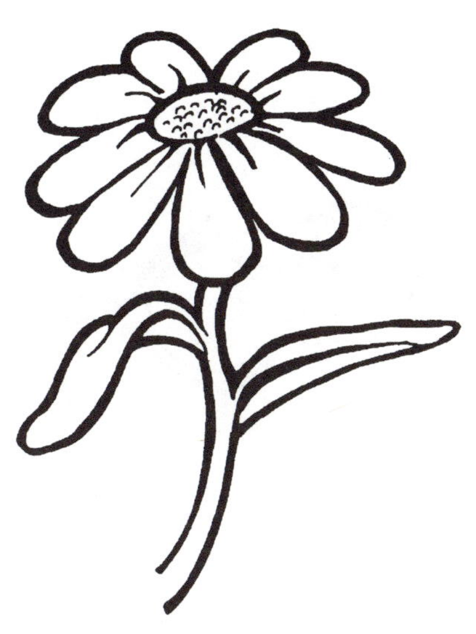

**flower**
*© 1994 Thinking Publications—Phonogroup*

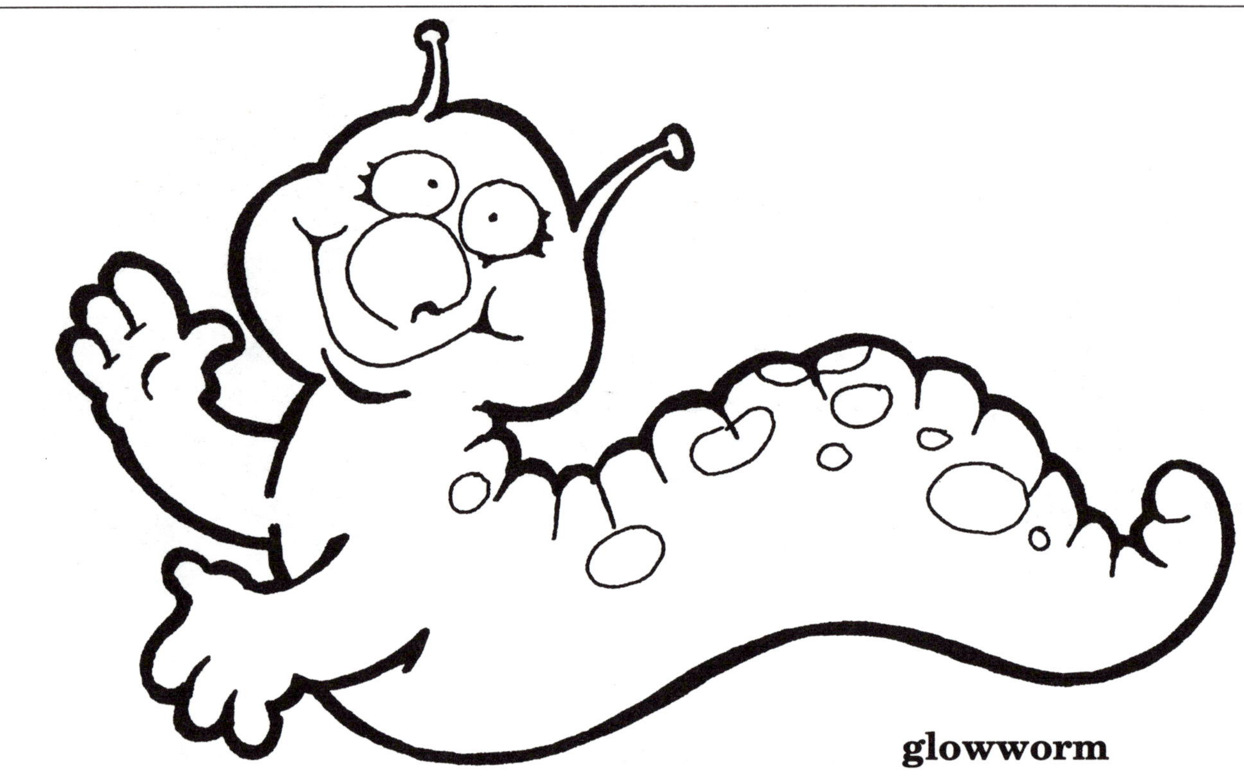

glowworm

© 1994 Thinking Publications—Phonogroup

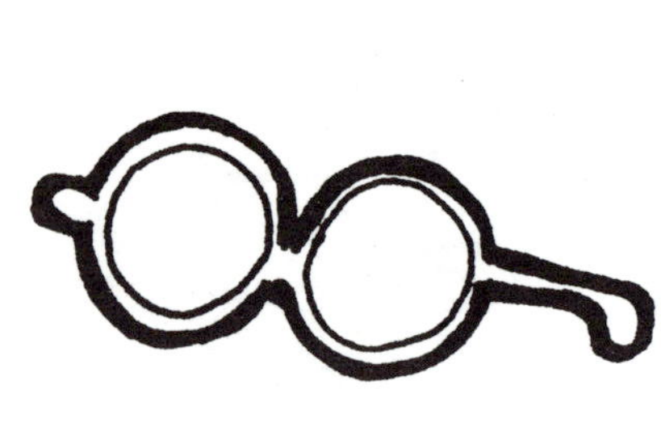

glasses



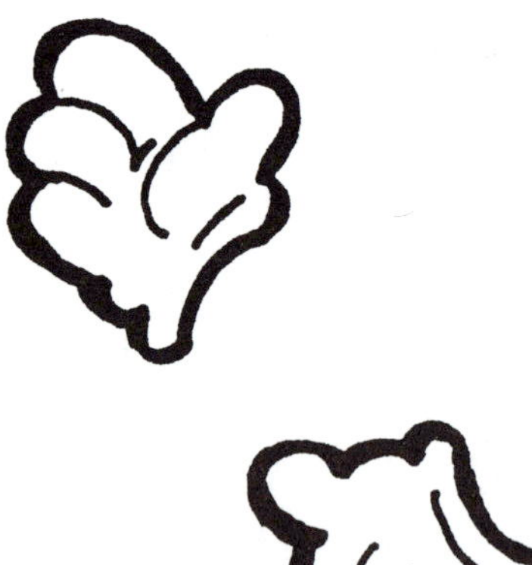

gloves



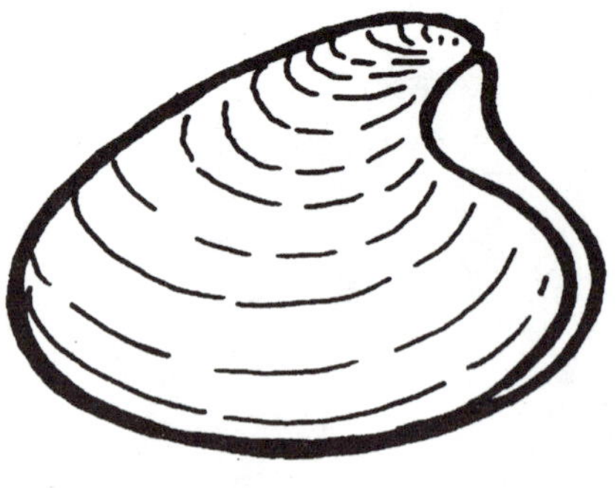

clam

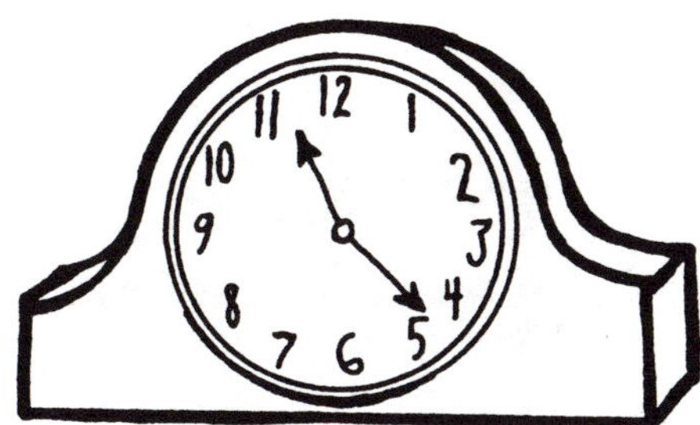

**clock**

**clouds**



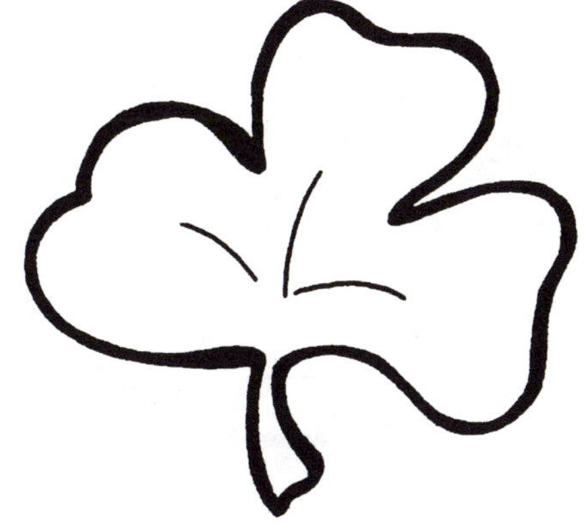

**clover**



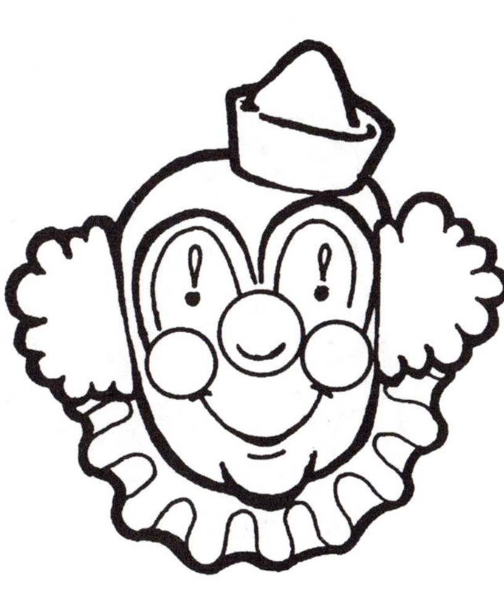

**clown**



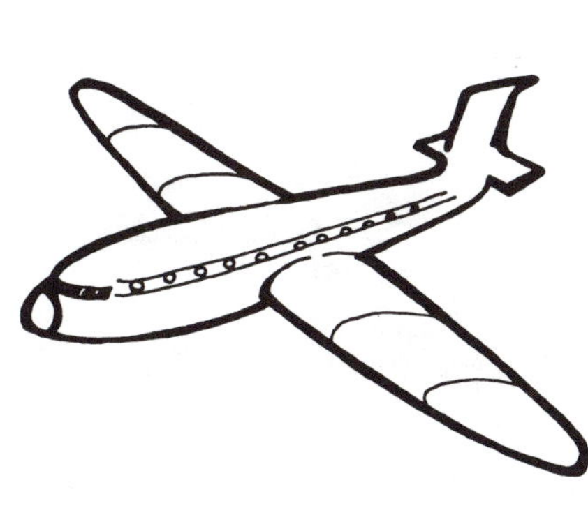

**plane**



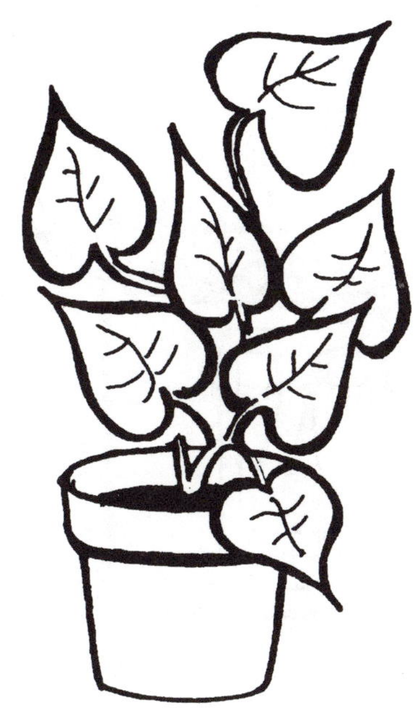

**plant**

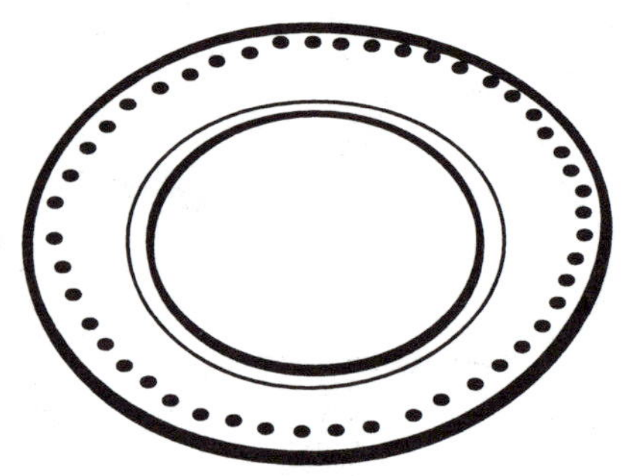

**plate**

*© 1994 Thinking Publications—Phonogroup*

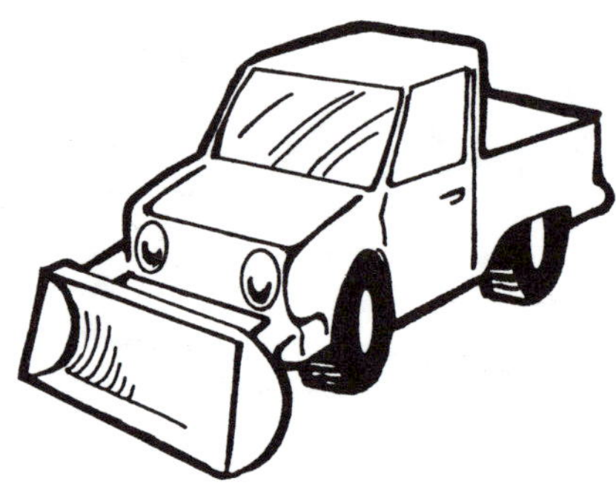

**plow**

*© 1994 Thinking Publications—Phonogroup*

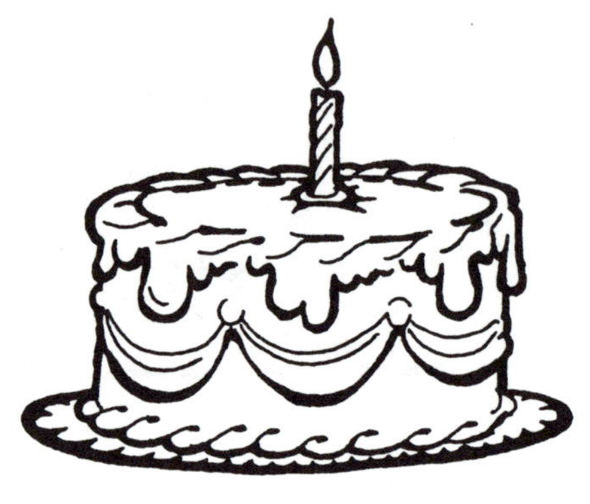

**cake**

*© 1994 Thinking Publications—Phonogroup*

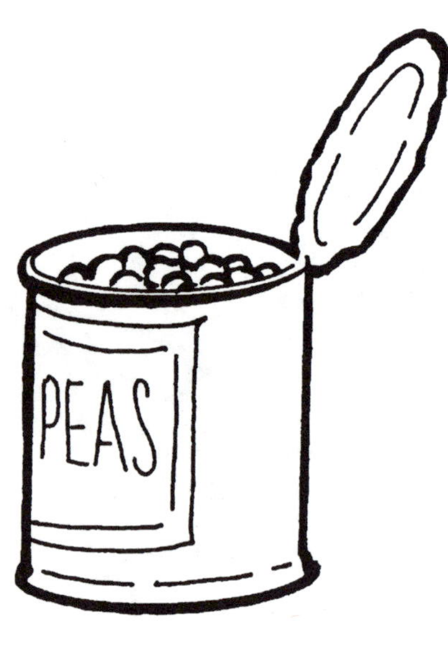


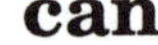

**can**

*© 1994 Thinking Publications—Phonogroup*

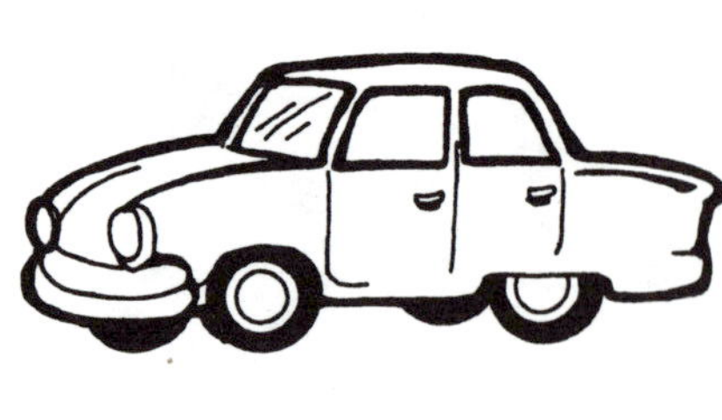

**car**

*© 1994 Thinking Publications—Phonogroup*

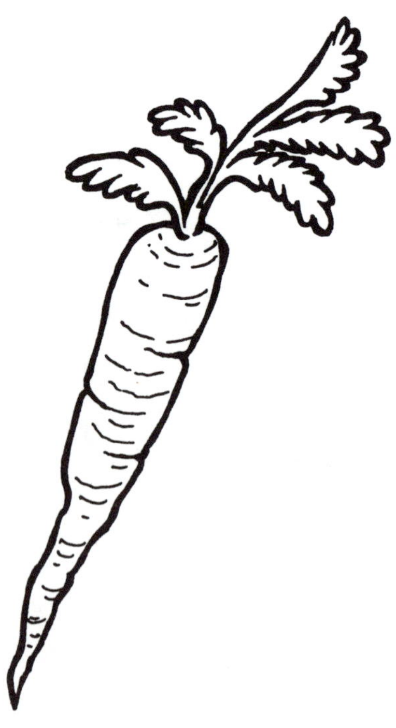

**carrot**

*© 1994 Thinking Publications—Phonogroup*

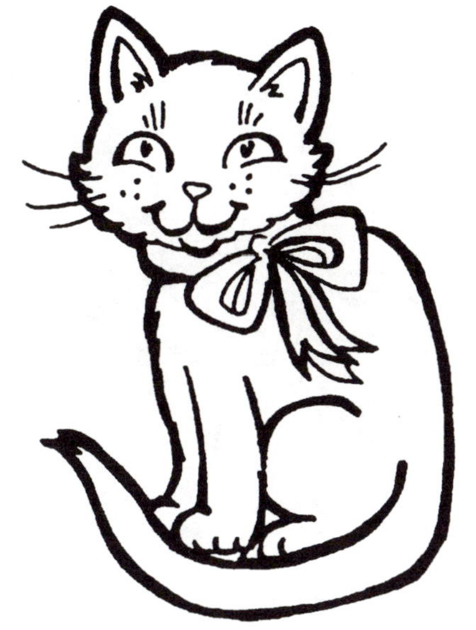

**cat**

© 1994 Thinking Publications—Phonogroup

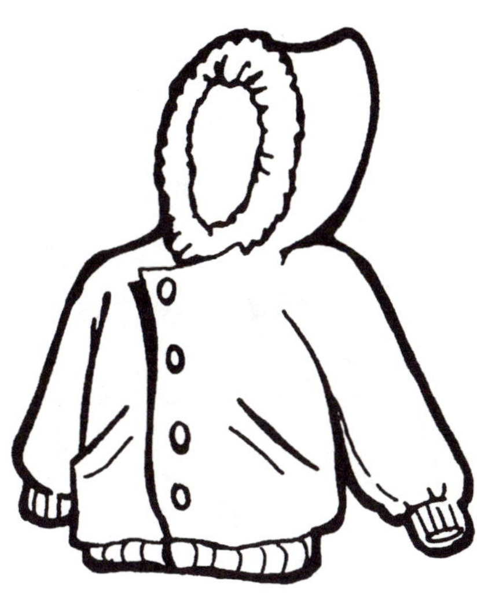

**coat**

© 1994 Thinking Publications—Phonogroup

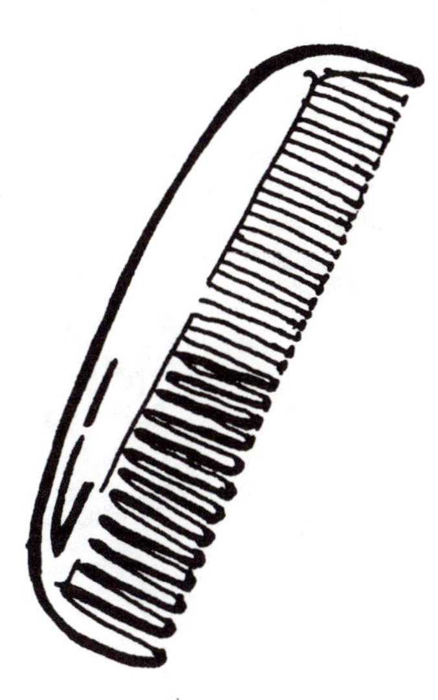

**comb**

© 1994 Thinking Publications—Phonogroup

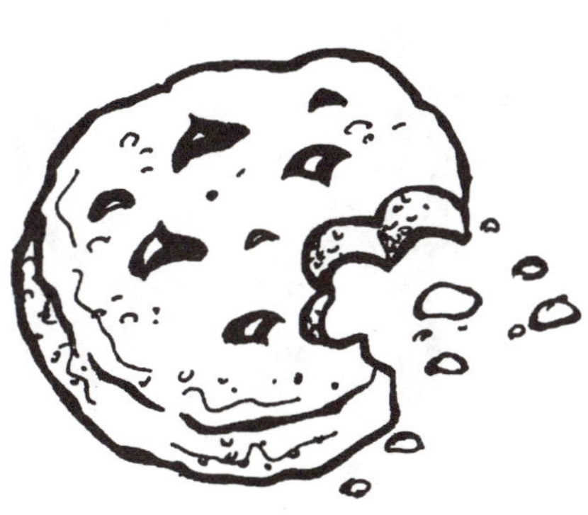

**cookie**

© 1994 Thinking Publications—Phonogroup

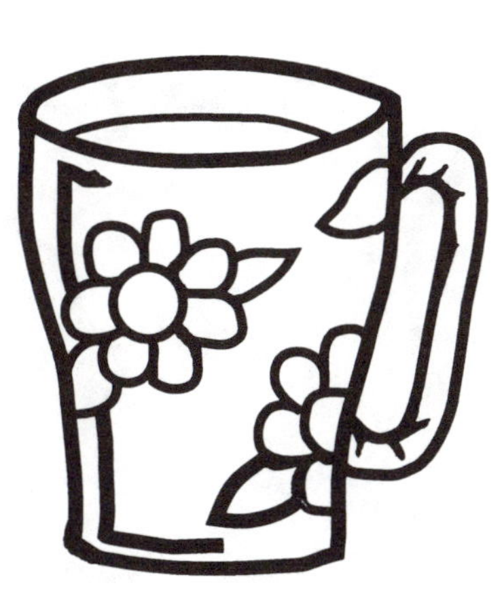

**cup**

© 1994 Thinking Publications—Phonogroup

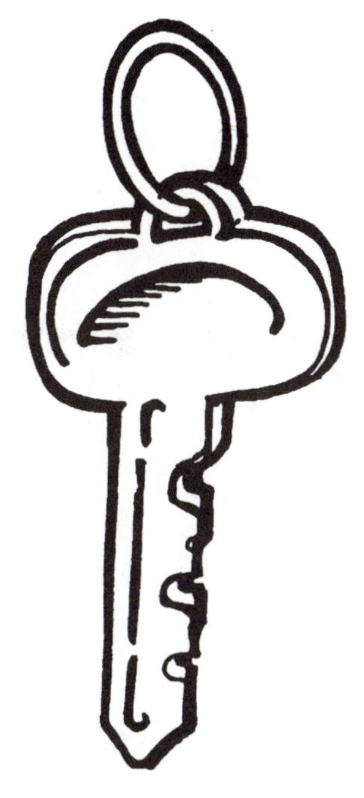

**key**

© 1994 Thinking Publications—Phonogroup

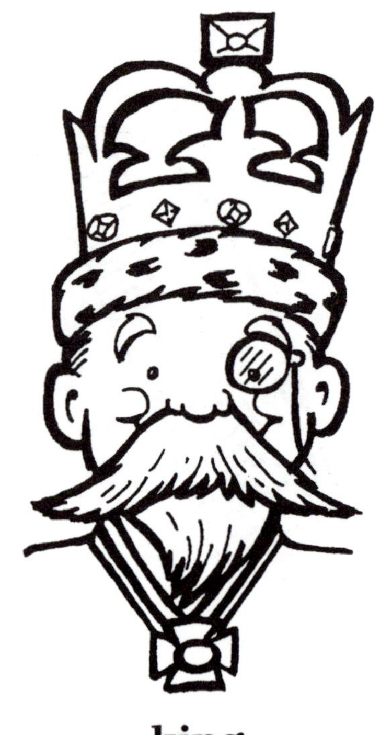

**king**



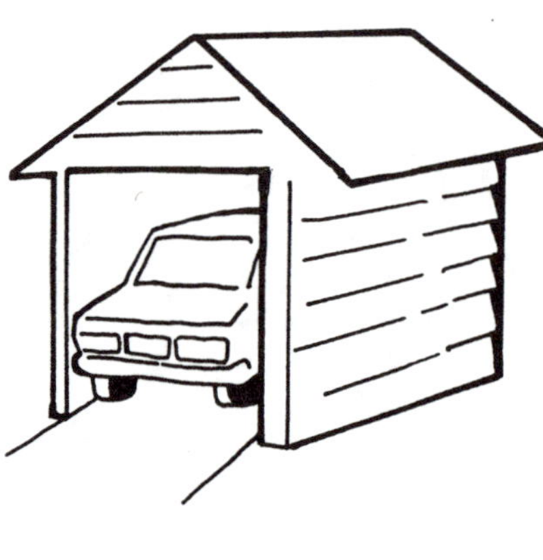

**garage**



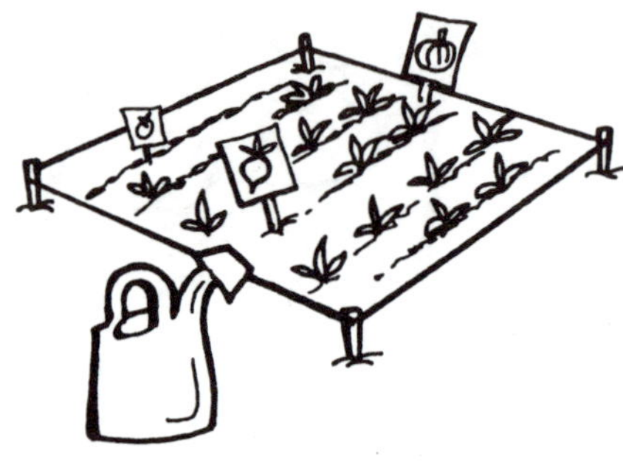

**garden**



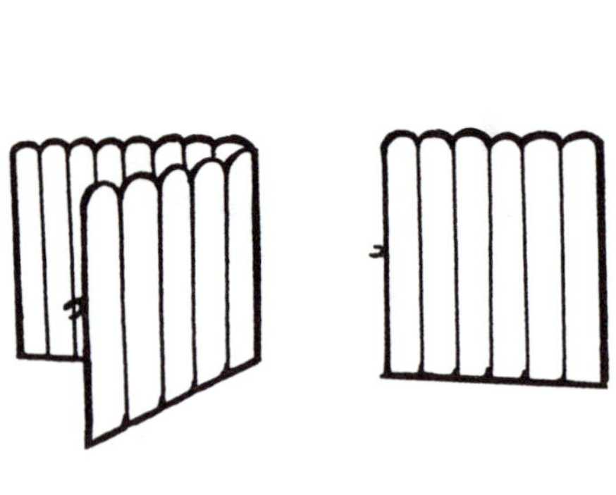
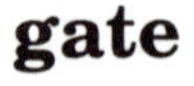

**gate**



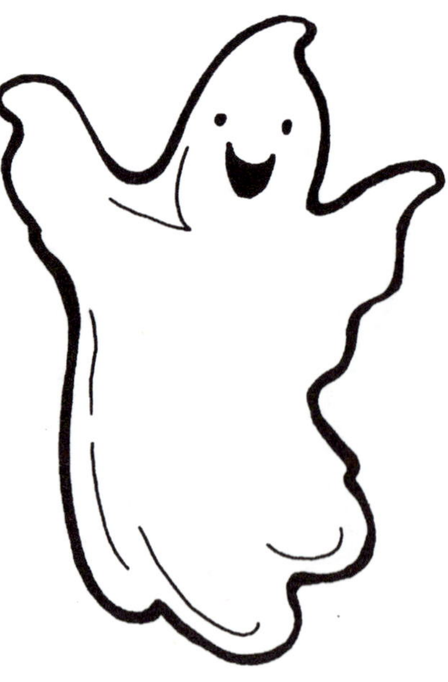

**ghost**



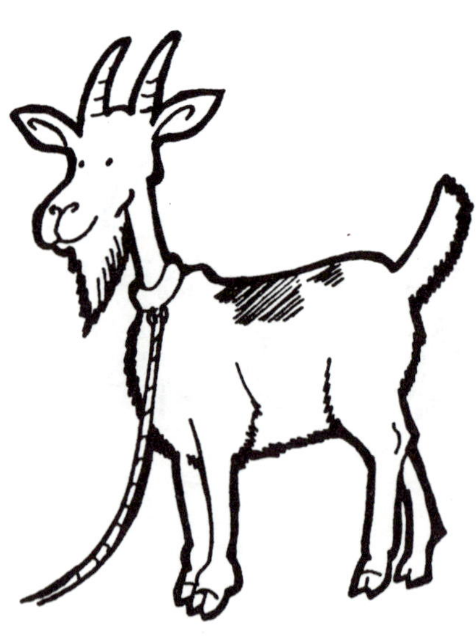

**goat**

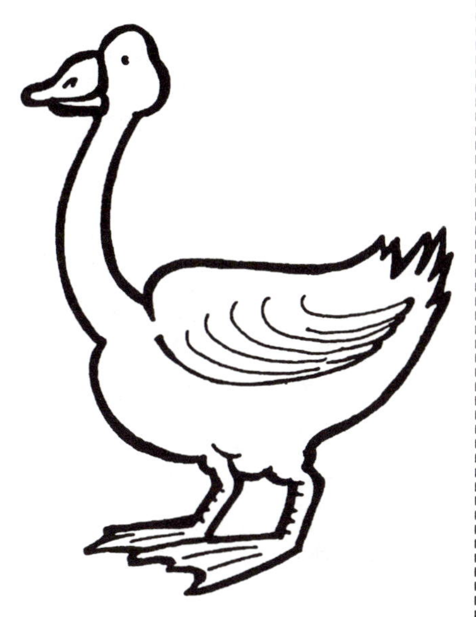

**goose**
*© 1994 Thinking Publications—Phonogroup*

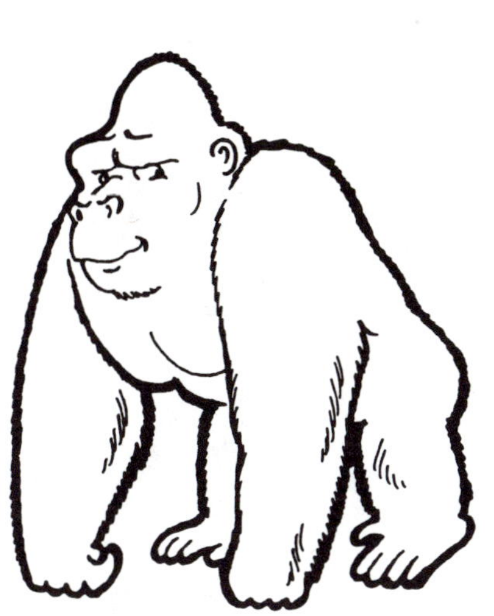

**gorilla**
*© 1994 Thinking Publications—Phonogroup*

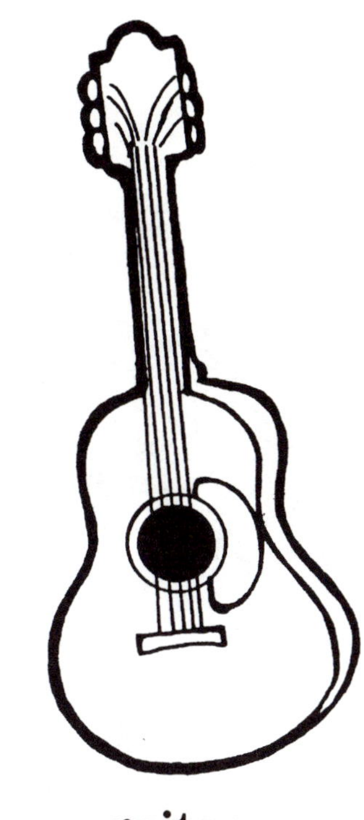

**guitar**
*© 1994 Thinking Publications—Phonogroup*

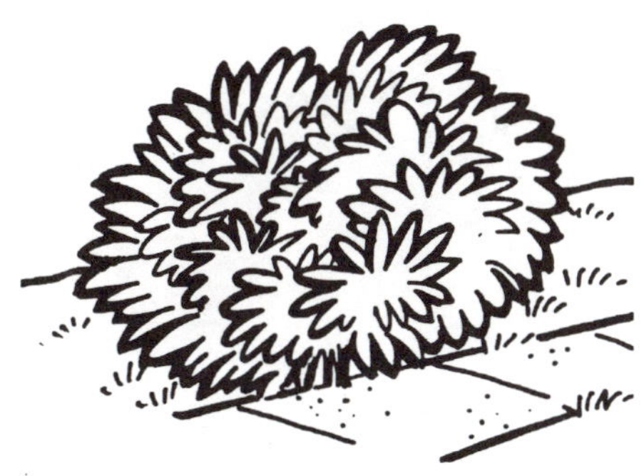

**bush**
*© 1994 Thinking Publications—Phonogroup*

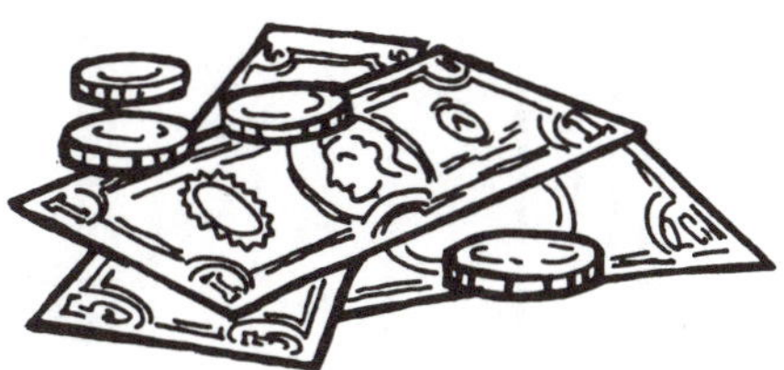

**cash**
*© 1994 Thinking Publications—Phonogroup*

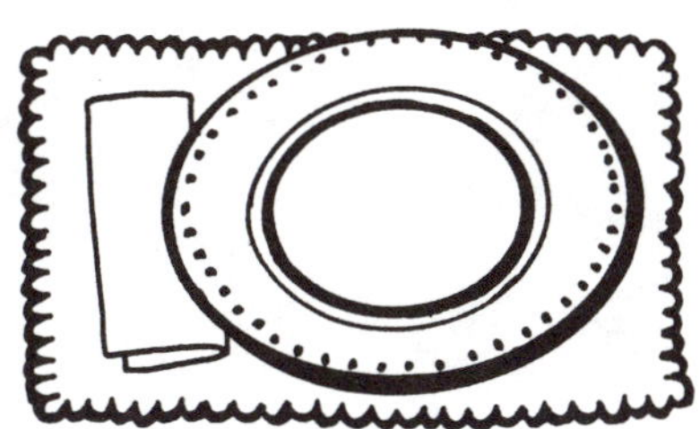

**dish**
*© 1994 Thinking Publications—Phonogroup*

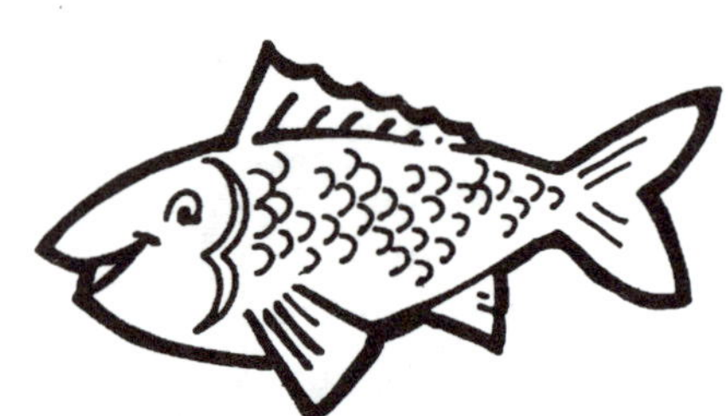

**fish**



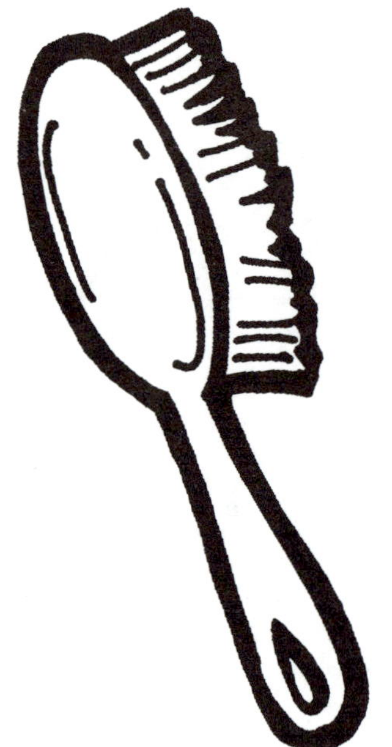

**hairbrush**



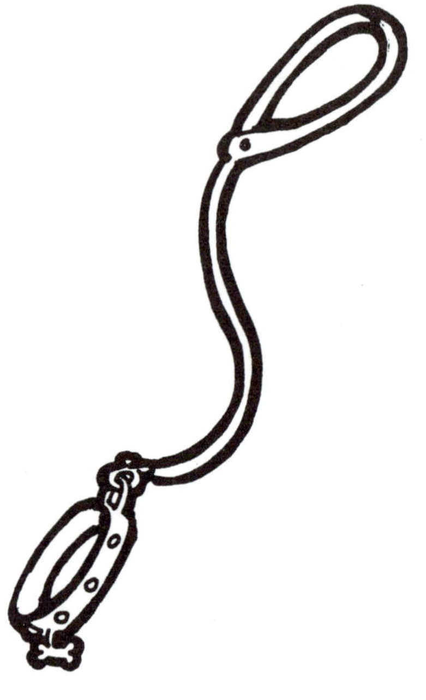

**leash**



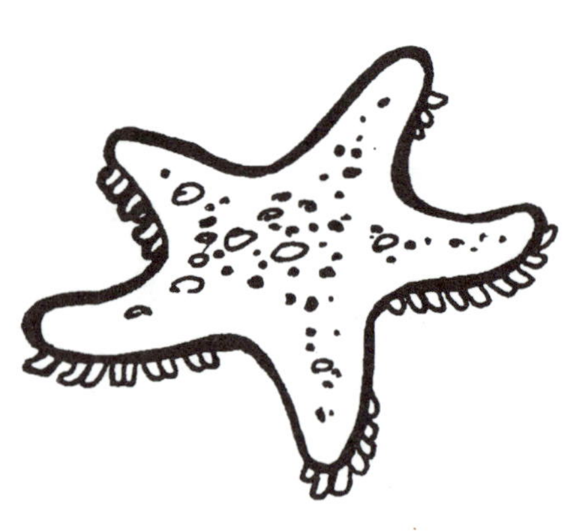

**starfish**

**trash**



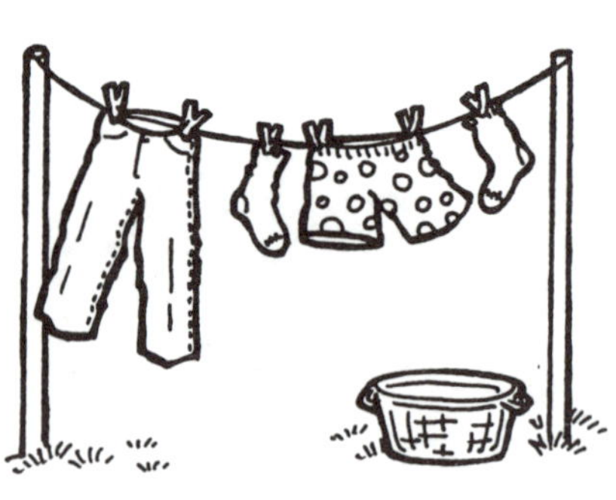

**wash**

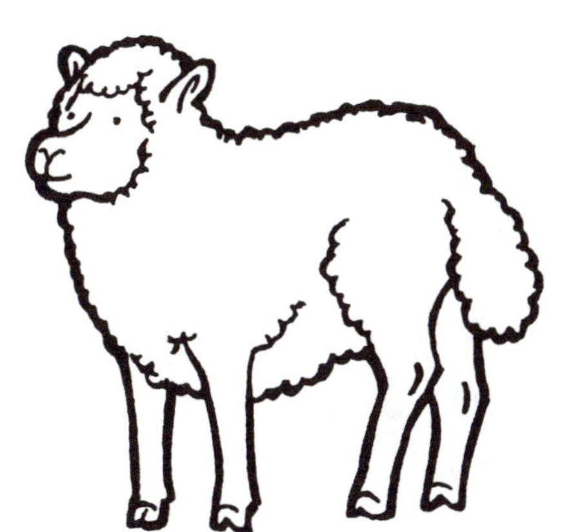

**sheep**
*© 1994 Thinking Publications—Phonogroup*

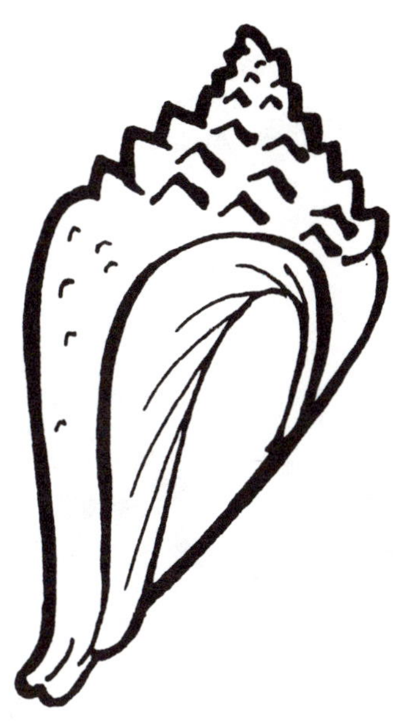

**shell**
*© 1994 Thinking Publications—Phonogroup*

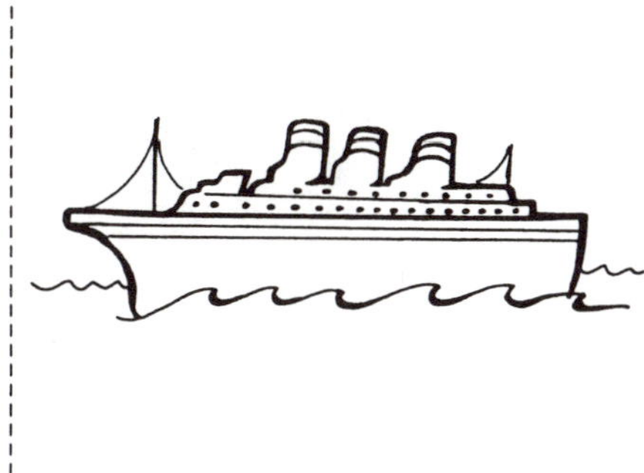

**ship**
*© 1994 Thinking Publications—Phonogroup*

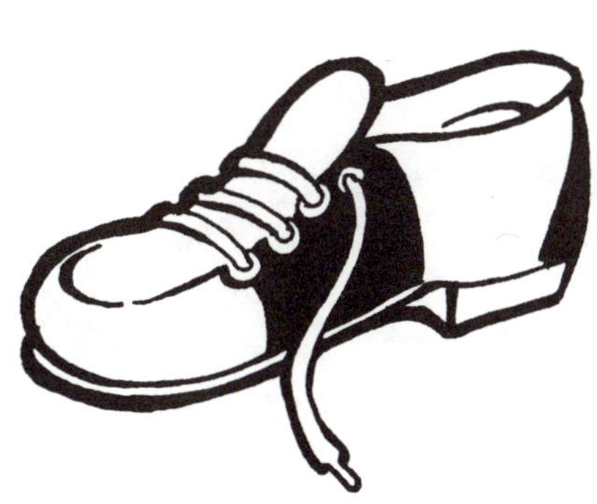

**shoe**
*© 1994 Thinking Publications—Phonogroup*

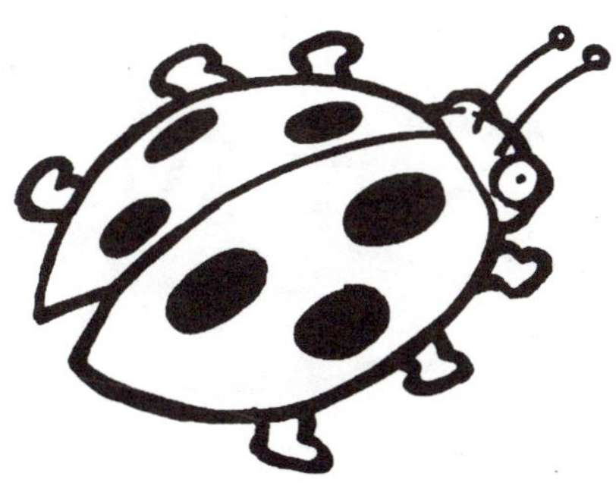

**ladybug**
*© 1994 Thinking Publications—Phonogroup*

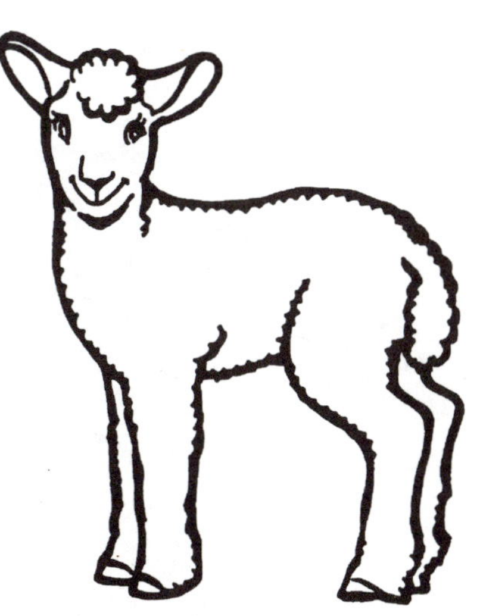

**lamb**
*© 1994 Thinking Publications—Phonogroup*

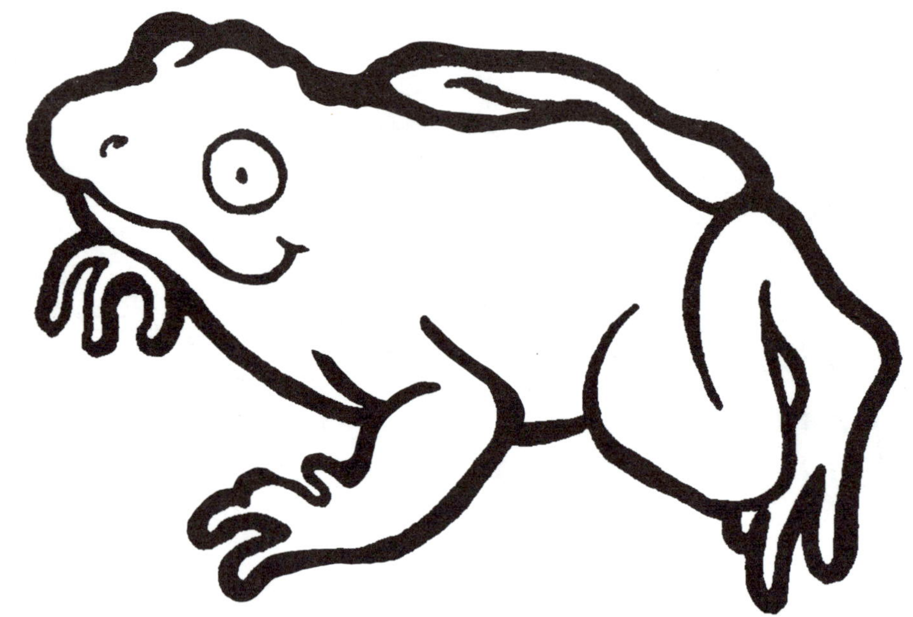

**leapfrog**

© *1994 Thinking Publications—Phonogroup*

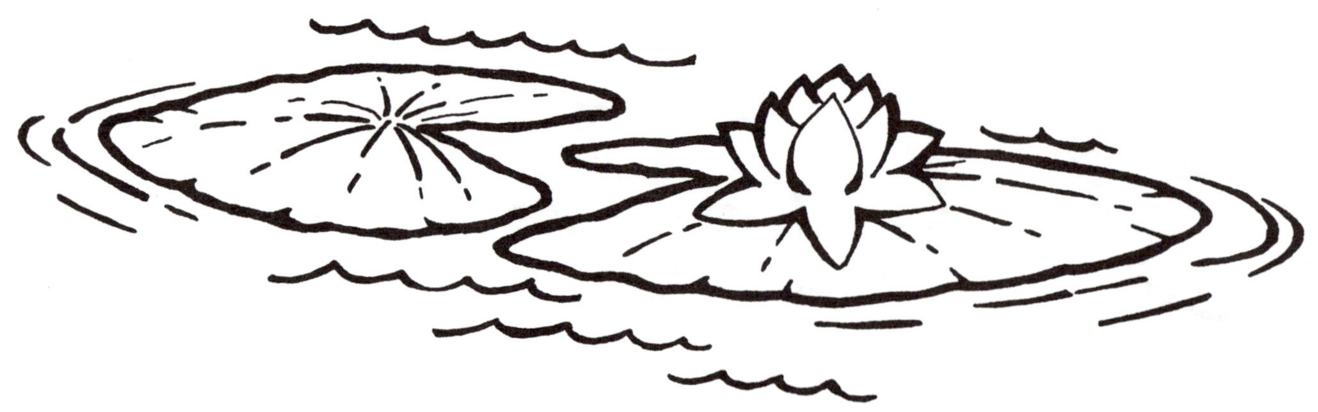

**lily pad**

© *1994 Thinking Publications—Phonogroup*

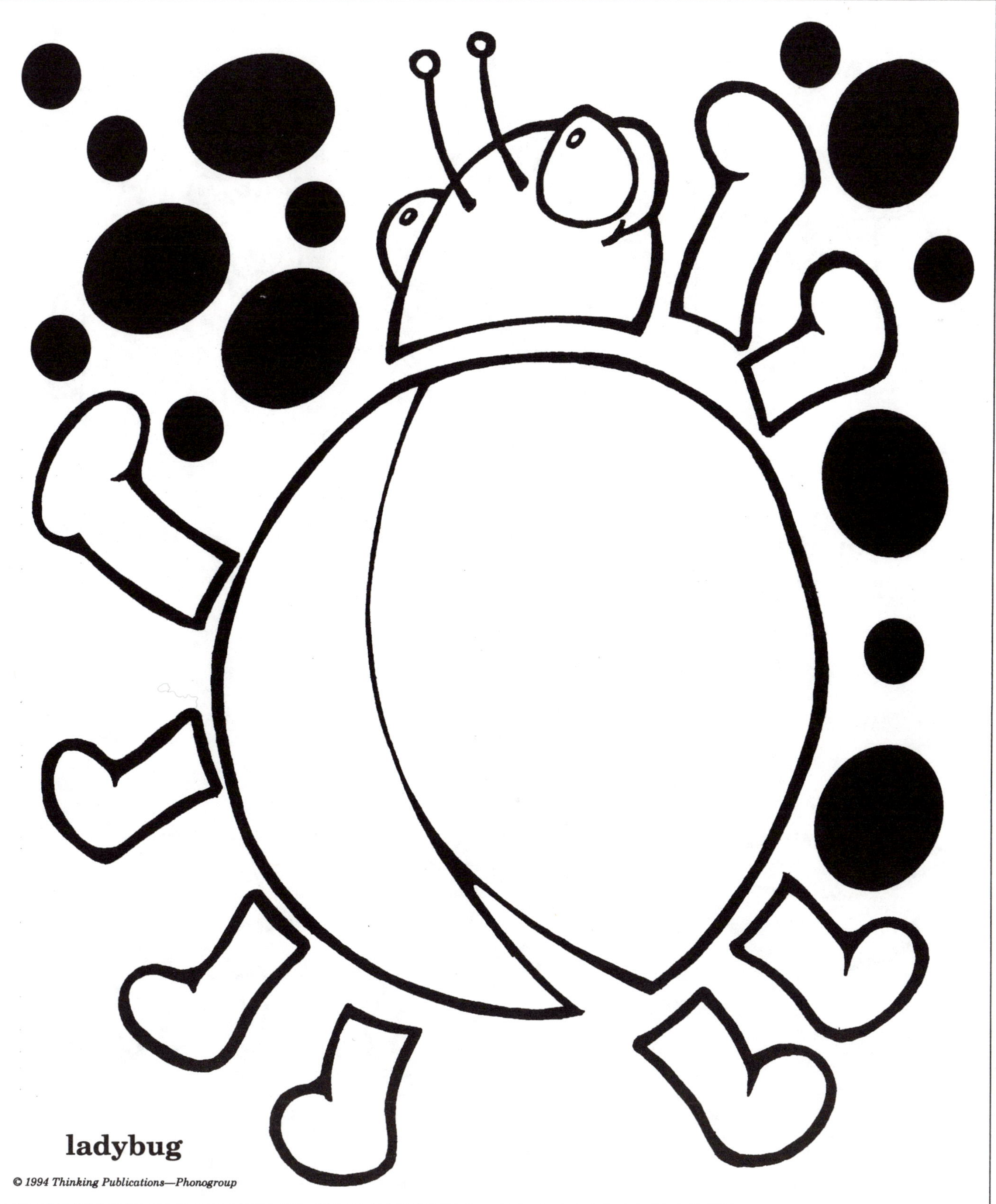

**ladybug**

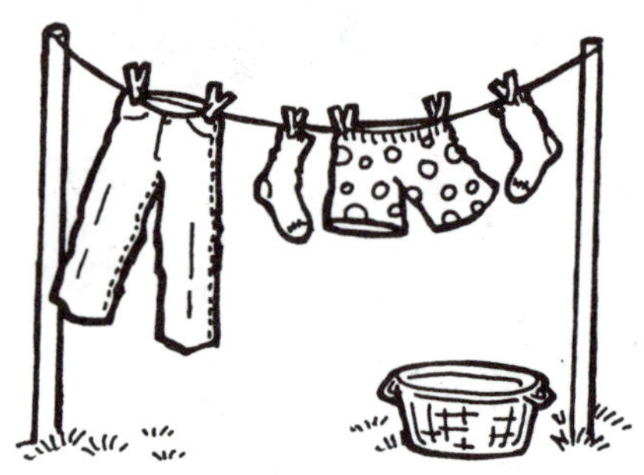

**laundry**

*© 1994 Thinking Publications—Phonogroup*

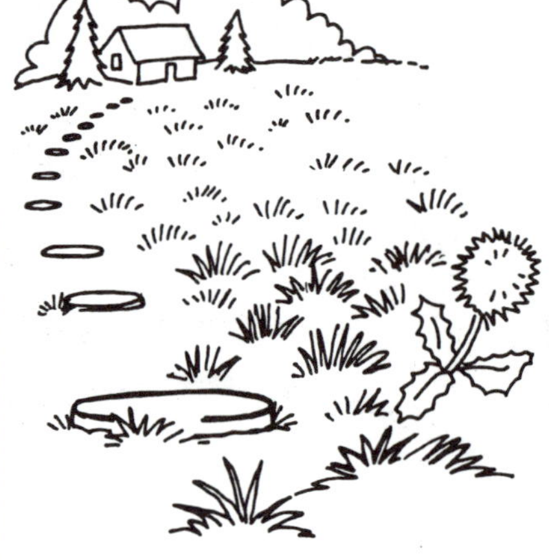

**lawn**

*© 1994 Thinking Publications—Phonogroup*

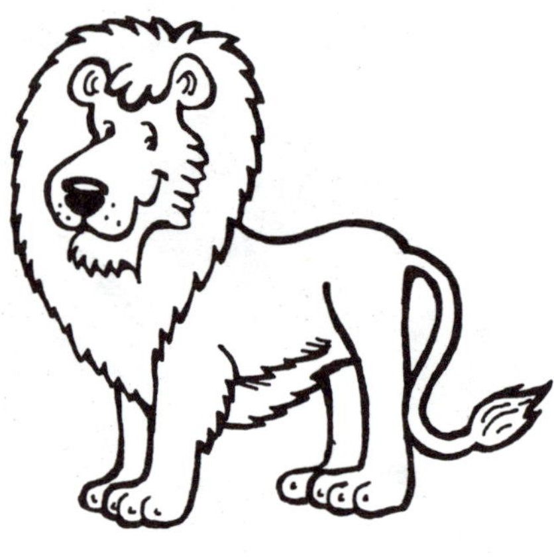

**lion**

*© 1994 Thinking Publications—Phonogroup*

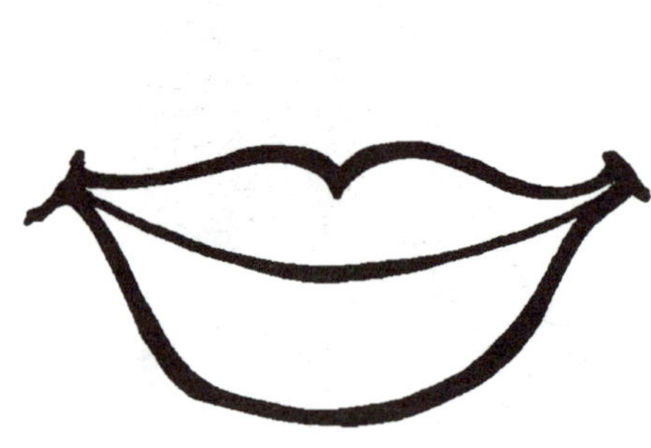

**lips**

*© 1994 Thinking Publications—Phonogroup*

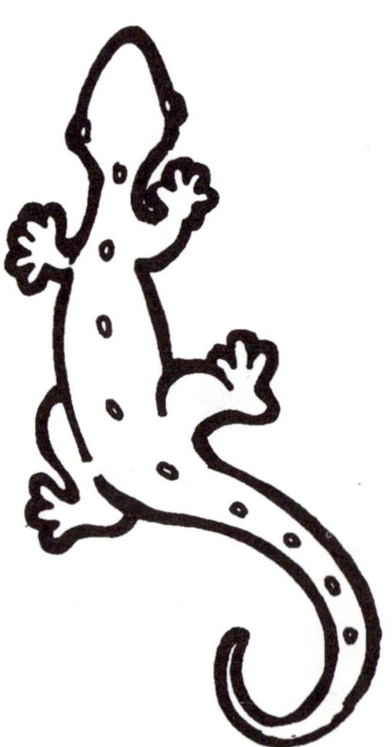

**lizard**

*© 1994 Thinking Publications—Phonogroup*

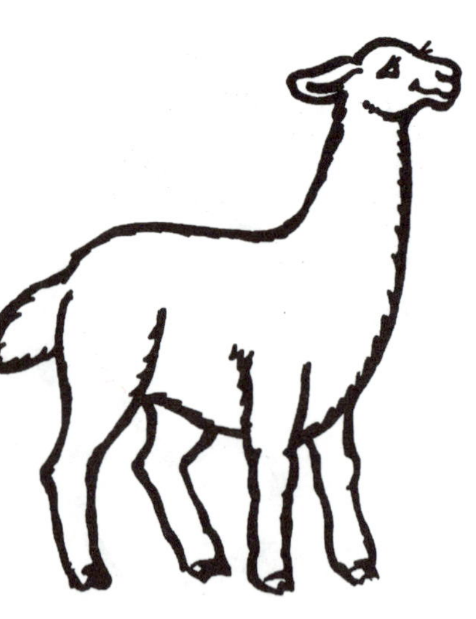

**llama**

*© 1994 Thinking Publications—Phonogroup*

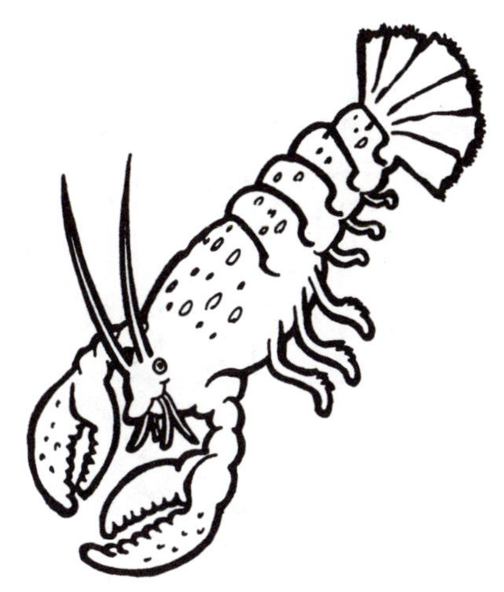

**lobster**

*© 1994 Thinking Publications—Phonogroup*

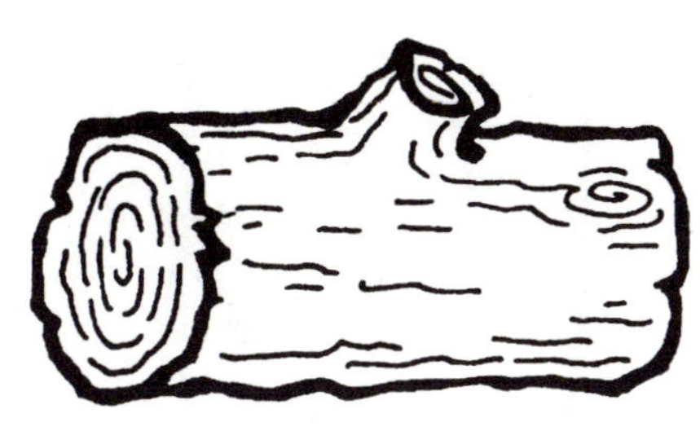

**log**

*© 1994 Thinking Publications—Phonogroup*

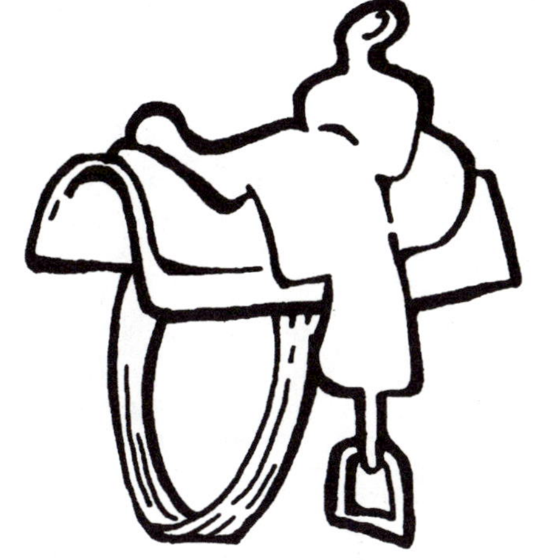

**saddle**

*© 1994 Thinking Publications—Phonogroup*

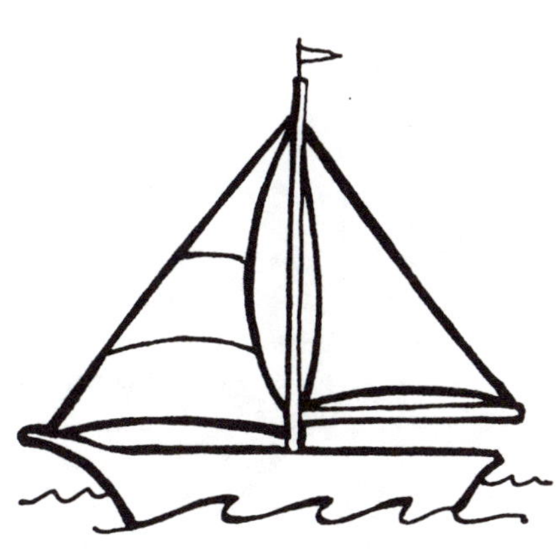

**sailboat**

*© 1994 Thinking Publications—Phonogroup*

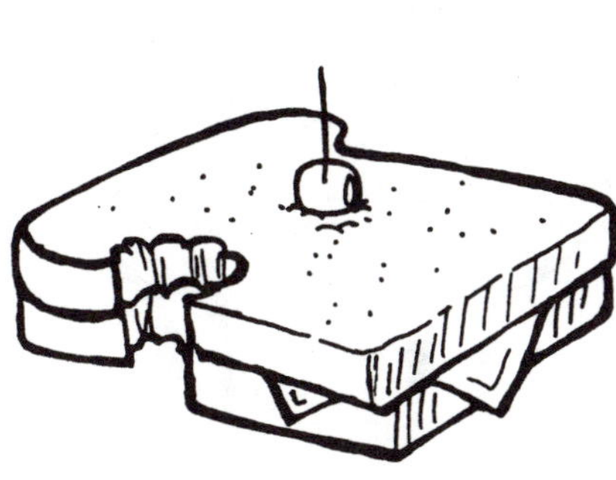

**sandwich**

*© 1994 Thinking Publications—Phonogroup*

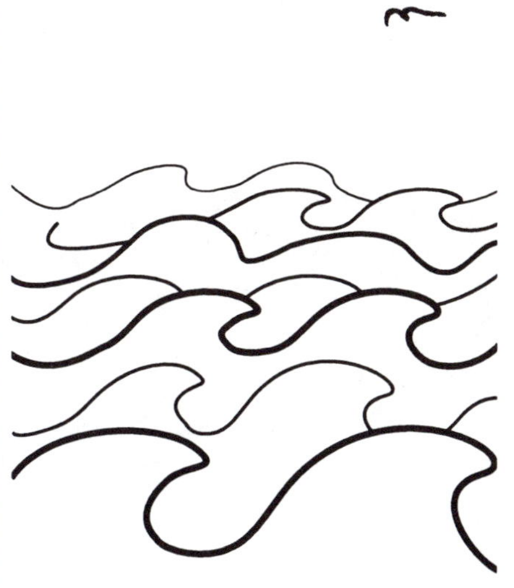

**sea**

*© 1994 Thinking Publications—Phonogroup*

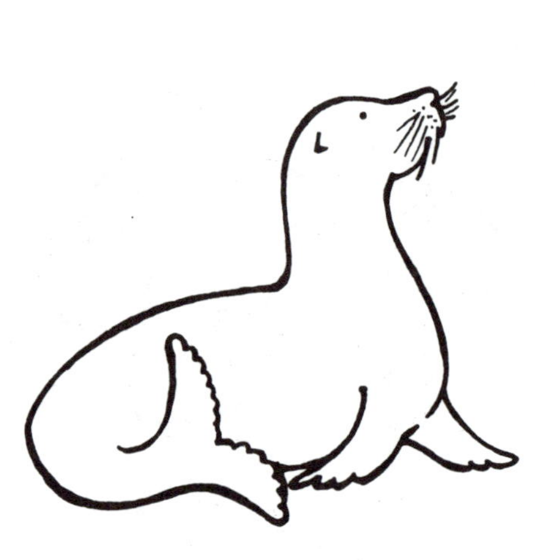

**seal**



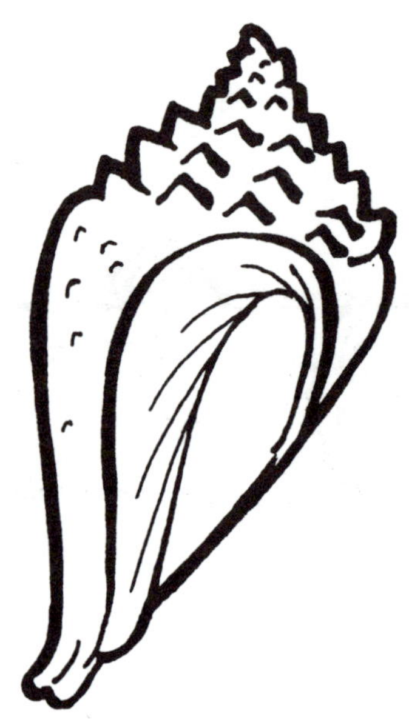

**seashell**



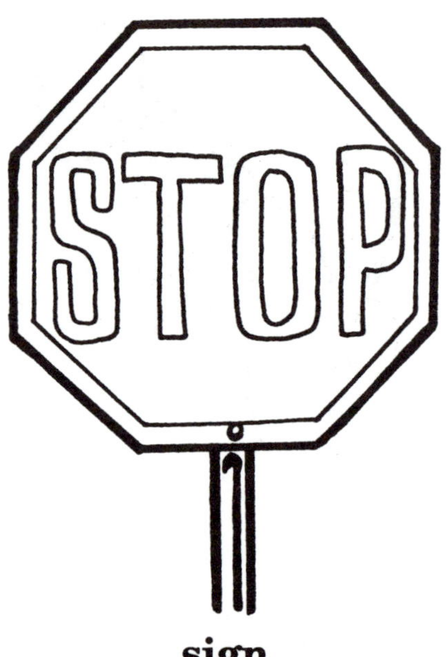



**sign**



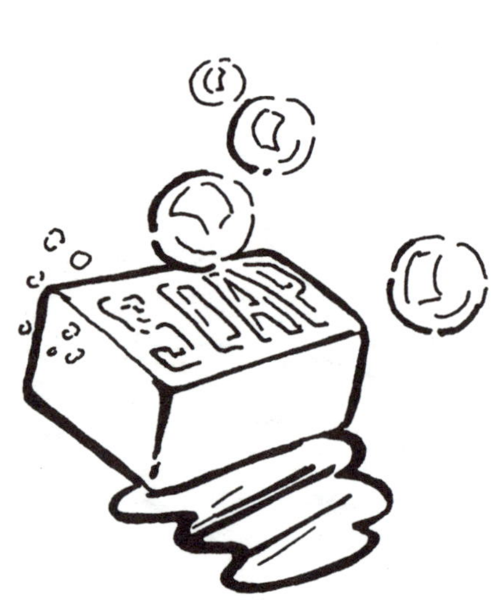



**soap**



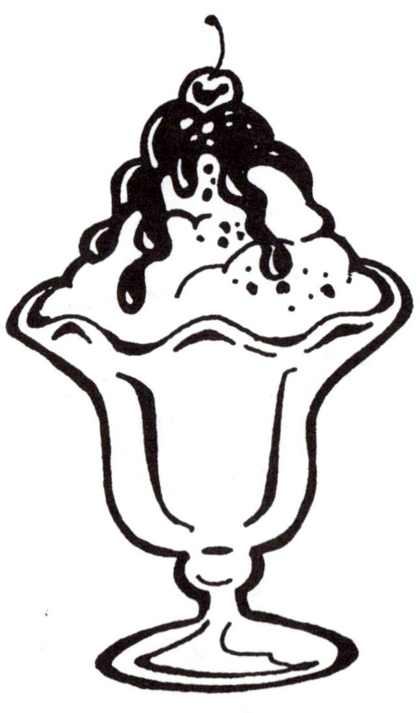

**sundae**



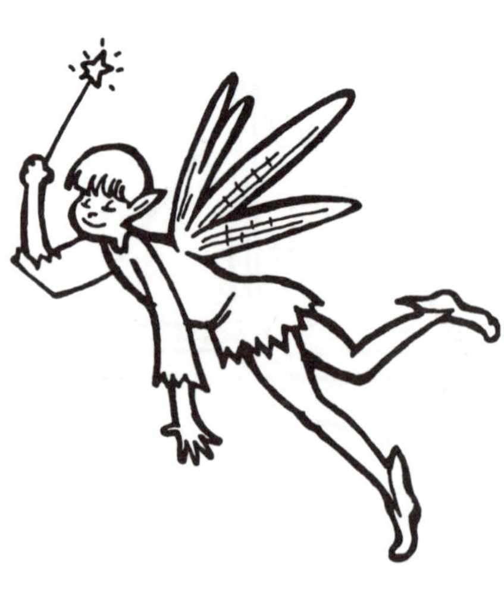

**fairy**

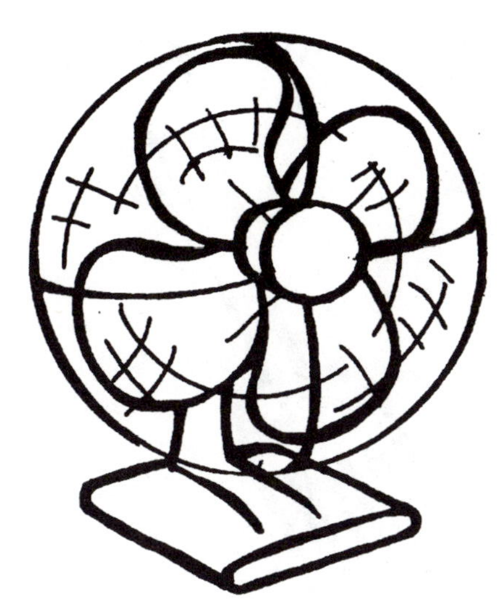

**fan**

© *1994 Thinking Publications—Phonogroup*

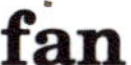

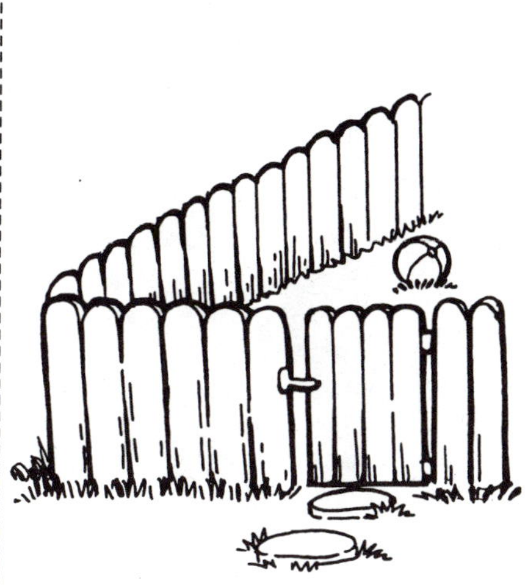

**fence**

© *1994 Thinking Publications—Phonogroup*

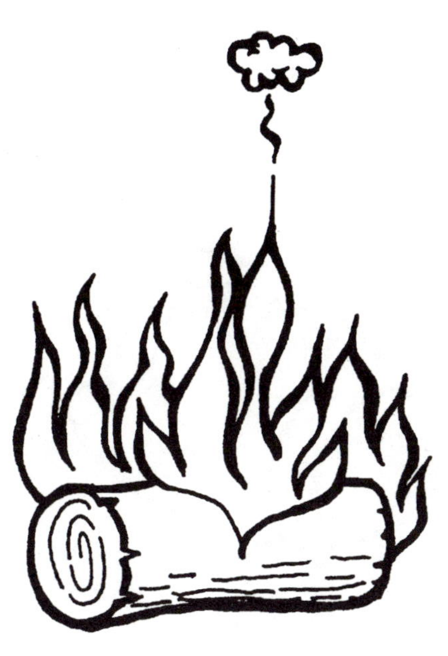

**fire**

© *1994 Thinking Publications—Phonogroup*

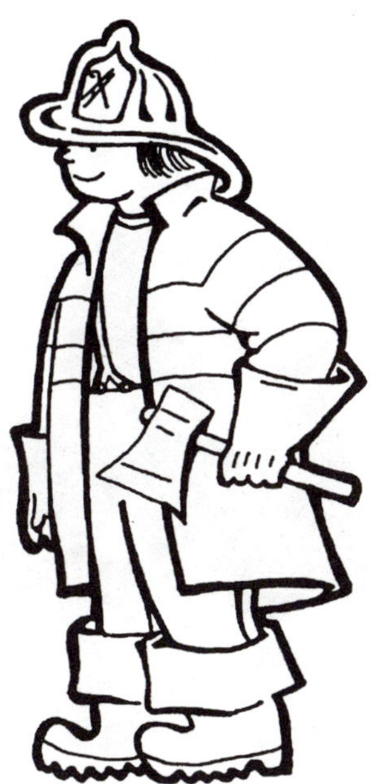

**firefighter**

© *1994 Thinking Publications—Phonogroup*

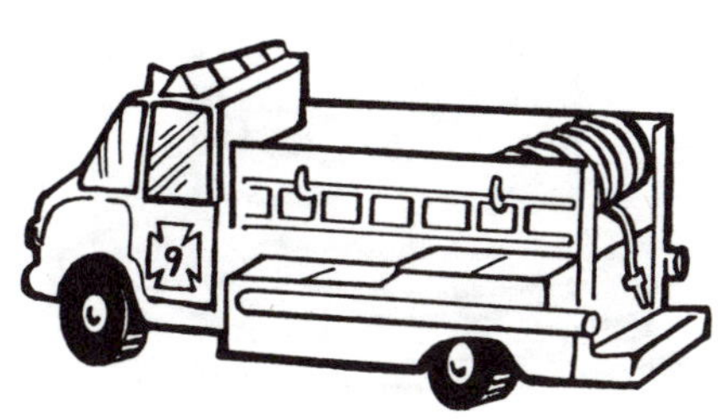

**fire truck**

© *1994 Thinking Publications—Phonogroup*

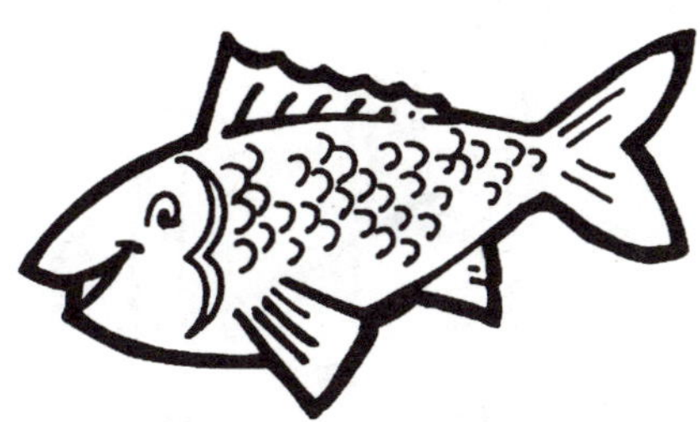

**fish**

© *1994 Thinking Publications—Phonogroup*

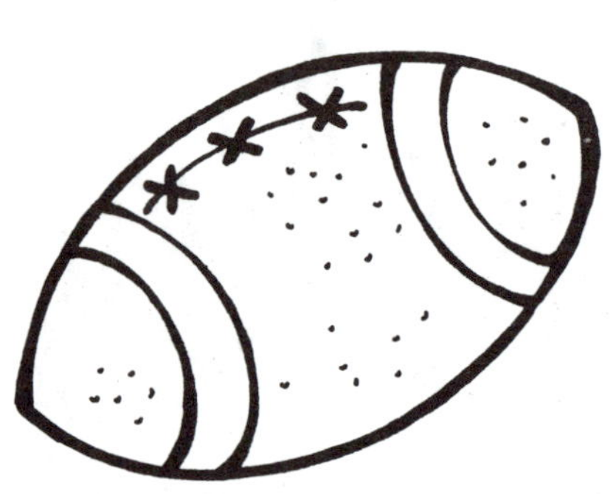

**football**



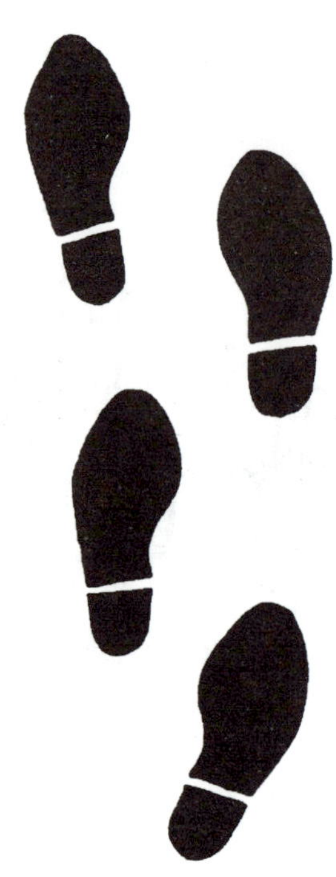

**footprints**



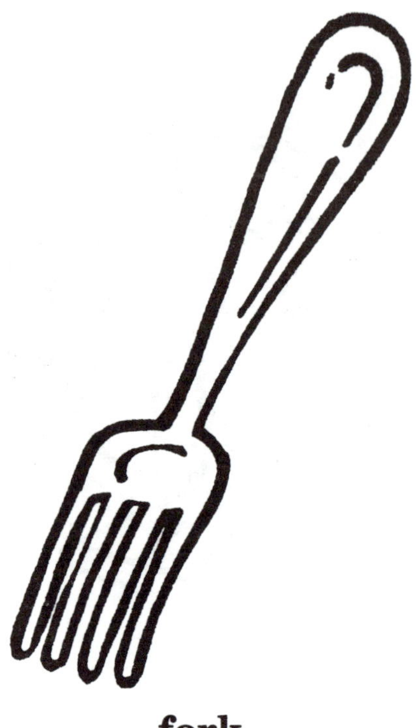

**fork**



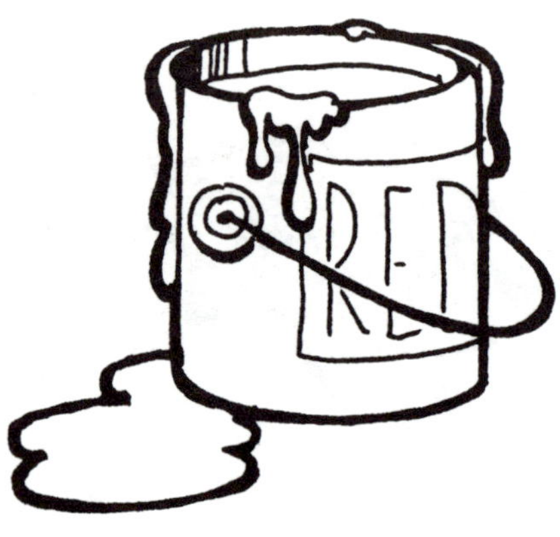

**paint**



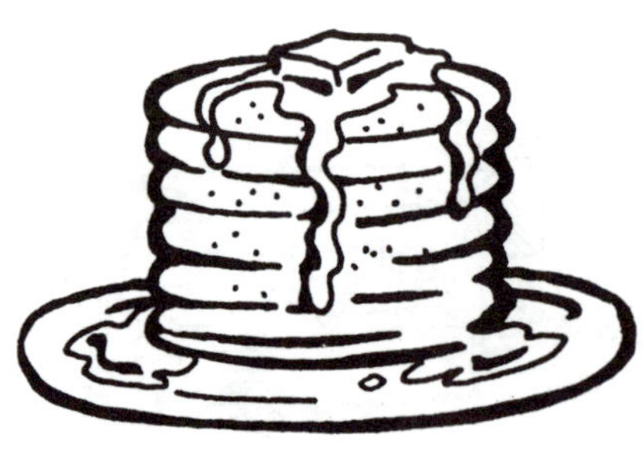

**pancakes**



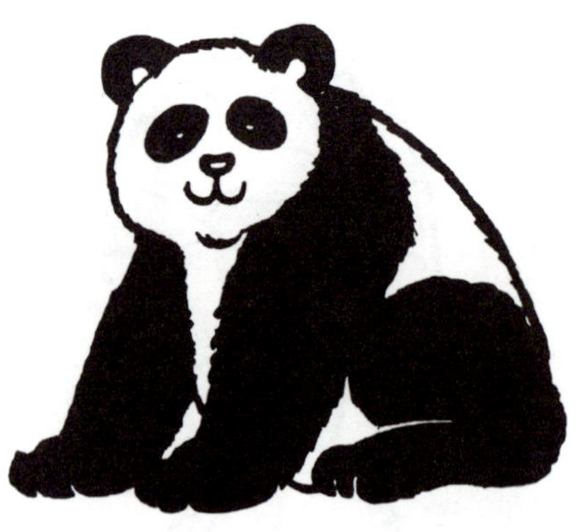

**panda**

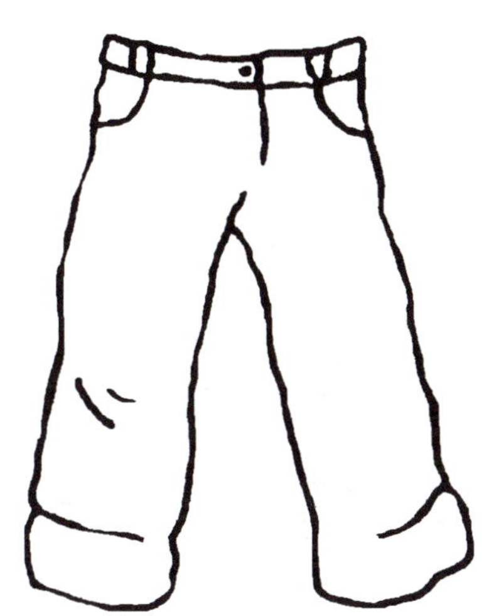

**pants**


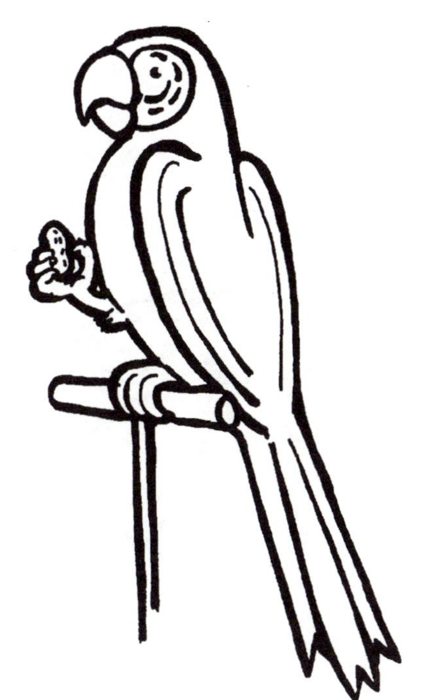

**parrot**


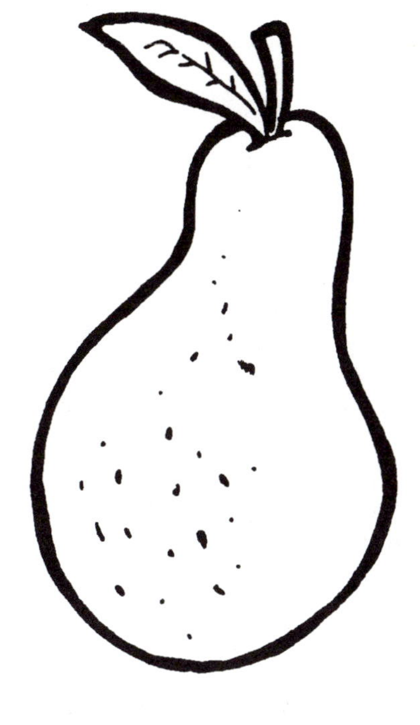

**pear**


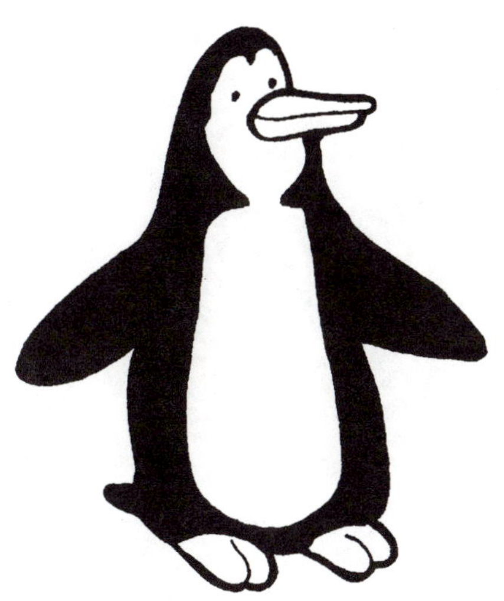

**penguin**


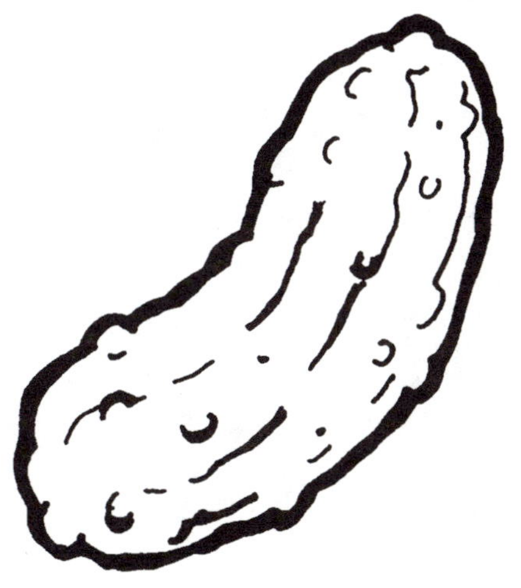

**pickle**


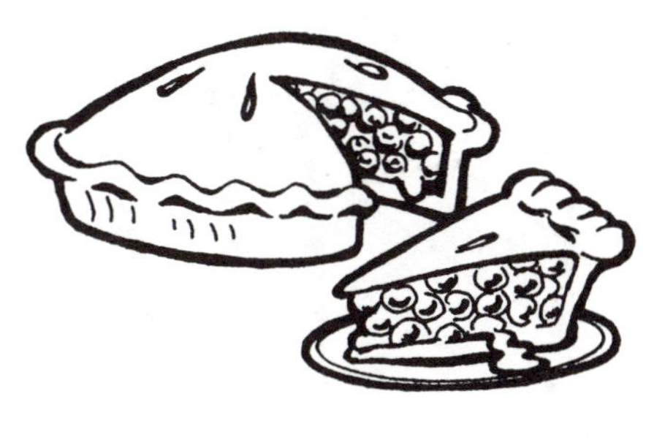

**pie**

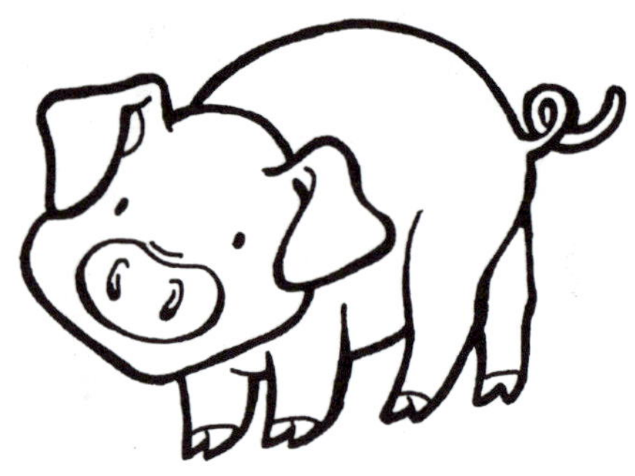

**pig**

© 1994 *Thinking Publications—Phonogroup*

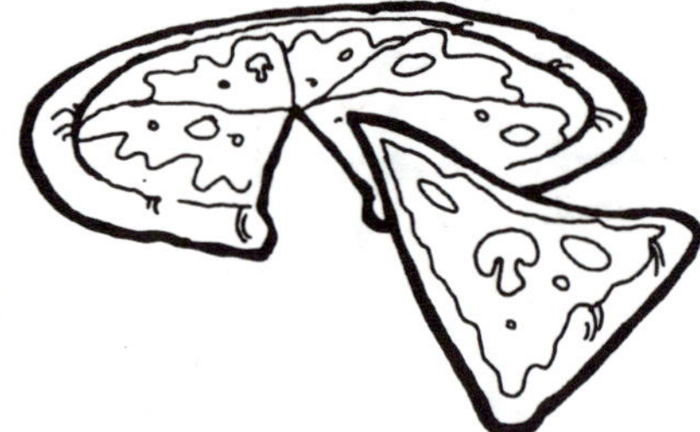

**pizza**

© 1994 *Thinking Publications—Phonogroup*

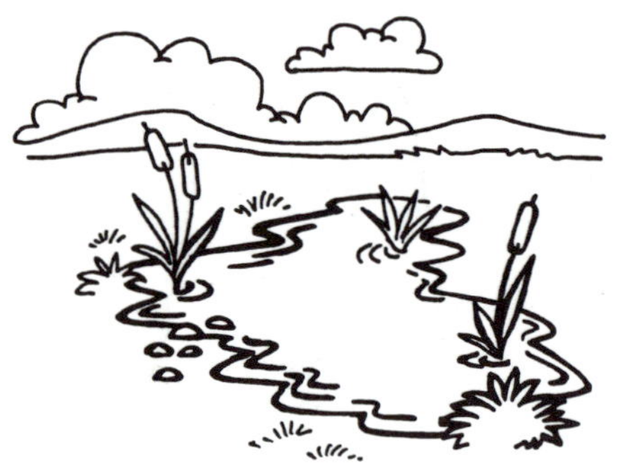

**pond**

© 1994 *Thinking Publications—Phonogroup*

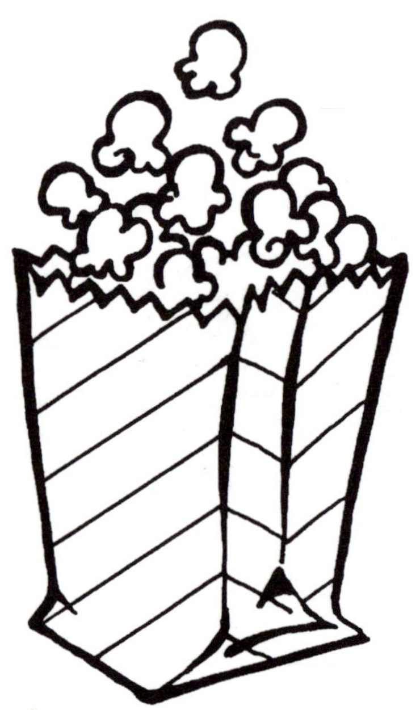

**popcorn**

© 1994 *Thinking Publications—Phonogroup*

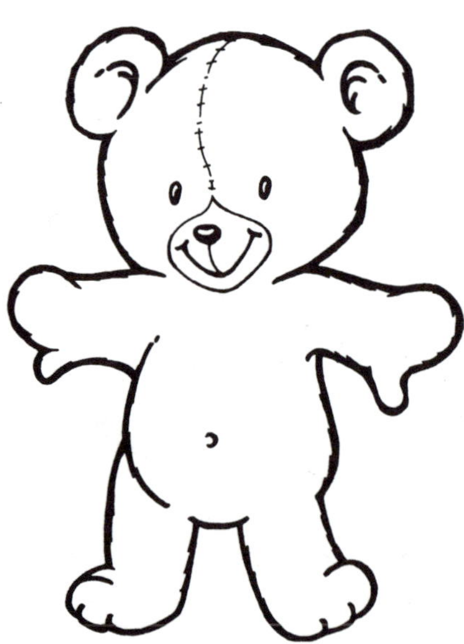

**teddy bear**

© 1994 *Thinking Publications—Phonogroup*

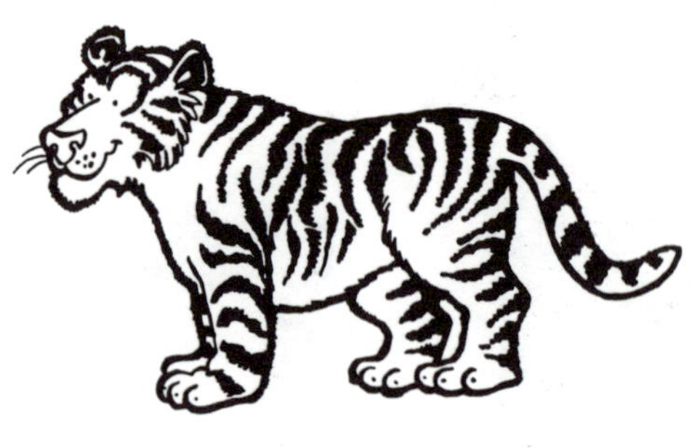

**tiger**

© 1994 *Thinking Publications—Phonogroup*

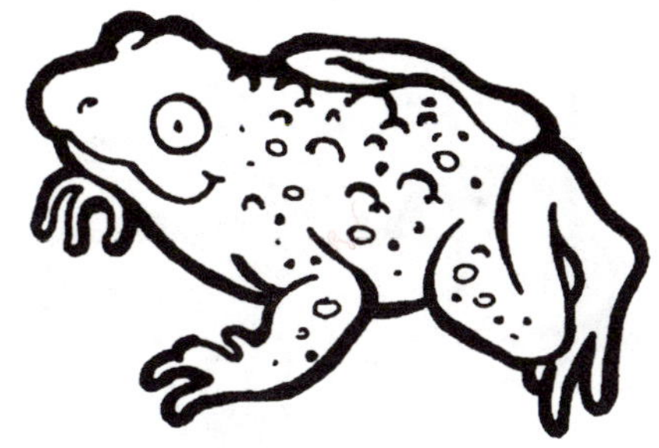

**toad**
© 1994 Thinking Publications—Phonogroup

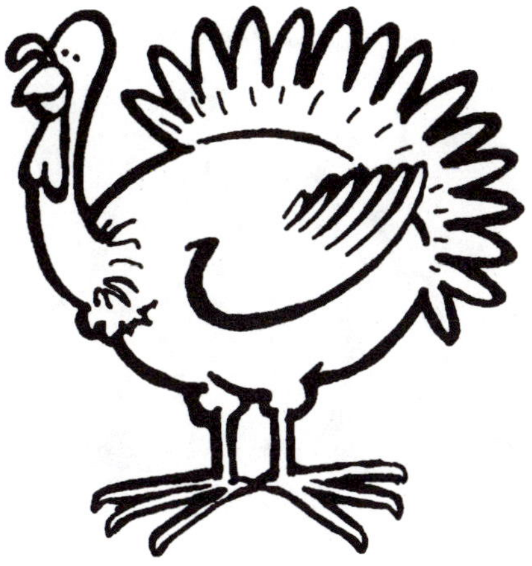

**turkey**
© 1994 Thinking Publications—Phonogroup

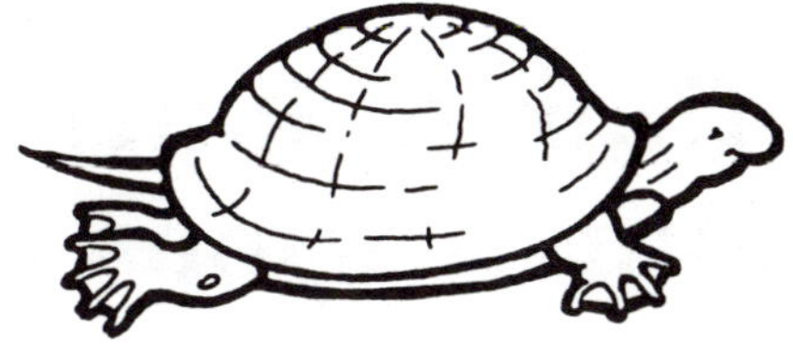

**turtle**
© 1994 Thinking Publications—Phonogroup

## Minimal Pairs Illustrations

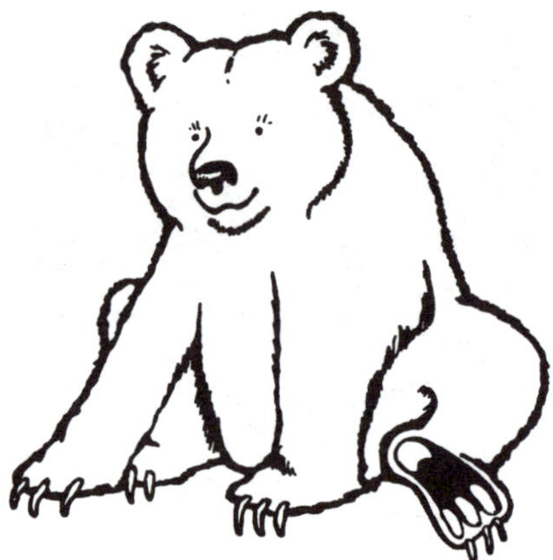

**bear**



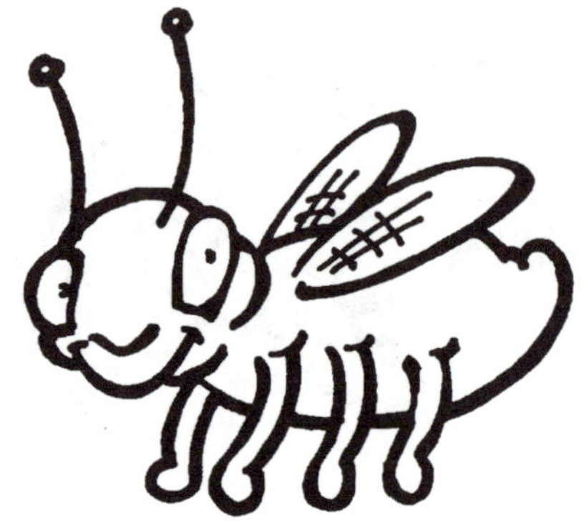

**bee**



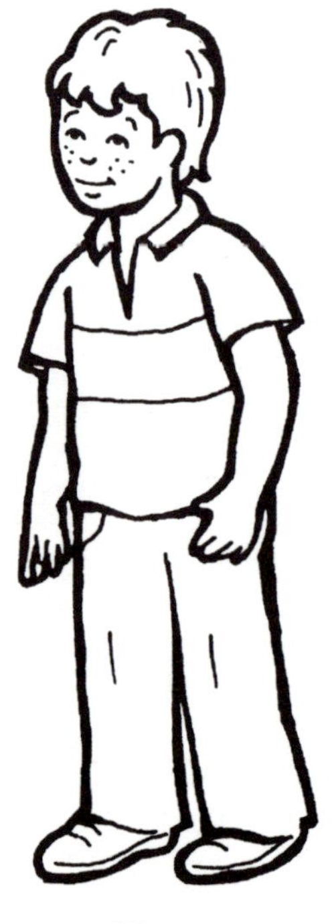

**Ben**



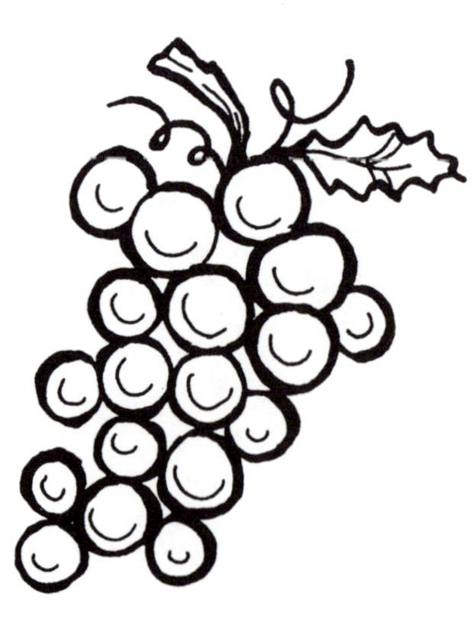

**bunch**



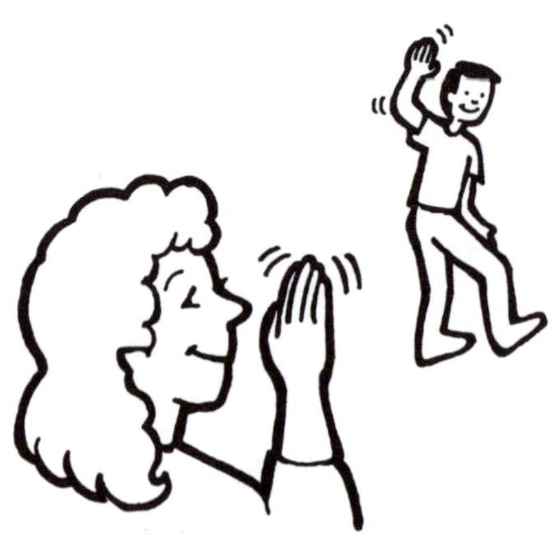

**bye**

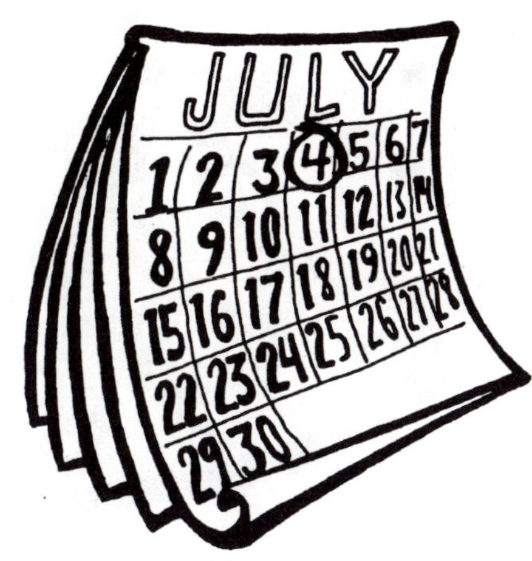

**date**



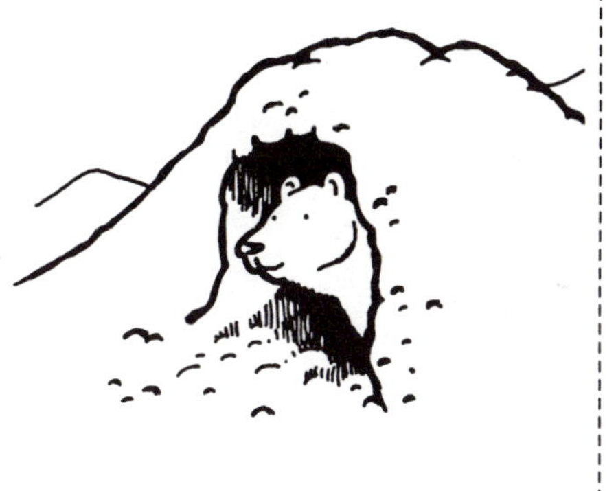

**den**

**dew**



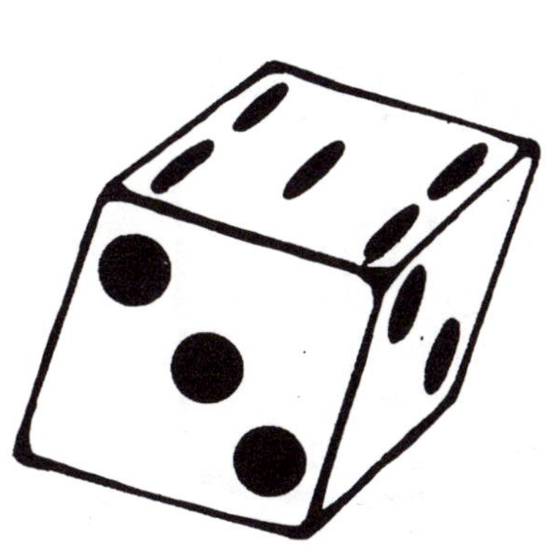

**die**



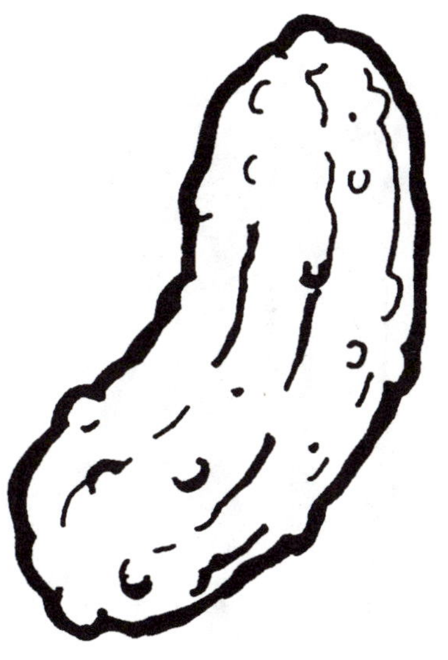

**dill**



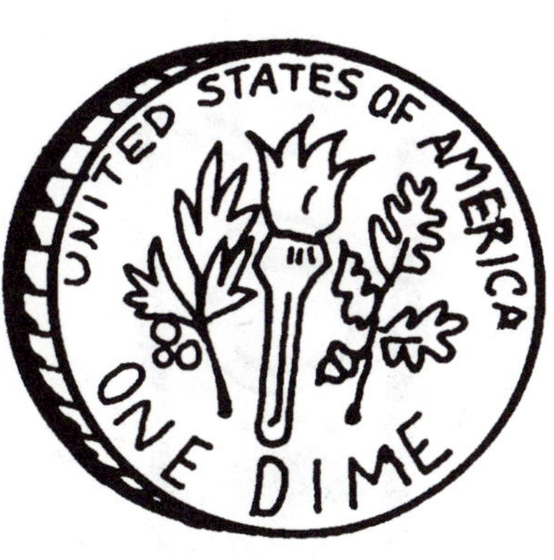

**dime**

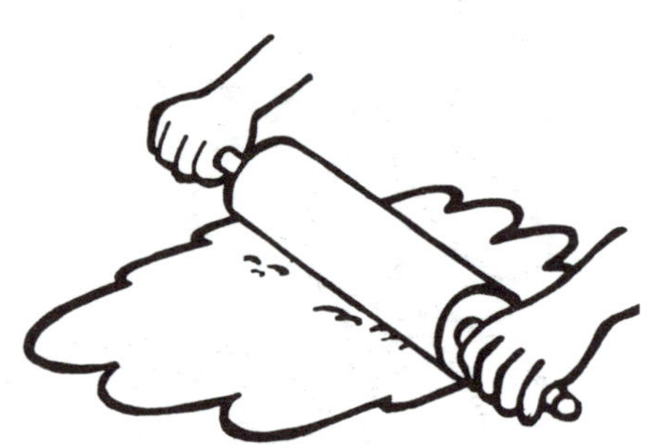

**dough**

© 1994 Thinking Publications—Phonogroup

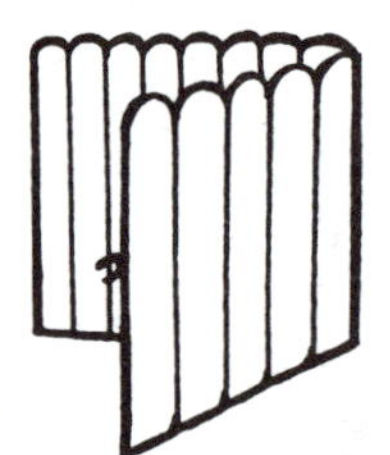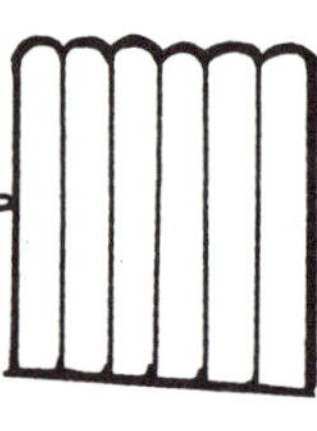

**gate**

© 1994 Thinking Publications—Phonogroup

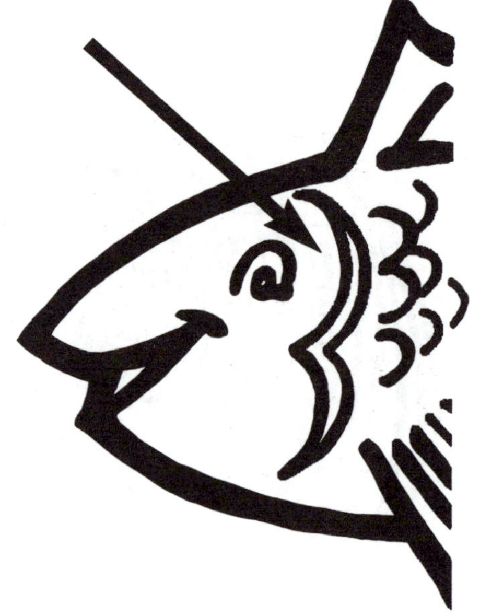

**gill**

© 1994 Thinking Publications—Phonogroup

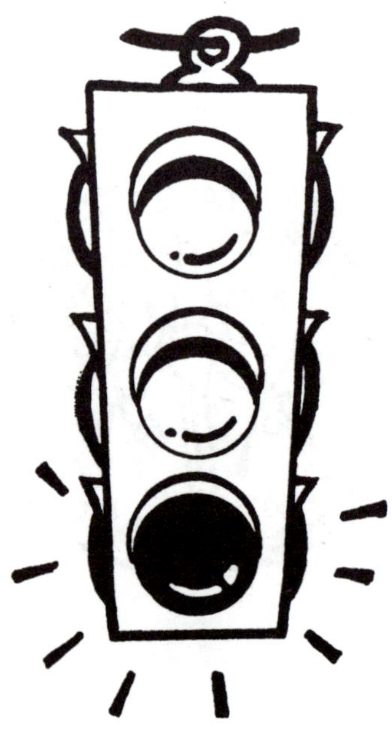

**go**

© 1994 Thinking Publications—Phonogroup

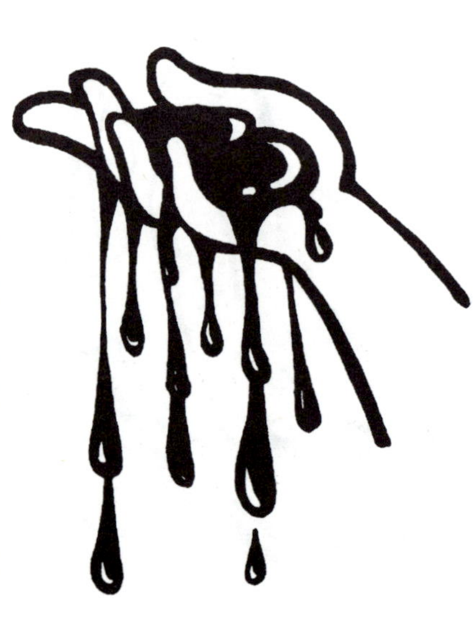

**goo**

© 1994 Thinking Publications—Phonogroup

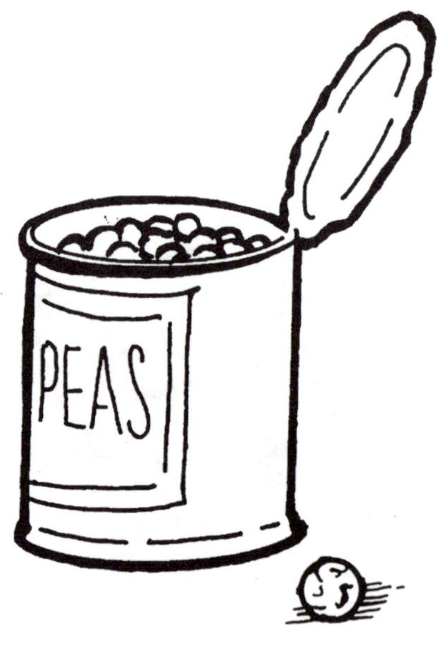


**pea**

© 1994 Thinking Publications—Phonogroup



© 1994 Thinking Publications. Duplication permitted for educational use only.

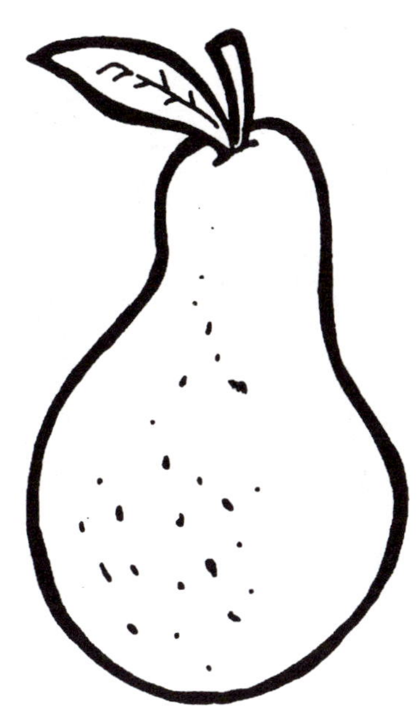

**pear**

**pen**



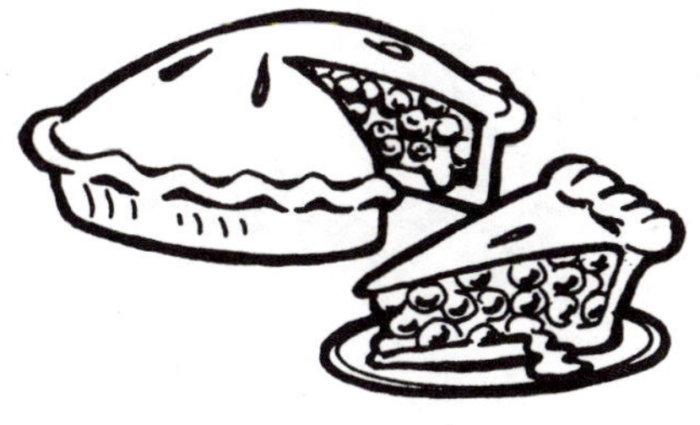

**pie**



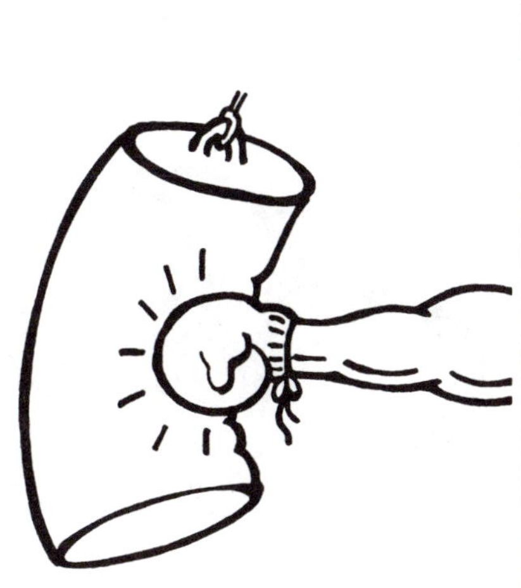

**punch**



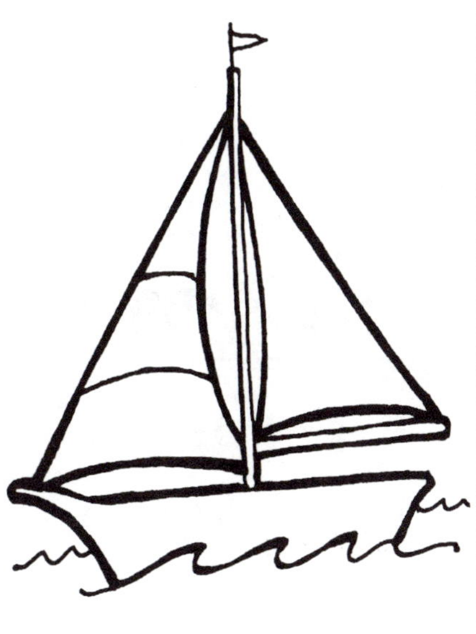

**sail**



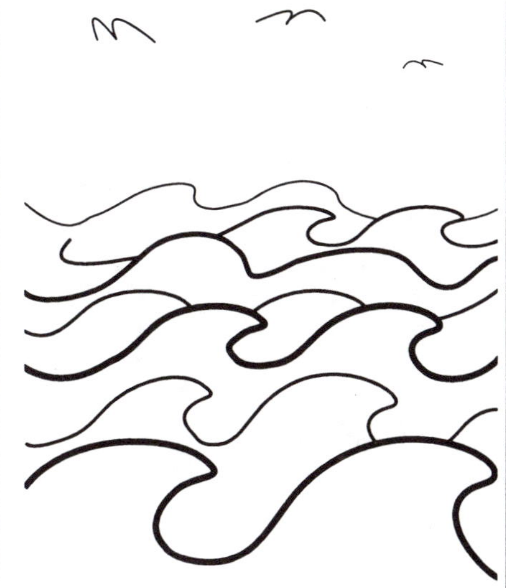

**sea**

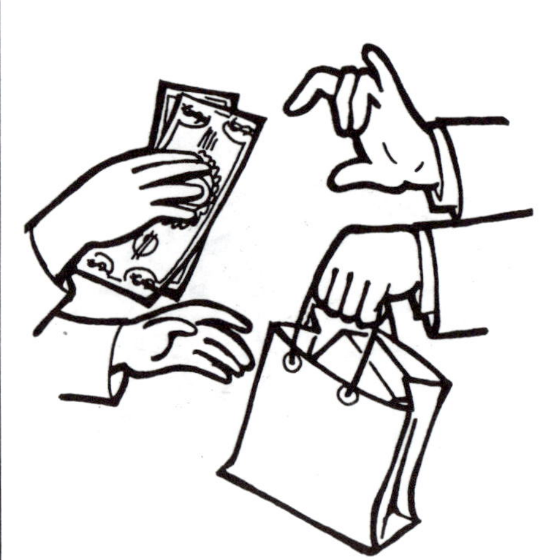

**sell**



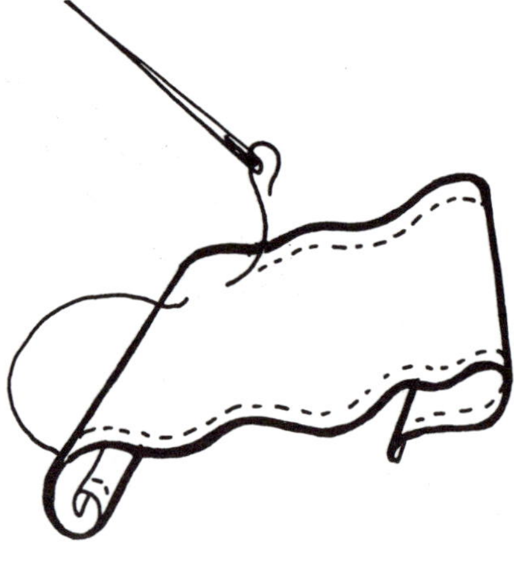

**sew**



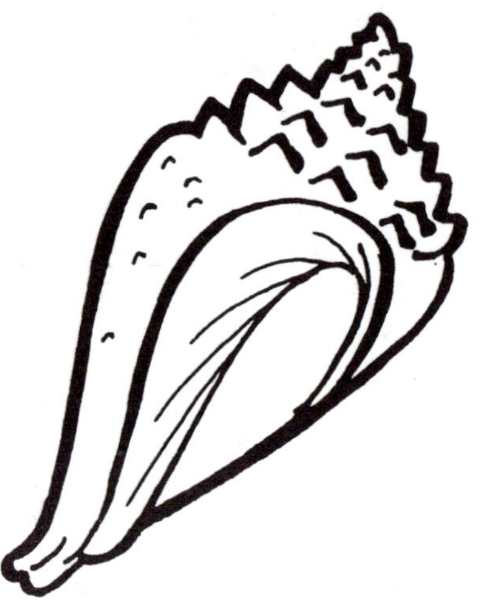

**shell**

**shine**



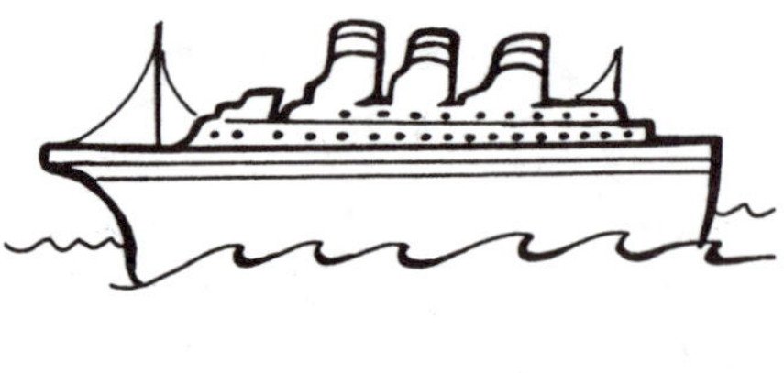

**ship**



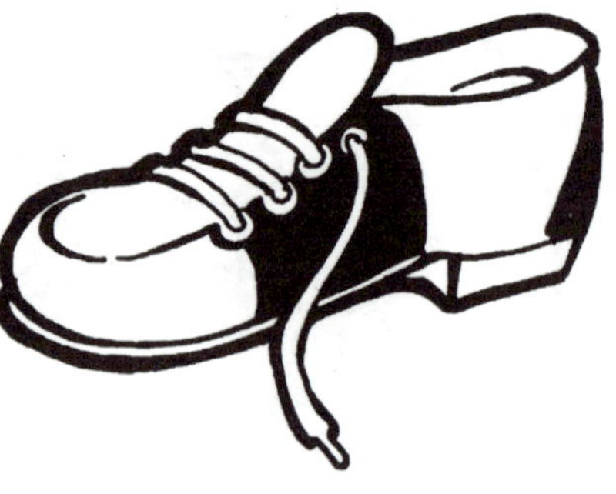

**shoe**

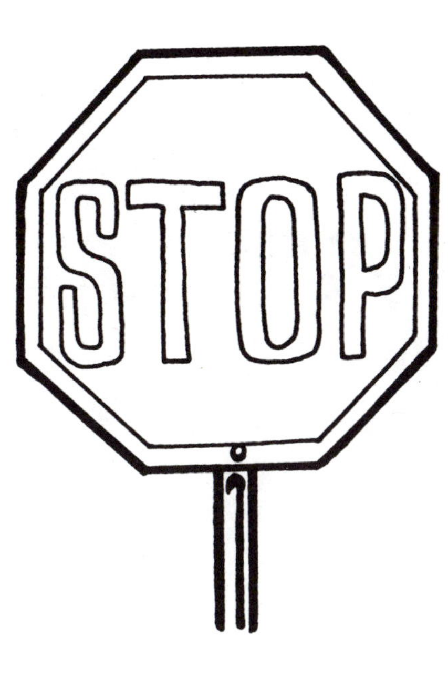
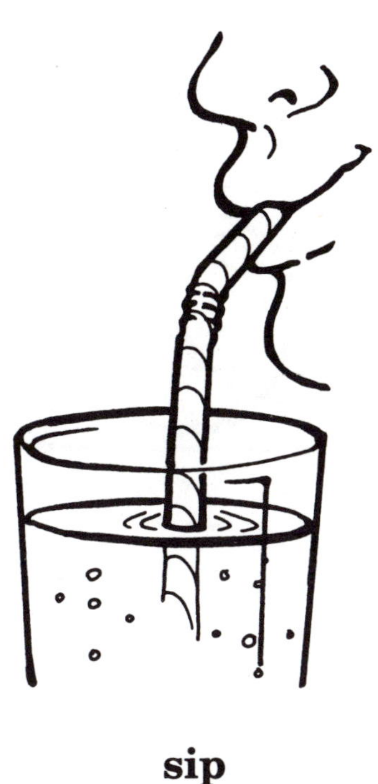
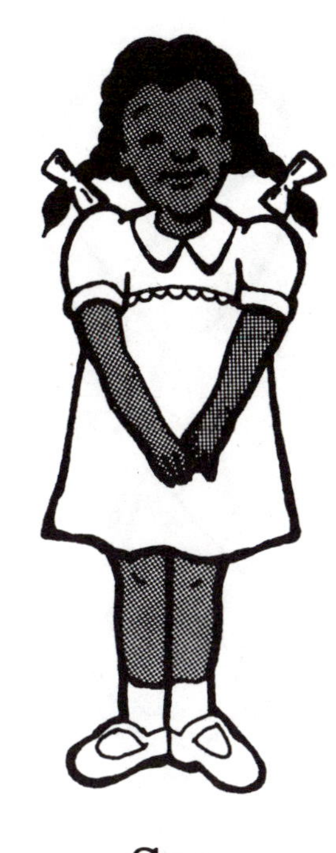

**sign**

*© 1994 Thinking Publications—Phonogroup*

**sip**

*© 1994 Thinking Publications—Phonogroup*

**Sue**

*© 1994 Thinking Publications—Phonogroup*

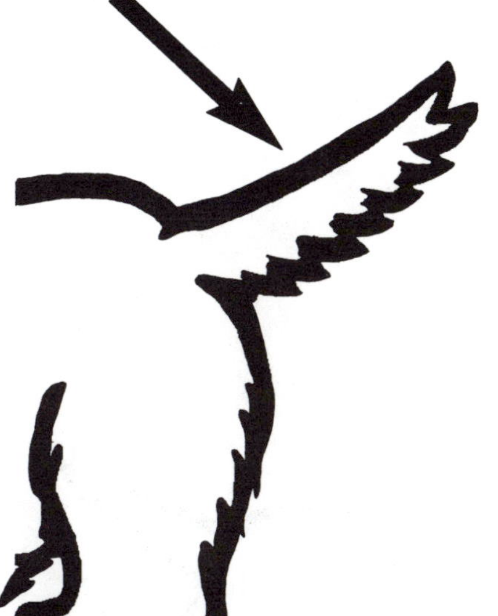
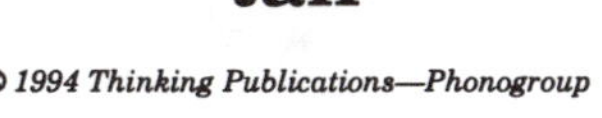
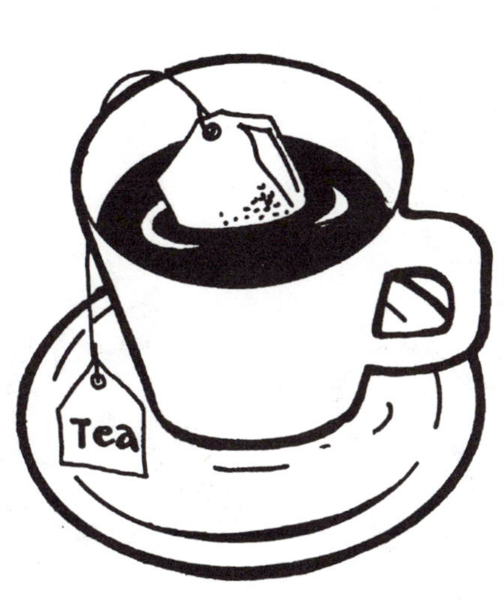
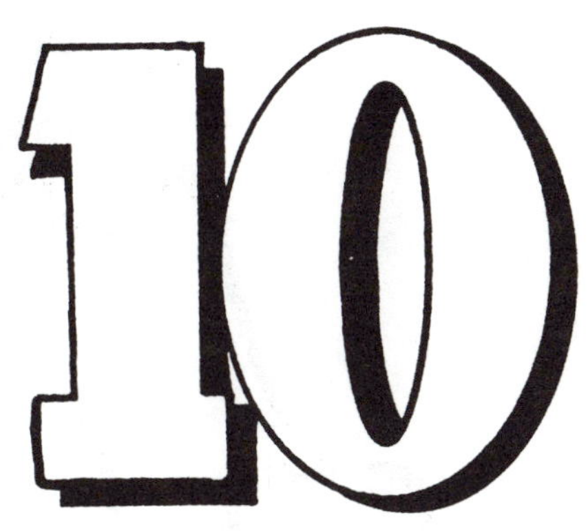

**tail**

*© 1994 Thinking Publications—Phonogroup*

**tea**

*© 1994 Thinking Publications—Phonogroup*

**ten**

*© 1994 Thinking Publications—Phonogroup*

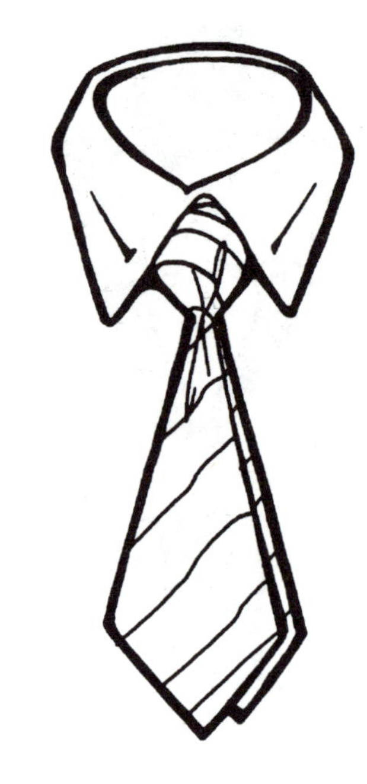

**tie**



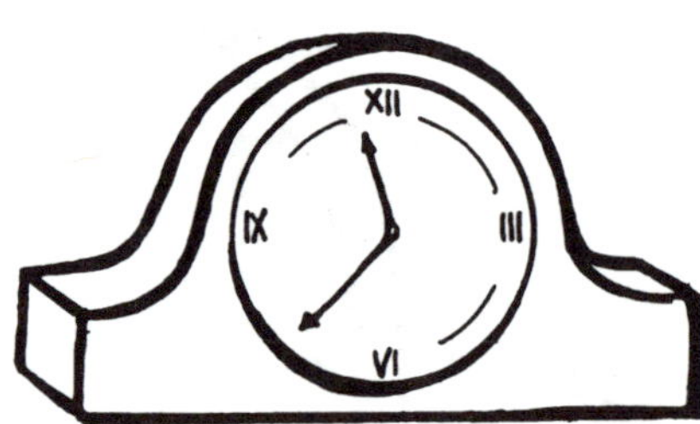

**time**



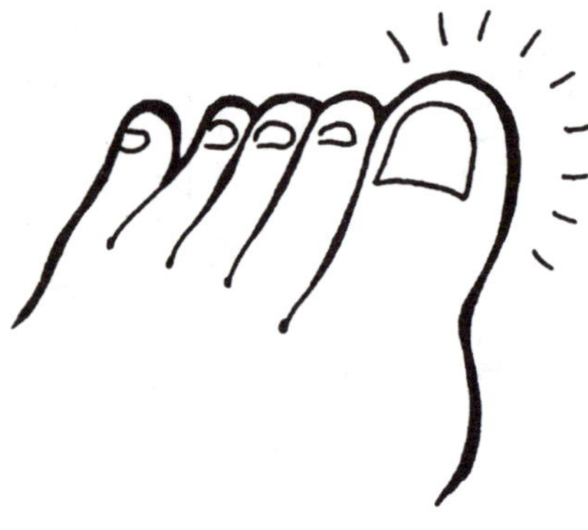

**toe**



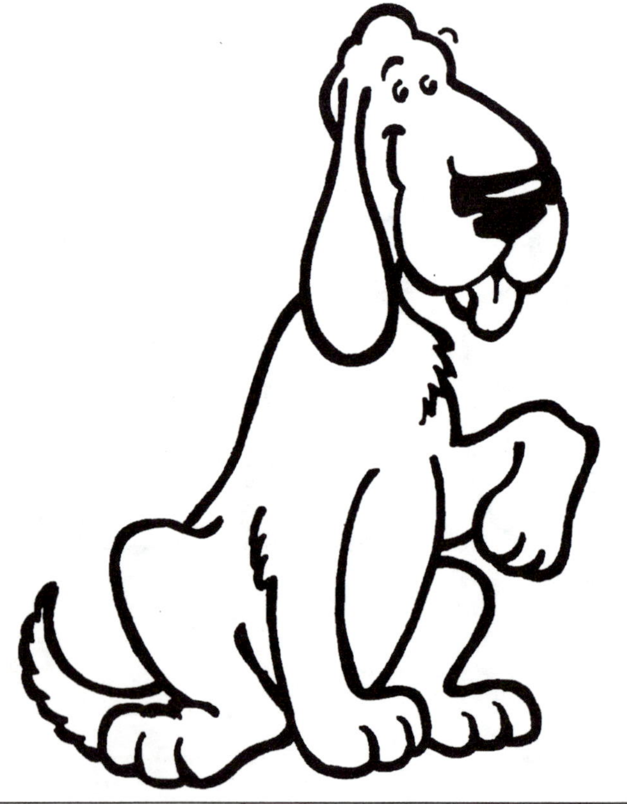

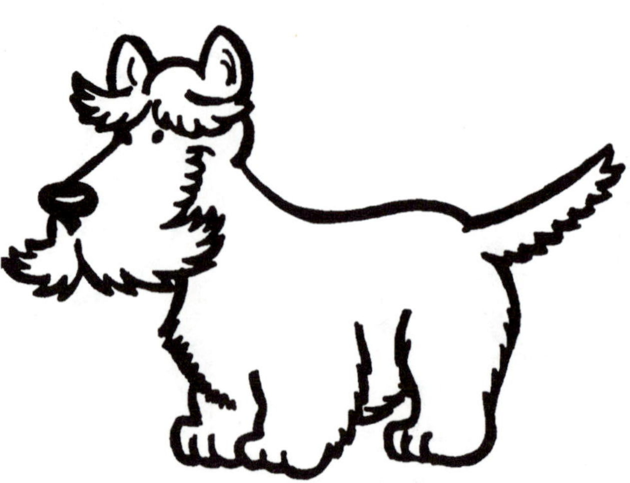

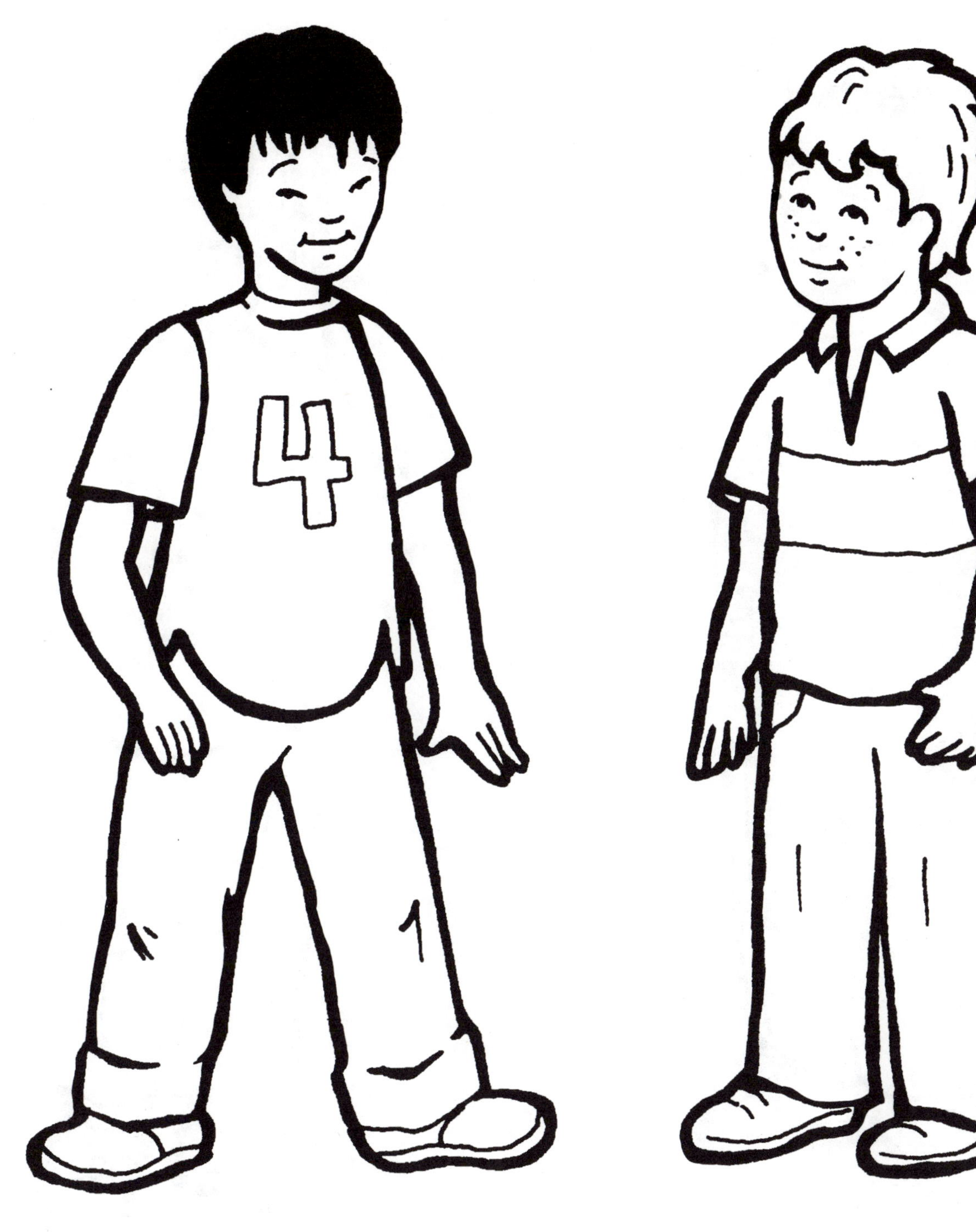

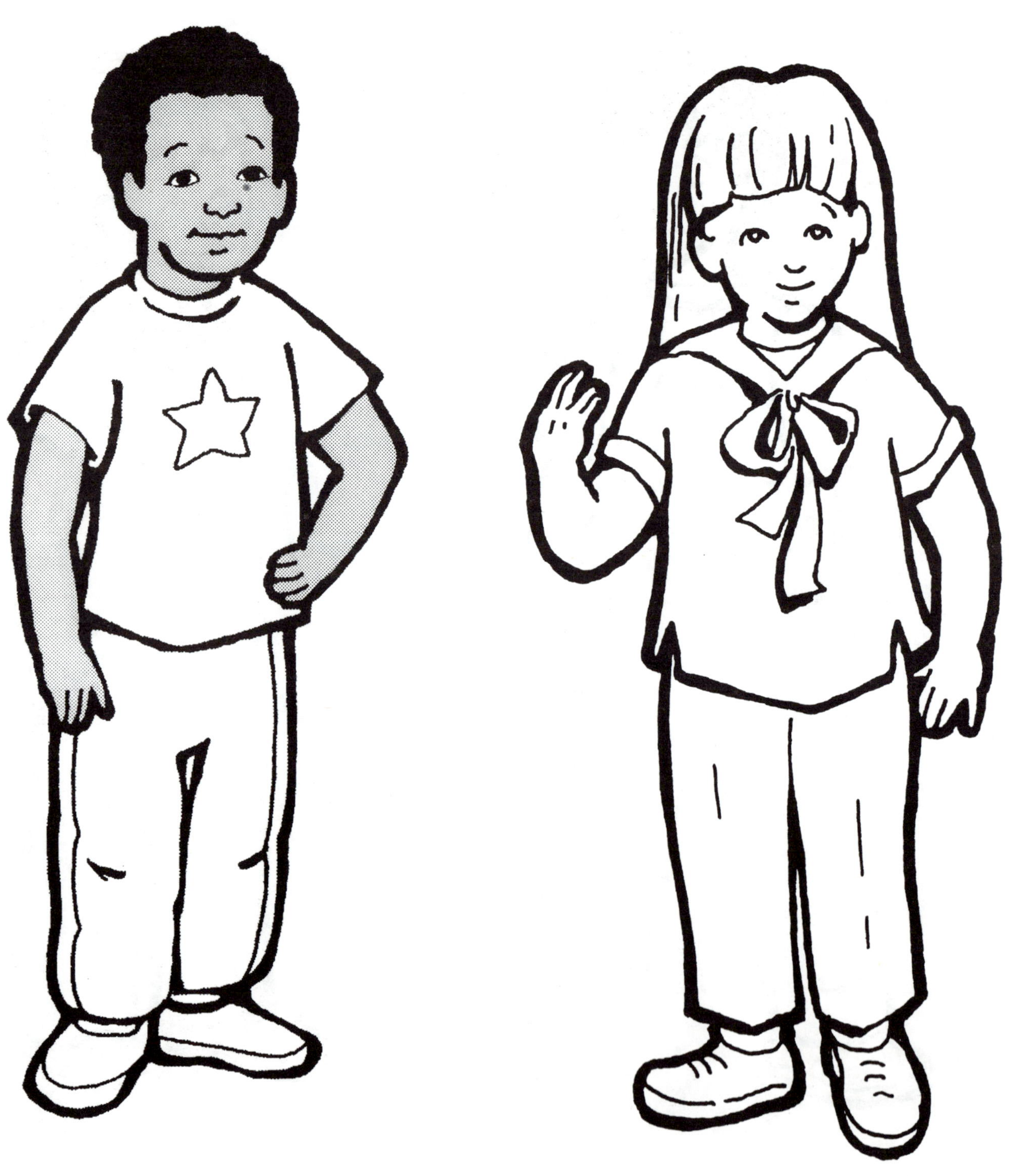



© 1994 Thinking Publications. Duplication permitted for educational use only.

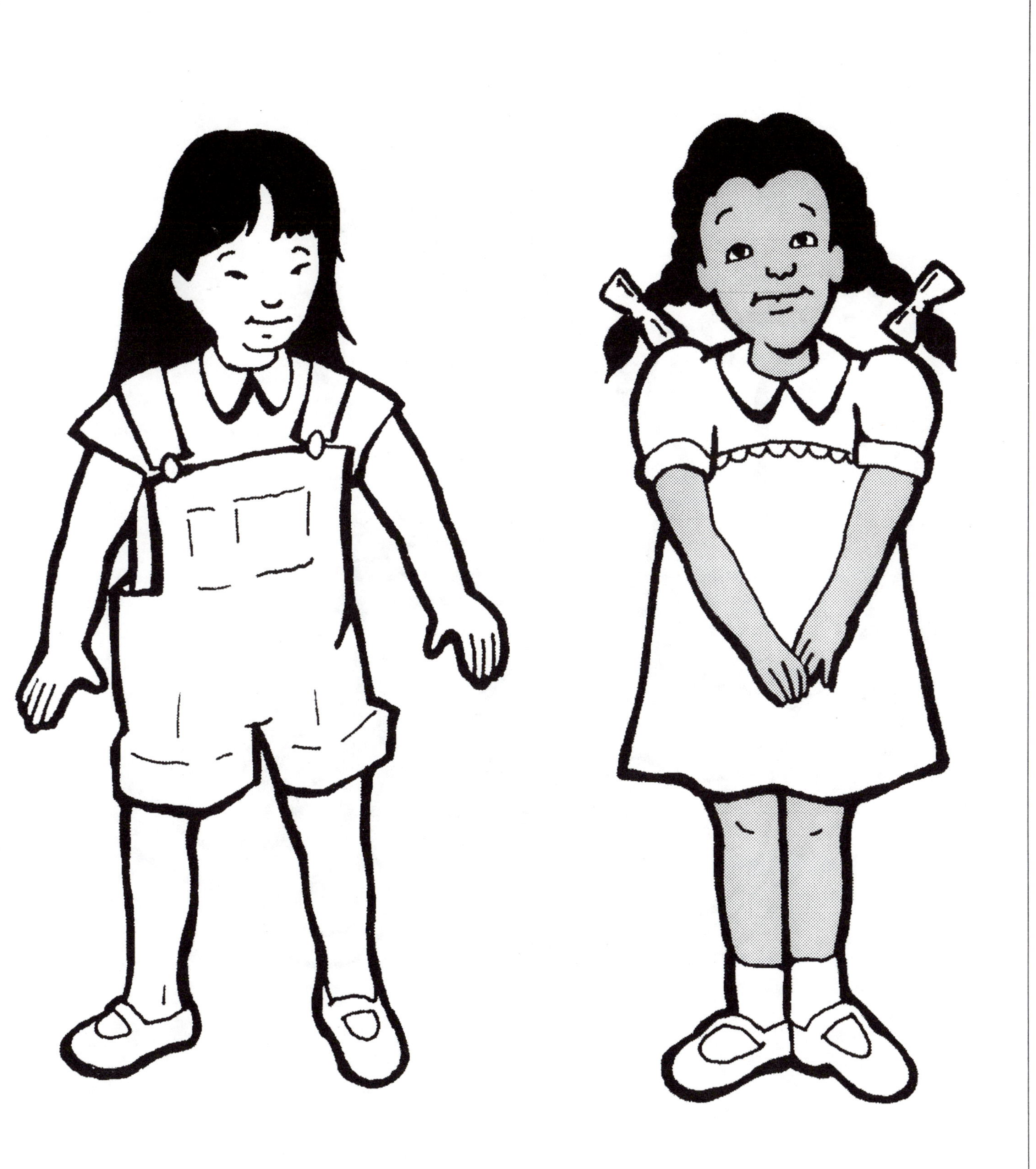

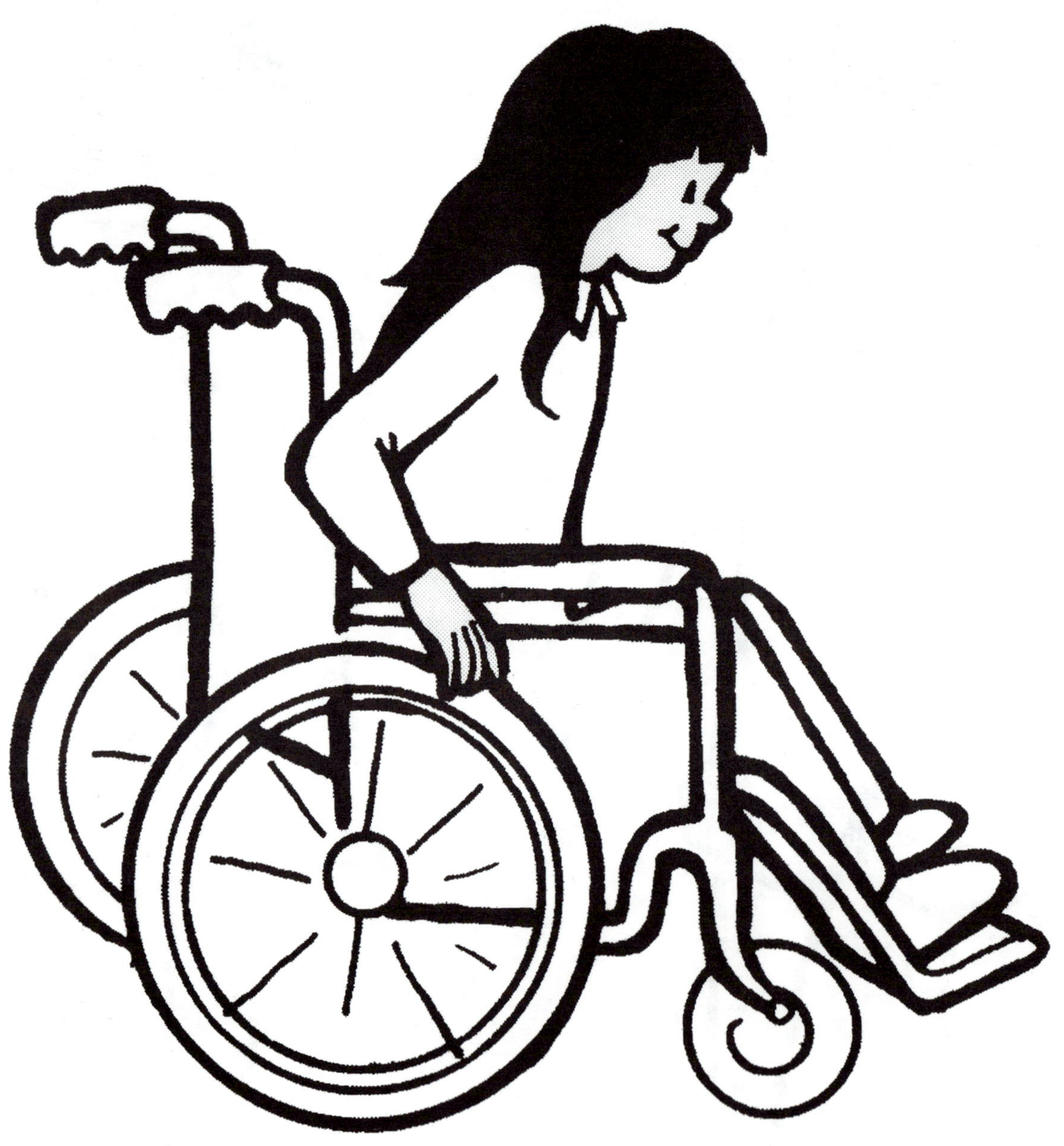

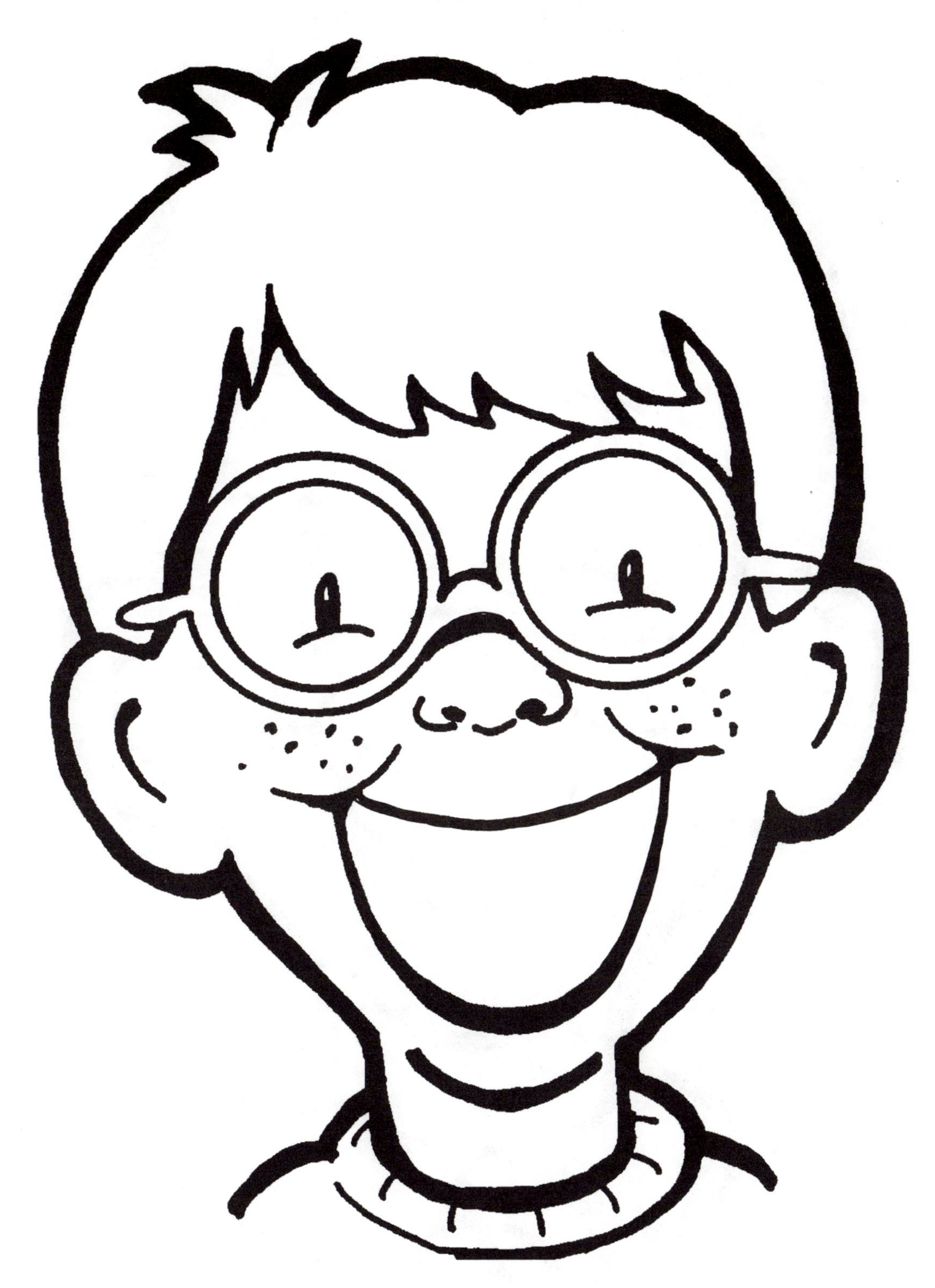

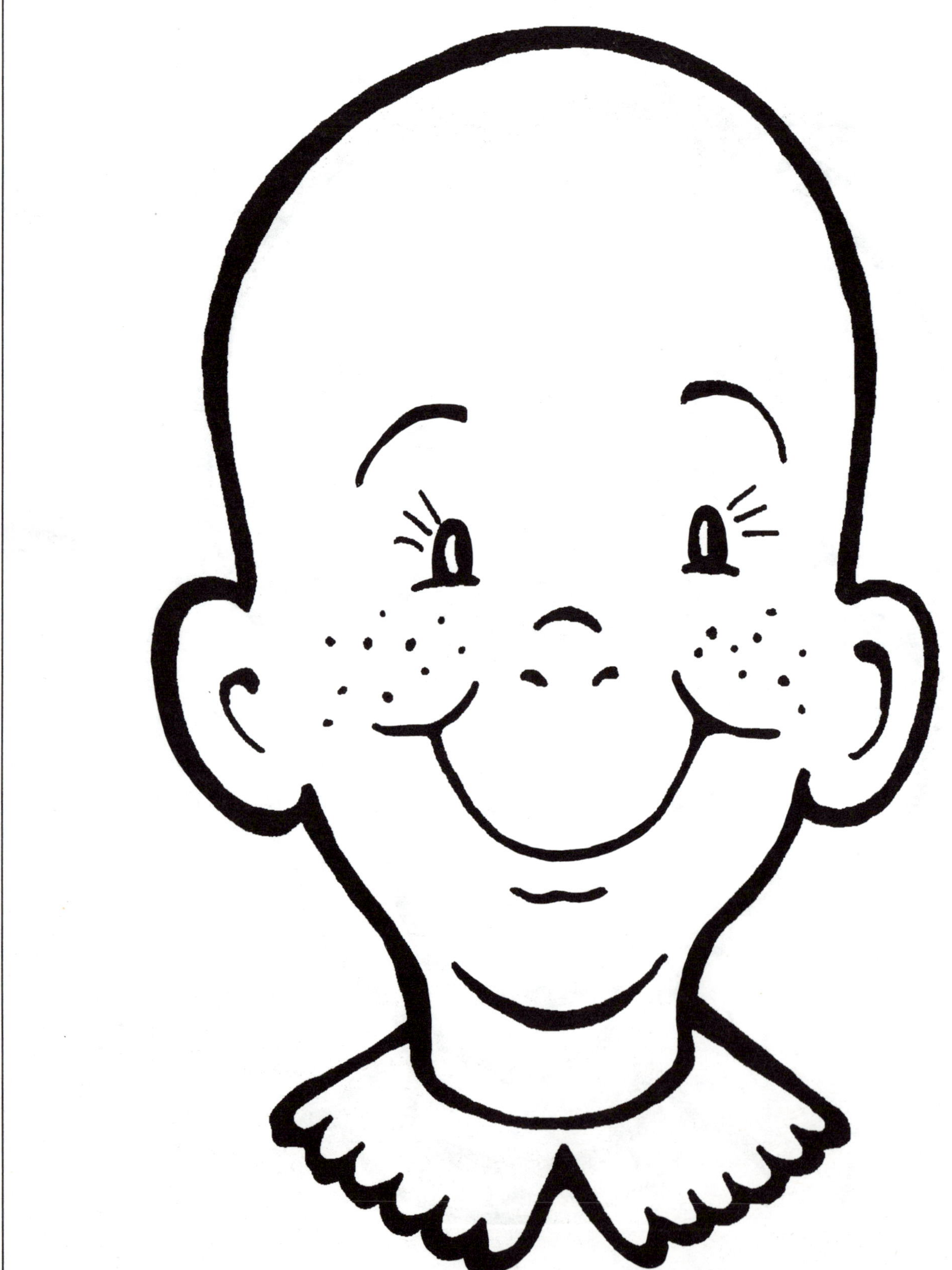